Promoting Behavioral Change to Improve Health Outcomes

Promoting Behavioral Change to Improve Health Outcomes

Guest Editors

John Parkinson
Javad Salehi Fadardi
Yuka Kotozaki

MDPI

Basel • Beijing • Wuhan • Barcelona • Belgrade • Novi Sad • Cluj • Manchester

Guest Editors
John Parkinson
Department of Psychology
Bangor University
Bangor
UK

Javad Salehi Fadardi
School of Community and
Global Health
Claremont Graduate
University
Claremont, CA
USA

Yuka Kotozaki
Department of Hygiene and
Preventive Medicine
Iwate Medical University
Iwate
Japan

Editorial Office
MDPI AG
Grosspeteranlage 5
4052 Basel, Switzerland

This is a reprint of the Special Issue, published open access by the journal *Behavioral Sciences* (ISSN 2076-328X), freely accessible at: https://www.mdpi.com/journal/behavsci/special_issues/800498Y26M.

For citation purposes, cite each article independently as indicated on the article page online and as indicated below:

Lastname, A.A.; Lastname, B.B. Article Title. *Journal Name* **Year**, *Volume Number*, Page Range.

ISBN 978-3-7258-4511-8 (Hbk)
ISBN 978-3-7258-4512-5 (PDF)
https://doi.org/10.3390/books978-3-7258-4512-5

Contents

Preface

This Special Issue focuses on research studying health behaviours and is particularly interested in the prevention agenda; that is, the way in which the adoption of healthy behaviours can delay or even prevent future illness and chronic disease. The studies reported herein span a diverse set of health behaviours, from addiction and physical activity sustainability to medical adherence, mental health, and sleep. The aim of bringing these papers together into a Special Issue is to demonstrate the power of theory-based behavioural research in supporting longevity and quality of life. The reprint will be of particular interest to researchers interested in behaviour change, and those looking for examples of how theory can be used effectively in both understanding complex challenges and in applied settings. The guest editors would like to thank all the authors who made contributions to the Special Issue and hope readers find the studies reported herein thought-provoking, interesting and valuable for their own work.

John Parkinson, Javad Salehi Fadardi, and Yuka Kotozaki
Guest Editors

behavioral sciences

MDPI

Editorial

Promoting Behavioral Change to Improve Health Outcomes

John A. Parkinson

Wales Centre for Behaviour Change, Department of Psychology, Bangor University, Gwynedd LL57 2AS, UK; j.parkinson@bangor.ac.uk

1. Introduction

The key to long-term mental and physical health, including a high quality of life without the burden of disease, is adopting and sustaining behaviors that prevent illness and promote resilient health. However, the prevalence of non-communicable diseases is increasing across the world, including obesity, type 2 diabetes, cardiovascular disease, mental health disorders, etc. Such a burden is unsustainable and reduces quality of life, productivity, and wellbeing across the board (Edwards, 2024; Olshansky, 2018). In the UK, where healthcare is free at the point of delivery, the National Health Service is struggling to manage this increased burden of disease across citizens (DHSC, 2018). Increasingly, arguments are being made for an emphasis on prevention and an understanding of the potential return on investment of acting early to prevent or reduce illness and promote wellbeing (Edwards, 2024; Masters et al., 2017; Musich et al., 2016).

By zooming out and viewing this health crisis from a distance, it seems clear that individuals, groups, and even entire populations need to change their behavior in order to promote better health outcomes. Adopting preventative habits, such as eating a healthy diet, exercising regularly, developing a healthy sleeping habit, and reducing or cutting out drug use (tobacco, alcohol, etc.), the burden of disease would be diminished, and the number of years a person lives disease-free (healthspan) would increase significantly. Currently, the opposite trend is true for many societies (Davoud¡-Monfared et al., 2024; DHSC, 2018; Wagner & Brath, 2012).

Sustained behavior change is challenging, not only because our good intentions are not always followed by good actions (Allan et al., 2008; Gould et al., 2024; Verplanken & Orbell, 2022). We have seemingly evolved with multiple brain mechanisms that make decisions and control our behavior in ways that are not always consistent or outwardly rational (Khalil & Amin, 2023; Lalani et al., 2023). As such, the particular value of behavioral science is in recognizing and understanding that non-conscious behavioral drivers can sometimes override deliberate intentions. Factors such as social norms, habits, and contextual elements—including physical architecture—play a crucial role in shaping behavior, often leading individuals to act contrary to their explicit intentions (Kahneman, 2013; Thaler & Sunstein, 2009).

This discrepancy between intention and action, commonly referred to as the "intention–action gap", is well-documented in the literature and can be traced back at least as far as Plato's *Republic*. A dual-process framework provides a theoretical lens through which this gap can be understood, suggesting that behavior is governed by two interacting pathways: one intuitive and automatic, and the other deliberative and controlled (Evans & Stanovich, 2013). Typically, these systems operate in concert to guide behavior, balancing automatic responses with intentional regulation. However, in certain contexts, these systems may come into conflict, and in such cases, Type 1 processes—characterized as evolutionarily older and more directly linked to behavioral execution at a neural level—are likely to dominate decision-making and action (Levant & Parkinson, 2014). Furthermore, with this insight, contemporary approaches to behavior change are more nuanced and cleverly designed to target the right systems for the right type of behavior. For example, the COM-B model, developed from Michie's Behavior Change Wheel (Cane et al., 2012; Michie et al., 2011) considers behavior through the lenses of capability, opportunity and motivation, acknowledging the myriad influences across contexts. Building upon this complexity, there is a growing recognition that system approaches are required to give a holistic view of how behavior is determined by the larger system within which it sits. This recognizes the importance of not only intervention at different levels (Bioethics, 2007; Chater & Loewenstein, 2023) but also understanding unintended consequences of interventions, as well as the need to map actors and behaviors within larger systems to fully understand the drivers and influencing factors (Gould et al., 2024; Parkinson et al., 2025; Reynolds, 2024).

Within this context, this Special Issue sought to bring together research that explored health-related behavior change, underpinned by contemporary theory, with the aim of promoting longer-term wellbeing and health across a number of domains and with a diversity of methodologies.

2. Research by Health Domain

The papers in this Special Issue span a diversity of domains and behaviors, demonstrating the far-reaching value of a behavioral science approach. For example, three studies focused on substance use. One used a brief motivational intervention to reduce excessive drinking in students (contribution 1) incorporating motivational interviewing and systematic motivational counseling. The intervention was successful, though there were gender differences around the specificity of efficacy for the interventions. The second study explored users' perceptions of therapeutic services for substance abuse to inform better experiences and outcomes for those enrolled (contribution 2). Users perceived the therapeutic context as distinct from the 'real world', and the authors emphasized the need for agency and empowerment to support the recovery process. The third study evaluated a novel acceptance and commitment therapy (ACT) intervention for substance users to better understand the process of change and recovery (contribution 3). The intervention was co-designed by people in recovery, and success was related to core ACT mechanisms at play.

In the context of physical exercise, one study focused on exercise intentions from the perspective of job-related factors (contribution 4), and identified certain high-risk groups. Recommendations for comprehensive work-based support were made. A second study considered exercise and its relationship to sleep quality with the added perspectives of self-control and mindfulness (contribution 5). As expected, exercise predicted sleep quality in college students, and the authors went on to explore the mediation and moderation of this relationship with self-control and mindfulness. Two studies had diet and weight management as a health focus. Shourche et al. (contribution 6) tested the Life Advancement and Enhancement Program (LEAP) in a group of overweight females. The results showed that adding LEAP to a weight management practice had a significant effect on improving outcomes. Exploring a different avenue, Halabi et al. (contribution 7) considered non-dairy alternatives in coffee drinkers from the perspective of health awareness and consumer's beliefs about the consequences of their actions. Based on the findings, the researchers made recommendations within the context of the Behavior Change Wheel framework, relating to fostering inclusivity, health awareness, and supporting environmental sustainability efforts.

Several studies considered medical adherence and/or the use of augmented medical devices. For example, one study sought to better understand home medication management practices in order to improve medical adherence (contribution 8) and proposed personalized guidance to patients from their healthcare providers. A second study explored attitudes and behaviors, including negative emotions such as fear and anxiety, towards vaccinations using a multicultural network analysis (contribution 9). A clear relationship was found between vaccination status and cognitive symptoms of fear and anxiety, suggesting novel routes for intervention to promote vaccine acceptance. Another study considered user intentions related to wearing augmented hearing aid devices (contribution 10) and found that functionality quality, perceived interaction speed, and perceived usability related to confidence in use of the novel devices.

Three studies focused on mental health. One looked at the role of guilt in mental health 'burnout' (contribution 11) and found that feelings of guilt appeared to drive psychosomatic symptoms during the burnout process. They recommend that future studies of burnout should encompass emotions including guilt as potentially important elements of the process. Two other studies focused on COVID-19. The first used a longitudinal design to track the mental health of university students over a two-year period during and after the initial COVID-19 epidemic (contribution 12). They found that distress and generalized anxiety remained high following the pandemic and argue that student mental health 'is still in crisis' with a need for further support for this cohort who are transitioning into the world of work. Another study looked at the potential role of 'behavioral fatigue' during the acute phase of COVID-19 (contribution 13) using a COM-B analysis and concluded that in order to maintain prolonged behavior change, capabilities, opportunities and motivation are all important for target behaviors. Continuing in the context of COVID-19, one experimental study explored risk behaviors from the perspective of psychological distance, testing an intervention designed to make COVID-19 feel more concrete and real (contribution 14). The authors demonstrated that participant risk perceptions were influenced by psychological distance (whether something is close/concrete or far/abstract) and were able to reduce the willingness of participants to engage in risky COVID-19 behaviors by making the concept of the COVID-19 virus more concrete.

To round off the diversity of behavioral domains, Hutchings et al. (contribution 15) evaluated data from an RCT trial of the KiVa anti-bullying school-based program in the UK. The results supported a social architecture model of bullying behavior and suggested further work to refine the model in addressing bullying as a public health challenge. Finally, Wetton et al. (contribution 16) used behavioral systems mapping to understand sustainability and waste management behaviors in Kenya. They developed a map which demonstrated key actors, sub-systems, and feedback loops that helped explain poor solid waste management practices and could be used to create systemic behavior change interventions in the future.

3. Research by Methodology and Approach

Across this Special Issue, two papers focused explicitly on prevention: one testing an intervention to reduce bullying, and the other exploring ways to promote COVID-19-safe behaviors (contribution 14; contribution 15). Additionally, eleven papers sought to use contemporary analyses in order to better understand a problem situation or behavior (contribution 2; contribution 4; contribution 5; contribution 7; contribution 8; contribution 9; contribution 10; contribution 11; contribution 12; contribution 13; contribution 16). Finally, three focused specifically on secondary prevention (Simeonsson, 1991) for either substance use or weight management (contribution 1; contribution 3; contribution 6).

Furthermore, of the approaches above, three papers based their study on the COM-B framework (contribution 7; contribution 13; contribution 16), whilst seven used questionnaires followed by a variety of modeling techniques, such as structural equation modeling (contribution 4; contribution 5; contribution 8; contribution 9; contribution 10; contribution 11; contribution 12). Finally, four employed intervention designs that were based on specific psychological (contribution 6; contribution 14; contribution 15) or therapeutic theories (contribution 1). Of these, only one paper explicitly incorporated dual-process theory (contribution 14).

4. Conclusions

This Special Issue showcases novel and impactful original research within the domain of promoting healthy behavior change. First and foremost, the research demonstrates the value of an approach based on behavioral science, particularly in demonstrating the value of integrating psychological theory, such as the dual-process approach (Evans & Stanovich, 2013), in developing interventions. The work herein also demonstrates the value of employing contemporary frameworks, such as COM-B (Michie et al., 2011), and testing them in the real world (Atkins et al., 2017).

Recently, we developed a high-level tool based on an integration of COM-B and dual-process theory ((Evans & Stanovich, 2013; Michie et al., 2011) to support health and wellbeing during the COVID-19 pandemic. The aim was to help those designing interventions to consider whether to target automatic (Type 1) or cognitive (Type 2) processes, and whether to focus on capability, opportunity, or motivation (see Figure 1, taken from (Gould et al., 2024). It also emphasizes that the moment of decision-making is often when behavior is most susceptible to influence. We hope that such an approach can improve the efficacy of behavioral interventions to promote positive and long-lasting health outcomes.

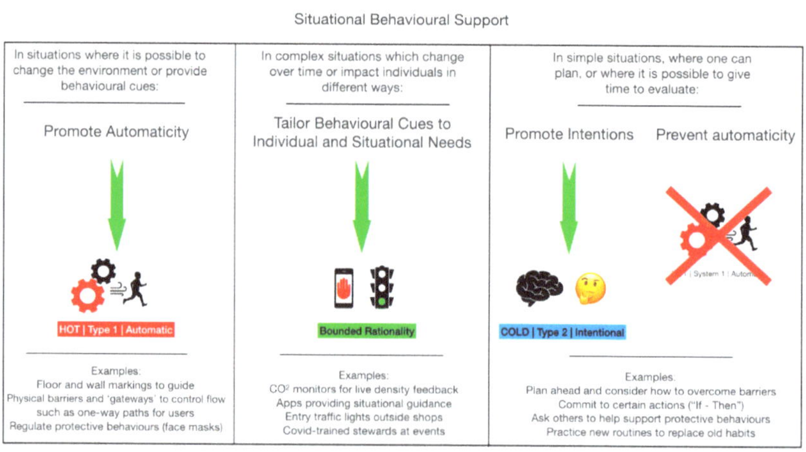

Figure 1. Taken from (Gould et al., 2024).

Ultimately, the combination of knowledge dissemination, targeted behavior change interventions, supportive environments, and strategic policies can lead to sustainable behavior change. The benefits of these interventions are twofold: individuals lead healthier, longer lives; and the societal costs associated with treating preventable diseases are considerably reduced. The field of health economics is becoming increasingly important in this regard, identifying the financial (and other) return on investment of implementing preventative and health-promoting interventions to build more human and social resilience to health challenges (Edwards, 2024; Whiteley et al., 2024). There is currently a paucity of research focused on identifying and utilizing dual-process theory in order to leverage the most effective behavior change techniques (Gould et al., 2024; Parkinson et al., 2014), particularly with regard to actually measuring behavioral outcomes rather than proxies such as attitudes or intentions (Murphy et al., 2023). Finally, given the complex nature of health challenges, future research will need to consider whole-system approaches, including system thinking, as well as considering at what level within a system an intervention is likely to have the largest benefit (Chater & Loewenstein, 2023; Parkinson et al., 2025; Reynolds, 2024).

Conflicts of Interest: The author declares no conflicts of interest.

List of Contributions:

1. Hogan, L. M., & Cox, W. M. (2024). Evaluating two brief motivational interventions for excessive-drinking university students. *Behavioral Sciences, 14*(5), 381. https://doi.org/10.3390/bs14050381.
2. Iudici, A., Berardelli, T., Fenini, D., Subissi, E., & Neri, J. (2024). The discursive configuration of the therapeutic community for substance users: Positioning and ethnopsychological processes concerning entry. *Behavioral Sciences, 14*(10), 951. https://doi.org/10.3390/bs14100951.
3. Shepley, E. L., Jackson, M. C., & Hogan, L. M. (2024). A qualitative exploration of the process and experience of change in moving on in my recovery: An acceptance and commitment therapy based recovery group for substance use disorder. *Behavioral Sciences, 14*(12), 1237. https://doi.org/10.3390/bs14121237.
4. Wang, W.-H., Hsu, W.-T., Cheng, H.-I., Li, R.-H., Huang, S.-L., & Tang, F.-C. (2024). Exploring job-related factors and exercise intentions in relation to overall physical activity and its subdivisions. *Behavioral Sciences, 14*(10), 912. https://doi.org/10.3390/bs14100912.
5. Li, X., Xu, C., Chen, W., & Tian, J. (2025). Physical exercise and sleep quality among chinese college students: The mediating role of self-control and the moderating role of mindfulness. *Behavioral Sciences, 15*(2), 232. https://doi.org/10.3390/bs15020232.
6. Shourche, R. M., Nematy, M., Cox, W. M., & Fadardi, J. S. (2024). Effectiveness of the life enhancement and advancement program for weight management in overweight and obese females. *Behavioral Sciences, 14*(8), 724. https://doi.org/10.3390/bs14080724.
7. Halabi, N., Hristova, V., & Vlaev, I. (2024). Milking the alternatives: Understanding coffee consumers' preferences for non-dairy milk. *Behavioral Sciences, 14*(7), 569. https://doi.org/10.3390/bs14070569.
8. Gualtieri, L., Steinfeldt, M., Shaveet, E., Estime, B., & Singhal, M. (2024). The impact of home medication management practices on medication adherence. *Behavioral Sciences, 14*(9), 804. https://doi.org/10.3390/bs14090804.
9. Malas, O., Boustani, N. M., Duradoni, M., Omotoso, D., Avşar, A. Ş., Shyroka, A., Colombini, G., & Tolsá, M. D. (2024). Links between vaccination fear-, anxiety-, alexithymia-, and type D personality-related vaccination decisions: A network analysis in a multicultural sample. *Behavioral Sciences, 14*(9), 761. https://doi.org/10.3390/bs14090761.
10. Deng, L., Chen, J., & Li, D. (2024). Factors influencing intentions of people with hearing impairments to use augmented reality glasses as hearing aids. *Behavioral Sciences, 14*(8), 728. https://doi.org/10.3390/bs14080728.
11. Gil-LaOrden, P., Carlotto, M. S., & Gil-Monte, P. R. (2024). The role of guilt feelings in the development of the burnout process: The influence on psychosomatic problems. *Behavioral Sciences, 14*(12), 1196. https://doi.org/10.3390/bs14121196.
12. Allen, R. E., Hochard, K. D., Kannangara, C., & Carson, J. (2024). The road to recovery: A two-year longitudinal analysis of mental health among university students during and after the COVID-19 pandemic. *Behavioral Sciences, 14*(12), 1146. https://doi.org/10.3390/bs14121146.
13. Khanal, S., Schmidtke, K. A., Haralampiev, K., & Vlaev, I. (2024). Considering the role of behavioural fatigue in the COVID-19 lockdown debates in Great Britain: A retrospective analysis of a national survey assessing the relationships between capability, opportunity, motivation, and behaviour. *Behavioral Sciences, 14*(9), 852. https://doi.org/10.3390/bs14090852.

14. Williams, C., Rauwolf, P., Boulter, M., & Parkinson, J. A. (2024). Closing the gap: How psychological distance influences willingness to engage in risky COVID behavior. *Behavioral Sciences, 14*(6), 449. https://doi.org/10.3390/bs14060449.
15. Hutchings, J., Pearson, R., Babu, M., Clarkson, S., Williams, M. E., Badger, J. R., Cannings-John, R., Hastings, R. P., Hayes, R., & Bowes, L. (2025). Participants' roles in bullying among 7–11 year olds: Results from a UK-wide randomized control trial of the KiVa school-based program. *Behavioral Sciences, 15*(2), 236. https://doi.org/10.3390/bs15020236.
16. Wetton, J. D., Santilli, M., Gitau, H., Muindi, K., Zimmermann, N., Michie, S., & Davies, M. (2025). Behavioural systems mapping of solid waste management in kisumu, kenya, to understand the role of behaviour in a health and sustainability problem. *Behavioral Sciences, 15*(2), 133. https://doi.org/10.3390/bs15020133.

References

Allan, J. L., Johnston, M., & Campbell, N. (2008). Why do people fail to turn good intentions into action? The role of executive control processes in the translation of healthy eating intentions into action in young Scottish adults. *BMC Public Health, 8*, 123. [CrossRef]

Atkins, L., Francis, J., Islam, R., O'Connor, D., Patey, A., Ivers, N., Foy, R., Duncan, E. M., Colquhoun, H., Grimshaw, J. M., Lawton, R., & Michie, S. (2017). A guide to using the theoretical domains framework of behaviour change to investigate implementation problems. *Implementation Science, 12*(1), 77. [CrossRef] [PubMed]

Bioethics, N. C. O. (2007). *Public health: Ethical issues*. C. P. Ltd. Available online: https://www.nuffieldbioethics.org/publications/public-health (accessed on 5 March 2025).

Cane, J., O'Connor, D., & Michie, S. (2012). Validation of the theoretical domains framework for use in behaviour change and implementation research. *Implementation Science, 7*(1), 37. [CrossRef] [PubMed]

Chater, N., & Loewenstein, G. (2023). The i-frame and the s-frame: How focusing on individual-level solutions has led behavioral public policy astray. *Behavioral and Brain Sciences, 46*, e147. [CrossRef]

Davoudi-Monfared, E., Mozafari, J. K., Keramatinia, A., Naimi, E., Amiri, P., Rahimpour, E., Ganji, S., Vejdani, M., & Mohseny, M. (2024). A review on lifestyle before and after COVID-19 pandemic: Four levels of prevention [short survey]. *International Journal of Body, Mind and Culture, 11*(4), 258–272. [CrossRef]

DHSC. (2018). *Prevention is better than cure: Our vision to help you live well for longer*. Available online: https://assets.publishing.service.gov.uk/media/5be00437e5274a6e174bdac1/Prevention_is_better_than_cure_5-11.pdf (accessed on 5 March 2025).

Edwards, R. T. (2024). *Health economics of well-being and well-becoming across the life-course*. Oxford University Press. [CrossRef]

Evans, J. S. T., & Stanovich, K. E. (2013). Dual-process theories of higher cognition: Advancing the debate. *Perspectives on Psychological Science, 8*(3), 223–241. [CrossRef]

Gould, A., Lewis, L., Evans, L., Greening, L., Howe-Davies, H., West, J., Roberts, C., & Parkinson, J. A. (2024). COVID-19 personal protective behaviors during large social events: The value of behavioral observations. *Behavioral Sciences, 14*(1), 63. [CrossRef]

Kahneman, D. (2013). *Thinking, fast and slow* (1st ed.). Farrar, Straus and Giroux.

Khalil, E. L., & Amin, A. (2023). The parallelism of cognitive economy and physiological economy: A rationality-based dual process theory. *Current Psychology, 42*(28), 24148–24162. [CrossRef]

Lalani, B., Gray, S., & Mitra-Ganguli, T. (2023). Systems Thinking in an era of climate change: Does cognitive neuroscience hold the key to improving environmental decision making? A perspective on climate-smart agriculture [perspective]. *Frontiers in Integrative Neuroscience, 17*, 1145744. [CrossRef]

Levant, B., & Parkinson, J. (2014). *Positive emotions and reward: Appetitive systems–Amygdala and striatum*. Elsevier.

Masters, R., Anwar, E., Collins, B., Cookson, R., & Capewell, S. (2017). Return on investment of public health interventions: A systematic review. *Journal of Epidemiology and Community Health, 71*(8), 827–834. [CrossRef]

Michie, S., van Stralen, M. M., & West, R. (2011). The behaviour change wheel: A new method for characterising and designing behaviour change interventions. *Implementation Science, 6*(1), 42. [CrossRef] [PubMed]

Murphy, C., Lim, W. W., Mills, C., Wong, J. Y., Chen, D. X., Xie, Y., Li, M. W., Gould, S., Xin, H. L., Cheung, J. K., Bhatt, S., Cowling, B. J., & Donnelly, C. A. (2023). Effectiveness of social distancing measures and lockdowns for reducing transmission of COVID-19 in non-healthcare, community-based settings. *Philosophical Transactions of the Royal Society A-Mathematical Physical and Engineering Sciences, 381*(2257), 20230132.

Musich, S., Wang, S., Hawkins, K., & Klemes, A. (2016). The impact of personalized preventive care on health care quality, utilization, and expenditures. *Population Health Management, 19*(6), 389–397. [CrossRef]

Olshansky, S. J. (2018). From lifespan to healthspan. *JAMA, 320*(13), 1323–1324. [CrossRef]

Parkinson, J. A., Eccles, K. E., & Goodman, A. (2014). Positive impact by design: The wales centre for behaviour change. *The Journal of Positive Psychology, 9*(6), 517–522. [CrossRef]

Parkinson, J. A., Gould, A., Knowles, N., West, J., & Goodman, A. (2025). Integrating systems thinking and behavioral science. *Behavioral Sciences*, *15*(4), 403. [CrossRef]
Reynolds, M. (2024). Systems thinking principles for making change. *Systems*, *12*(10), 437. [CrossRef]
Simeonsson, R. J. (1991). Primary, secondary, and tertiary prevention in early intervention. *Journal of Early Intervention*, *15*(2), 124–134. [CrossRef]
Thaler, R. H., & Sunstein, C. R. (2009). *Nudge: Improving decisions about health, wealth, and happiness*. Penguin Books.
Verplanken, B., & Orbell, S. (2022). Attitudes, habits, and behavior change. *Annual Review of Psychology*, *73*(1), 327–352. [CrossRef]
Wagner, K.-H., & Brath, H. (2012). A global view on the development of non communicable diseases. *Preventive Medicine*, *54*, S38–S41. [CrossRef]
Whiteley, H., Parkinson, J., Hartfiel, N., Makanjuola, A., Lloyd-Williams, H., Lawrence, C., & Edwards, R. T. (2024). Evaluating the well-being benefits and social value of volunteer gardening: Health economics meets behavioral science. *Behavioral Sciences*, *14*(12), 1233. [CrossRef]

behavioral sciences

MDPI

Article

Evaluating Two Brief Motivational Interventions for Excessive-Drinking University Students

Lee M. Hogan [1,2,*] and W. Miles Cox [3]

1 North Wales Clinical Psychology Programme, Bangor University, Bangor LL57 2DG, UK
2 Substance Misuse Services, Betsi Cadwaladr University Health Board, Rhyl LL18 3EY, UK
3 School of Psychology and Sport Sciences, Bangor University, Bangor LL57 2DG, UK; m.cox@bangor.ac.uk
* Correspondence: lee.hogan@bangor.ac.uk

Abstract: Objective: Two brief computerized motivational interventions for excessive-drinking university students were evaluated. Method: Participants (N = 88, females = 61.5%, mean age = 21.05 years) were randomly assigned to a control group or one of two experimental groups: Computerized Brief Intervention (CBI) or Computerized Brief Intervention-Enhanced (CBI-E). CBI followed the principles of Motivational Interviewing to motivate participants to change their drinking behavior. CBI-E additionally used the principles of Systematic Motivational Counseling to identify and discuss with participants their dysfunctional motivational patterns that were interfering with their attainment of emotional satisfaction. At baseline and a three-month follow-up, the participants completed a battery of measures of alcohol consumption and related problems. Results: At baseline, the participants were confirmed to be heavy drinkers with many drink-related negative consequences. Males and females responded differently to the interventions. During follow-up, males' alcohol use was ordered: CBI-E < CBI < Controls. The females in all three groups reduced their alcohol use, but there were no significant group differences. Conclusions: Males responded to the interventions as expected. For females, the assessment itself seemed to serve as an effective intervention, and there were no post-intervention differences among the three groups. Suggestions for future research using CBI and CBI-E are discussed.

Keywords: alcohol consumption; computerized brief intervention; gender difference; motivation; university students

1. Introduction

University students' excessive consumption of alcohol (drinking more than 14 units of alcohol per week), often in binges ("drinking heavily over a short space of time" or "drinking to get drunk"; National Health Service), is a major problem [1–5]. When students drink in a hazardous or harmful manner, this can lead to a variety of short-term and long-term academic, economic, medical, psychological, and social consequences [4,6]. Some excessive-drinking students will eventually resolve their problems with alcohol. Other students, however, will risk developing into dependent drinkers [7]. Clearly, therefore, interventions are needed to tackle the problem of university students' drinking. Over the years, various programs have, in fact, been developed to help students control their drinking, but issues have emerged concerning whether the intended techniques have been properly implemented [8,9], and the problems associated with university students' drinking persist.

Many interventions for university students' drinking were designed to utilize the principles of Motivational Interviewing [10–13]. In the spirit of client-centered counseling [14], Motivational Interviewing is a nonconfrontational, supportive approach to counseling. When used with problem drinkers, Motivational Interviewing and its variants (Motivational Enhancement Therapy and the Drinker's Check-Up) seek to support clients in choosing the drinking goal that is best for them. Specifically, these techniques (a) express empathy for the client's feelings; (b) develop a discrepancy between where the client is now with respect to drinking and where the client would like to be; (c) roll with resistance, i.e., when the client resists the counselor's suggestions, the counselor reflects on the client's views and avoids argumentation; and (d) support clients' self-efficacy by attempting to instill in them a feeling of self-worth and of being in control [15].

Evaluations of the effectiveness of MI and of MET for helping drinkers resolve their problematic use of alcohol have shown that both MI [16–20] and MET [21] are more effective than no treatment and are as effective as other treatments. Brief interventions with university students, which typically use Motivational Interviewing, most frequently report using change strategies that provide personal drinking summaries (including Blood Alcohol Concentration estimates), normative comparisons, consideration of the negative consequences of drinking, risk factors, and behavioral strategies [22], each of which was used in the interventions described in the present study.

Systematic Motivational Counseling (SMC) [23], on the other hand, is based on the motivational model of alcohol use [24–28]. SMC and its briefer variant—the Lifestyle Enrichment and Advancement Program [29,30]—start by assessing drinkers' goals and concerns in various areas of their life (e.g., education, employment, finances, relationships) that might have an impact on their motivation to use alcohol. The technique seeks to identify and alter drinkers' maladaptive motivational patterns that are sources of frustration or a determent to attaining emotional satisfaction without the use of alcohol. As Miller and Rollnick [11] described, "The structured goal attainment counseling procedures . . . nicely complement our more problem-focused discussions of motivational interviewing" (p. 188).

Systematic Motivational Counseling (SMC) begins by assessing participants' motivational structure, using the Motivational Structure Questionnaire or one of its variants [28,31] to identify maladaptive motivational patterns that prevent drinkers from achieving emotional satisfaction, thereby propelling them to seek satisfaction by drinking alcohol. The faulty motivational patterns then become the focus of change during SMC. SMC has been shown to be effective in a variety of formats (with individuals, in groups, as self-help) and with a variety of samples of participants, including university students [29] and patients with diagnoses in addition to an alcohol use disorder [23,28].

The present study utilized the principles of both Motivational Interviewing and Systematic Motivational Counseling to address the problem of university students' excessive use of alcohol. To do so, two computerized brief interventions were developed. One intervention—the Computerized Brief Intervention (CBI)—is based on the principles of Motivational Interviewing. The other intervention—the Computerized Brief Intervention-Enhanced (CBI-E)—is an enhanced version of the first intervention that includes (additional to the CBI intervention) components of Systematic Motivational Counseling (SMC). The addition of the SMC components for dealing with participants' maladaptive motivation was important to include because maladaptive motivation is positively correlated with the amount of alcohol that university students consume [32,33]. As Miller and Rollnick [11] stated, the SMC goal-attainment procedures complement the alcohol-specific focus of MI.

The decision to use a researcher-delivered intervention employing a computer-assisted method was to ensure that (a) immediate graphic and printed feedback could be given, and (b) each participant would receive the same intervention method, albeit personalized for each person.

The impact of each intervention on students' drinking was compared with a control group. The purpose of the study was to evaluate the impact of two computerized motivational interventions compared to a control condition. We hypothesized that (a) compared to the control condition, reductions in drinking would be achieved with both CBI and CBI-E, and (b) the reductions achieved with CBI-E would be greater than those achieved with CBI. Because the overwhelming majority of prior studies evaluating alcohol use interventions for university students have not found gender differences (see [8,9,22,34], we did not expect to find gender differences and gender differences were not hypothesized.

2. Materials and Methods

2.1. Participants

A power analysis indicated that with an expected attrition rate of 15% and an effect size of $f = 0.36$, and to achieve a statistical power of 0.80 and $p < 0.05$ with three groups of participants, an initial sample of approximately 90 participants was needed. Miller et al. [22] reported medium-to-large effect sizes ($\eta^2 = 0.12$ to 0.23) in their review of brief interventions with university students (i.e., proportionate to the Cohen's f effect size of 0.36 selected for this study). Accordingly, 90 participants were recruited from students at Bangor University through an offer of either course credit (one hour of research credit for each hour that they participated) or a modest cash payment of GBP 10. The inclusion criteria were that men should drink more than 21 units of alcohol per week or 8 or more units on one occasion at least weekly, and women should drink more than 14 units per week or 6 or more units on one occasion at least weekly. Each UK unit of alcohol represents 10 mL or 8 g of pure alcohol. The participants were randomly assigned to one of the three groups: Computerized Brief Intervention (CBI), Computerized Brief Intervention-Enhanced (CBI-E), or the Control group. The final sample who completed the first session included 88 students, 54 (61.5%) of whom were female, and their mean age was 21.05 years ($SD = 4.42$). Seventy-five participants completed the follow-up session; 60% of them were female. In the CBI group ($n = 27$), 16 (60%) of the participants were female; in the CBI-E group ($n = 22$), 15 (68%) were female; in the Control group ($n = 26$), 14 (54%) were female. The three groups, therefore, were balanced with regard to gender. The mean age of participants who completed the follow-up session was 21.24 years ($SD = 4.7$).

2.2. Baseline Assessment

At baseline, the participants were individually administered the following measures:

Quantity/Frequency Alcohol Consumption Questionnaire. The Quantity/Frequency (QF) Alcohol Consumption Questionnaire [35,36] is a simplified version of the Alcohol Timeline Followback (TLFB) [37] method for measuring alcohol consumption. The QF was used to record participants' alcohol consumption during the 12 weeks prior to their inclusion in the study. Like the TLFB, the QF uses a calendar to assist the respondent in recalling the amounts of alcohol consumed in a given time period. Unlike the TLFB, the QF focuses on weekly drinking instead of daily drinking. The participant was asked to estimate (a) the usual amount of alcohol consumed during each week and the number of days this usual amount was consumed, and (b) the largest amount of alcohol consumed during each week and the number of days this largest amount was consumed.

Drinker's Inventory of Consequences: The Drinker's Inventory of Consequences (DrInC–2R) [38] is a 50-item questionnaire that measures a variety of negative consequences of drinking that occurred during the prior three months. From respondents' answers, both a total score and scores on five subscales depicting adverse consequences of drinking (physical, intrapersonal, social responsibility, interpersonal, impulse control) can be derived. The internal and test–retest reliability of the DrInC–2R has been confirmed [38].

Short Alcohol Dependency Data Questionnaire: The Short Alcohol Dependency Data Questionnaire (SADD) [39] is a 15-item questionnaire designed to estimate respondents' level of alcohol dependency from their current drinking habits. Based on their total scores, respondents are classified as low, medium, or high in terms of dependency. Various studies [39,40] have confirmed the validity of the SADD.

Readiness to Change Questionnaire: The Readiness to Change Questionnaire (RTCQ) [41] is a 12-item questionnaire designed to assess respondents' level of commitment to changing their drinking. Respondents are assigned to one of three stages of change—precontemplation, contemplation, or action—according to their highest total score. The total score is obtained from the respondent's answers to the 12 items after reverse-scoring the answers to the precontemplation items [42]. Both the internal consistency and test–retest reliability of the RTCQ have been confirmed [43].

Short Tridimensional Personality Questionnaire: The Short Tridimensional Personality Questionnaire (Short–TPQ) is a 44-item questionnaire that measures three personality dimensions: Novelty Seeking (NS), Harm Avoidance (HA), and Reward Dependence (RD) [44]. The internal consistency and test–retest reliability of the three subscales were reported as good [44].

2.3. Computer Software

The computerized brief interventions used in the study were created on a Microsoft Excel 97–2004 Workbook (.xls) [45], which allowed various algorithms and images to be inserted into the program.

2.4. Follow-Up Assessment

At follow-up, the participants were individually administered the Alcohol Timeline Followback [37], which retrospectively estimated their daily drinking during the prior three months with the use of a calendar to help respondents recall the amount of alcohol consumed each day. In addition, the participants were re-administered the DrInC–2R.

2.5. Procedure

At baseline, each participant was interviewed individually in a quiet experimental room at Bangor University. On arrival, the participant read and signed a consent form. In order to protect the anonymity and confidentiality of the participants, each person was assigned a number and data were kept securely in locked file cabinets in a locked office. The participants were randomly assigned to each group following a predetermined list according to the order in which they volunteered for the study. The participants' alcohol consumption in all three groups was assessed with the QF, and they completed the other measures in the baseline battery before participants in the Control group were then dismissed and participants in the CBI group and the CBI-E group individually completed the computerized intervention. These participants received a printed summary of the results of the intervention.

Approximately 12 weeks (M = 85.1 days, SD = 7.8) later, all participants were interviewed about their drinking during the prior 12-weeks with the use of the Alcohol Timeline-Followback method, and they were also re-administered the DrInC–2R. Participants in the Control group were then offered the opportunity to complete the CBI intervention. Each participant was thanked, debriefed, and dismissed. The procedure that was implemented is shown in Figure 1. No data were missing from any of the questionnaires.

2.6. Interventions

2.6.1. Computerized Brief Intervention

The participants were introduced to the CBI as a computer-assisted interview during which they would receive personalized and objective feedback about their drinking. The CBI aimed to motivate participants to change their current use of alcohol through the use of the following components: First, participants were given objective feedback about their drinking. Second, the discrepancy between participants' current drinking and their drinking goal was highlighted. Third, participants were asked to consider the implications of not changing their current level of alcohol use. The CBI achieved these objectives in approximately 30 min through the use of 12 computer screens.

Screen 1: Welcome Page. Screen 2: Calculating Your Blood Alcohol Concentration. Screen 3: Your Weekly Alcohol Consumption (in comparison with other people's drinking using gendered norms). Screen 4: Listing the Good Things About Drinking. Screen 5: Listing the Not-So-Good Things About Drinking. Screen 6: Weighing Up the Good Things and the Not-So-Good Things About Drinking. Screen 7: Future Consequences of Continuing to Drink in this Manner. Screen 8: Would You Like to Change Your Use of Alcohol? (yes, no, maybe). Screen 9: Your Drinking Goal (to cut down, stop, or stay the same). Screen 10: Strategies for Cutting Down or Stopping Drinking. Screen 11: Positive

Action (to take today). Screen 12: Feedback Sheet (summarized the information from the previous screens).

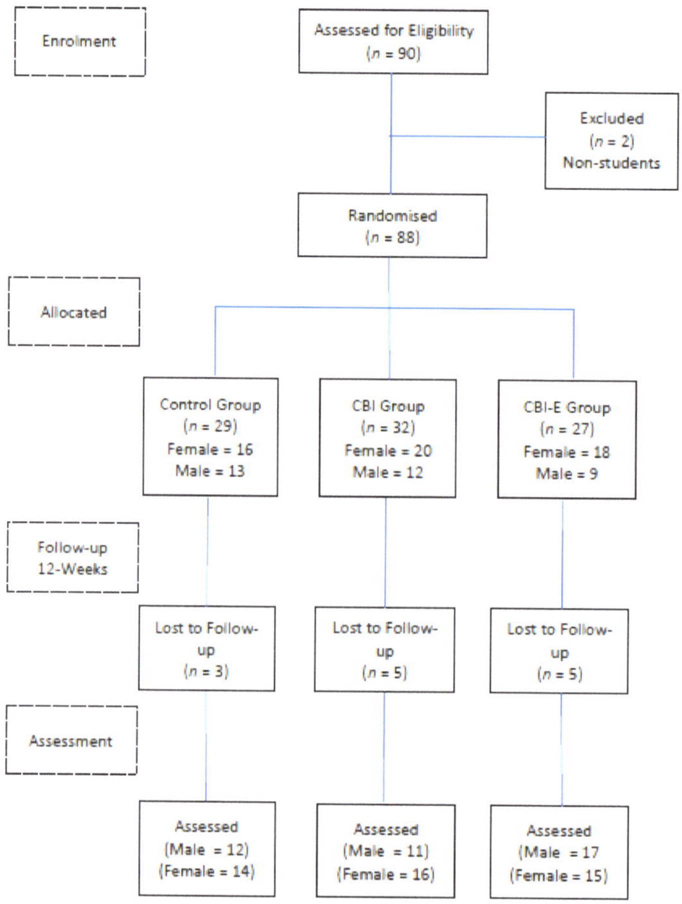

Figure 1. Flow diagram of implemented study procedure.

2.6.2. Enhanced Computerized Brief Intervention

Participants were introduced to the Enhanced Computerized Brief Intervention (CBI-E) as a computer-assisted task that was designed to give them both (a) personalized and objective feedback about their drinking, and (b) feedback about their concerns in other areas of their life that might have an impact on their drinking. The first 12 screens of the CBI-E were the same as those for the CBI. The number of additional screens was variable and depended on the number of concerns the participant named in the other areas; however, on average the additional screens took an additional 30 min to complete.

After completing the CBI, the participant was introduced to the Personal Concerns Inventory (PCI) [23,46], its rationale, and the steps necessary for completing it. The participants were then asked to select the PCI life areas (e.g., Home and Household; Employment and Finances; Relationships) in which they had concerns and to briefly describe each concern and their goal for resolving it. In subsequent screens, they rated each of their goal pursuits on ten rating scales (Commitment, Importance, How Likely to Succeed, Expected Joy, etc.). Doing so revealed the structure of the participant's motivation (i.e., the degree to which it was adaptive or maladaptive), which was shown to the participant in graphical format. Thereafter, the interviewer provided feedback by calling attention to maladaptive patterns (e.g., pursuing unrealistic goals or goals that were unlikely to succeed or unlikely to be emotionally satisfying) and discussing with the participant ways to change faulty motivational patterns into adaptive ones. The suggestions were based on one of the 12 components of SMC [23]. Each suggestion aimed to help the participant find more adaptive ways to resolve important concerns that impacted his or her motivation to achieve emotional satisfaction by drinking alcohol or abstaining from drinking. For instance, it seemed best for some participants to disengage from goal pursuits that were unlikely to succeed or unlikely to be satisfying, even if successful. Some participants needed suggestions for finding pleasurable goals to pursue as an alternative to drinking alcohol. Other participants needed help in dividing their long-range goals into interim steps, whose achievement would bring a feeling of success. Still others seemed to benefit simply from receiving feedback about how their excessive drinking was interfering with their achievement of appropriate and realistic goals that they were already pursuing.

The interventions were conducted by the first author, who was an advanced Ph.D. student in clinical and health psychology. He was trained and supervised (a) in the delivery of the MI components by members of the counseling staff at Cyngor Alcohol Information Services, and (b) in the delivery of the SMC components by the second author, who is the co-developer of SMC.

2.7. Analysis

To analyze participants' baseline characteristics, descriptive statistics, ANOVAs, Tukey post hoc tests, and *t*-tests were conducted. Similarly, to analyze changes in participants' alcohol consumption following the interventions, ANOVAs and *t*-tests were used.

3. Results

3.1. Baseline Characteristics

At baseline, the male and female participants' mean weekly alcohol consumption was 35.0 (SD = 22.7) units and 25.9 (SD = 18.1) units, respectively ($t(86) = 2.097, p < 0.039$). The mean number of binge episodes during the previous 12 weeks (defined as eight or more units on one occasion for males and six or more units for females) was 23.5 (SD = 12.7) for males and 22.61 (SD = 16.0) for females ($t(86) < 1.0$, *NS*). Table 1 displays the participants' mean weekly alcohol consumption, along with the number of binge episodes and negative drinking consequences for each group.

Table 1. Means and standard deviations of weekly alcohol consumption, number of binges, and drink-related problems at baseline (t1) and follow-up (t2) for males and females in the control, CBI, and CBI-E groups.

	Control				CBI				CBI-E			
	Male (n = 12)		Female (n = 14)		Male (n = 11)		Female (n = 16)		Male (n = 7)		Female (n = 15)	
Variable	M	SD	M	SD	M	SD	M	SD	M	SD	M	SD
Weekly units, t1	37.3	33.1	23.3	12.1	35.1	17.1	25.3	20.9	37.4	13.0	23.0	9.9
Weekly units, t2	29.3	18.3	15.7	8.2	22.7	14.4	12.1	7.2	14.6	7.4	17.6	12.6
Binge † total, t1	20.1	13.5	19.7	9.0	25.0	12.8	23.4	21.0	27.7	12.8	20.2	8.1
Binge † total, t2	18.9	12.7	15.1	10.3	17.5	10.7	10.4	9.0	9.8	6.5	16.0	13.3
DrInC total, t1	20.8	14.9	25.3	14.5	18.4	7.8	22.9	19.0	23.3	13.5	21.4	12.4
DrInC total, t2	20.3	13.3	15.4	8.2	19.4	11.5	14.6	11.6	19.1	10.6	18.8	12.1

Note: † Binge criteria were that males consumed eight units or more on one occasion, and females, six units or more on one occasion.

The mean number of drinking-related negative consequences was 20.7 (SD = 11.5) for males and 23.2 (SD = 15.4) for females ($t(86) < 1.0$, *NS*). Had a hangover (at 95%) and felt bad about myself because of my drinking (at 66%) were the most frequently reported negative consequences. On the DrInC subscales, the participants scored highest on negative physical consequences, and next highest on adverse consequences related to social responsibility, impulse control, intrapersonal consequences, and interpersonal consequences.

To determine whether participants' level of alcohol consumption was related to the number of alcohol-related problems they had experienced, they were allocated to one of three groups (low-risk drinkers, hazardous drinkers, or harmful drinkers), based on the UK's public health guidelines [47]. A one-way analysis of variance indicated that the three groups differed significantly ($F(2,87) = 8.240$, $p < 0.001$). Tukey's HSD post hoc tests showed that the low-risk drinkers had significantly lower DrInC total scores ($M = 15.45$, $SD = 9.40$) than both the hazardous drinkers ($M = 21.46$, $SD = 11.65$, $p < 0.022$) and the harmful drinkers ($M = 33.81$, $SD = 18.82$ $p < 0.001$), but the hazardous and harmful drinkers did not differ from each other. The participants' scores on the SADD indicated that the majority of them (59.7%) were at the low level of alcohol dependence; 37.5% were at the medium level; and 3.4% were at the high level.

The three groups (CBI, CBI-E, Control) were also compared on each of the other baseline measures, but there were no baseline differences. It is noteworthy, however, that females ($M = 11.37$, $SD = 5.94$) as a whole were significantly higher than males ($M = 5.70$, $SD = 3.30$) on the Harm Avoidance scale of the Short Tridimensional Personality Questionnaire ($t(68) = 5.22$, $p < 0.001$). The distribution of the three groups on the three stages of change (precontemplation, contemplation, action) from the Readiness to Change Questionnaire did not differ (χ^2 (4, $n = 88$) = 2.34, $p > 0.05$). The majority of the participants were in either the precontemplation stage or the contemplation stage; only 22% of them were in the action stage.

3.2. Changes in Drinking at Follow-Up

The rate of attrition for the three groups was as follows: Control, $n = 3$ (10.3%); CBI $n = 5$; (15.6%); and CBI-E, $n = 5$ (17.2%). The mean weekly alcohol consumption of the participants who were retained in the study ($M = 29.01$, $SD = 19.72$) and those who dropped out ($M = 30.62$, $SD = 23.06$) did not differ ($t(88) < 1.0$, *NS*), and there was no apparent relationship between participants' drop-out rates and their level of drinking at baseline. Reductions in mean weekly alcohol consumption from baseline to the three-month follow-up were examined for differences among the groups and, unexpectedly, differences between the male and female participants were detected. Consequently, for ease of interpretation, the three groups' mean weekly alcohol consumption at baseline and during the follow-up period are shown separately for males and females in Figure 2 and Figure 3, respectively.

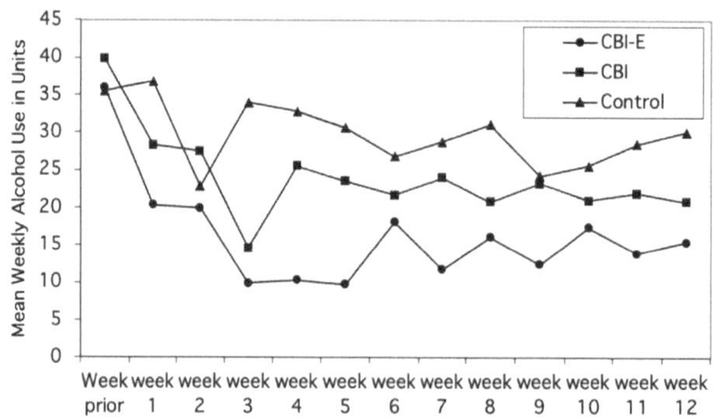

Figure 2. Mean weekly alcohol consumption of males in the CBI-E, CBI, and Control group during the week prior to being included in the study and during each of the 12 weeks following the intervention.

For males, after a steady reduction in drinking during the first three weeks after being included in the study, the weekly consumption of each of the groups stabilized. Individuals in the CBI-E group drank less alcohol than the other two groups, and the CBI group drank less than the Control group. For females, however, the post-intervention pattern of drinking was quite different. First, the female participants in all three groups considerably reduced their consumption just after they completed the baseline assessment. Second, the reductions were maintained throughout the 12 weeks of follow-up. Third, the differences in consumption among the three groups were less distinct than for the males.

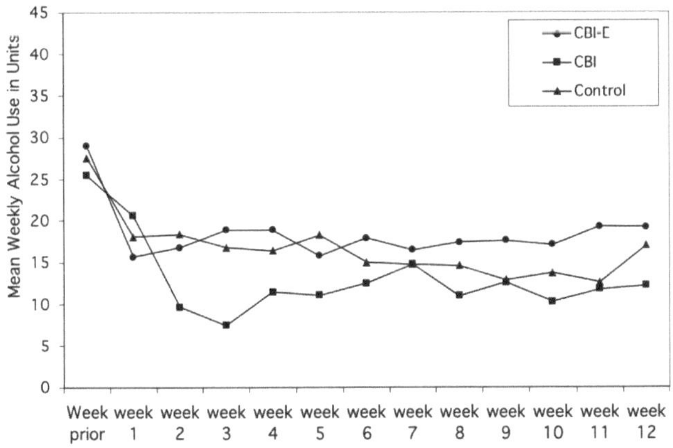

Figure 3. Mean weekly alcohol consumption of females in the CBI-E, CBI, and Control group during the week prior to being included in the study and during each of the 12 weeks following the intervention.

Prior to analyzing the results statistically, the distributions of the variables were examined for deviations from normality, and any deviations were corrected with logarithmic or square root transformations. Thereafter, mean alcohol consumption during the 12 weeks prior to the interventions (baseline) was compared with mean consumption during the 12 weeks following the interventions (follow-up). A repeated-measures ANOVA that included groups (CBI, CBI-E, Control) and gender (females, males) as the between-participants factors and time of testing (baseline, follow-up) as the within-participants factor showed that the participants reduced their consumption from baseline ($M = 29.0$, $SD = 19.7$) to follow-up ($M = 18.4$, $SD = 12.9$, $F(1,69) = 51.59$, $p < 0.001$). There was also (a) a groups-by-time interaction ($F(2,69) = 3.67$, $p < 0.04$), indicating differential reductions among the three groups, and (b) a groups-by-time-by-gender interaction ($F(2,69) = 3.26$, $p < 0.044$).

To identify the source of the three-way interaction, repeated-measures ANOVAs were conducted separately for males and females. In each analysis, group was the between-participants factor, and time was the within-participants factor. For males, there was a main effect for time ($F(1,27) = 23.92$, $p < 0.001$), and a groups-by-time interaction ($F(2,27) = 4.42$, $p < 0.022$). The source of the two-way interaction was identified using paired-samples t-tests. For male participants in the CBI-E group, there was a significant reduction in alcohol consumption from baseline ($M = 37.4$, $SD = 13.0$) to follow-up ($M = 14.6$, $SD = 7.4$, $t(6) = 3.69$, $p = 0.01$). For male participants in the CBI group, there was also a significant reduction in alcohol consumption from baseline ($M = 35.1$, $SD = 17.1$) to follow-up ($M = 22.7$, $SD = 14.4$, $t(10) = 3.07$, $p = 0.012$). The male participants in the Control group, however, did not significantly reduce their consumption from baseline ($M = 37.3$, $SD = 33.1$) to follow-up ($M = 29.3$, $SD = 18.3$), $t(11) = 0.96$, $p = 0.357$. Additionally, the mean weekly consumption of the males who received the CBI-E intervention was below the UK Department of Health's recommended limit of 21 units per week for each of the 12 weeks following the intervention. The males in the CBI group were below this limit during just four of these weeks. The males in the Control group, on the other hand, exceeded this limit during each of the 12 weeks.

Females also reduced their consumption from baseline ($M = 23.9$, $SD = 14.9$) to follow-up ($M = 15.1$, $SD = 9.5$, $F(1,42) = 29.081$, $p < 0.001$). However, the groups-by-time interaction ($F(2,42) = 1.36$, $p = 0.27$) was not significant, indicating that the three groups did not differ in the amount they reduced from baseline (CBI-E group: $M = 23.0$, $SD = 9.9$; CBI group: $M = 25.3$, $SD = 20.9$; Control group: $M = 23.3$, $SD = 12.1$) to follow-up (CBI-E group: $M = 17.6$, $SD = 12.3$; CBI group: $M = 12.1$, $SD = 7.2$; Control group $M = 15.7$, $SD = 8.2$).

3.3. Reductions in Binge Drinking

A repeated-measures ANOVA was also used to evaluate the changes in the number of binge-drinking episodes from baseline to follow-up. The participants as a whole reduced the number of binge episodes from baseline ($M = 22.2$, $SD = 13.6$) to follow-up ($M = 14.7$, $SD = 11.1$, $F(1,69) = 30.46$, $p < 0.001$). Because the groups-by-time interaction closely approached significance ($F(2,69) = 3.07$, $p < 0.053$), paired-samples t-tests were run to identify the source of the interaction. The participants in the CBI-E group reduced the number of binge episodes from baseline ($M = 22.59$, $SD = 10.17$) to follow-up ($M = 13.95$, $SD = 11.81$, $t(21) = 3.86$, $p = 0.001$). Likewise, the participants in the CBI group reduced the number of binge episodes from baseline ($M = 24.04$, $SD = 17.86$) to follow-up ($M = 13.30$, $SD = 10.16$, $t(26) = 4.17$, $p < 0.001$). The participants in the Control group, however, did not significantly reduce the number of binge episodes from baseline ($M = 19.88$, $SD = 11.07$) to follow-up ($M = 16.85$, $SD = 11.40$, $t(25) = 1.44$, $p = 0.16$). Neither the time-by-gender interaction ($p = 0.688$) nor the three-way interaction ($p = 0.139$) was significant.

Changes in the number of negative consequences of drinking from baseline to follow-up were also examined for differences between groups and between genders. A repeated-measures ANOVA yielded a significant main effect for time, indicating that the number of negative consequences decreased from baseline ($M = 22.1$, $SD = 14.1$) to follow-up ($M = 17.6$, $SD = 11.2$, $F(1,67) = 11.08$, $p < 0.001$). There was also a gender-by-time interaction ($F(1,67) = 4.25$, $p < 0.043$). Males did not change ($M = 20.5$ ($SD = 12.1$) between baseline and ($M = 19.7$, $SD = 11.7$) at follow-up ($t(28) = < 1.0$, NS). By contrast, females decreased from $M = 23.1$ ($SD = 15.4$) at baseline to $M = 16.3$ ($SD = 10.8$) at follow-up ($t(43) = 3.99$, $p < 0.001$).

4. Discussion

Two brief interventions aimed at reducing university students' excessive use of alcohol were evaluated. The Computerized Brief Intervention (CBI) utilized the principles of Motivational Interviewing to directly address students' excessive use of alcohol and motivate them to change their drinking. The Enhanced Computerized Brief Intervention (CBI-E) additionally addressed students' concerns in other life areas that affected their motivation to drink alcohol. Consistent with Value X Expectancy theory [27,48–50], the aim was to help students form goals that both held value for them and for which they had a realistic expectancy of successful goal attainment. We hypothesized that both CBI and CBI-E would induce a reduction in consumption and that CBI-E would bring about a greater reduction than CBI.

Unexpectedly, distinct differences between the male and female participants' responsiveness to the two interventions were revealed. The results obtained with male participants supported the research hypotheses. Unlike male participants in the Control group, those in both the CBI-E group and the CBI group reduced their consumption, and the reduction in the CBI-E group exceeded that of the CBI group. The post-intervention pattern of drinking of the female participants was, however, quite different. The females in all three groups (CBI-E, CBI, Control) reduced their consumption, and the reduction was relatively stable throughout the post-intervention period.

The gender difference in responsiveness to the two interventions can be accounted for in the following way: at the baseline assessment, the participants in each of the three groups answered detailed questions about their alcohol consumption during the preceding three months. The assessment is likely to have made participants acutely aware of how much alcohol they were drinking; the negative consequences they had experienced because of their excessive drinking; and the need to cut down. The explanation for why only the female participants reacted to the assessment by reducing their drinking appears to lie in a personality difference between the male and female participants. Consistent with the findings of other studies [51,52], the female participants in this study scored higher on harm-avoidance than the male participants. Harm-avoidant individuals use protective behavioral strategies to avoid engaging in harmful behaviors when they become aware of them. Therefore, for the female participants, the assessment itself appeared to serve as a brief intervention that induced them to reduce their alcohol consumption.

In previous studies, a gender difference in university students' responsiveness to a brief intervention for excessive drinking has often not been found [8,9,22,34,53,54]. Nevertheless, within other samples the gender difference that we found is not without precedent. Specifically, the World Health Organization's study of brief interventions [55] reported that females in both the control group and the intervention group reduced their alcohol consumption. Males, on the other hand, reduced their alcohol consumption only if they received a brief intervention. Similarly, Chang [56] reviewed prior studies of brief interventions with females and concluded that brief interventions were not consistently more helpful for females than a control condition. Other studies [57,58] have found a gender difference in changes in drinking, although the changes were not a function of the intervention received.

The results of this initial evaluation of CBI and CBI-E are promising for two reasons. First, it is noteworthy that for the female participants, the comprehensive assessment of their drinking habits was sufficient to cause a stable reduction in consumption, and this was apparently due to the females' stronger use of protective behavioral strategies. Second, the study also demonstrated that when used with male university students, both CBI and CBI-E were effective, but CBI-E was more effective than CBI. The improved outcome with CBI-E was theoretically expected because the enhanced intervention addressed both participants' problematic use of alcohol and their maladaptive motivational patterns that undergirded their motivation to drink alcohol.

Limitations

Despite these encouraging results, the limitations of the current study should be addressed in future evaluations of the two motivational interventions. First, although a power analysis indicated that the sample size was sufficient for testing the main hypotheses, the unexpected need to divide the sample into subgroups in order to evaluate gender differences resulted in relatively small subgroups. Second, in future studies, it would be advisable to use additional controls, particularly a sham intervention to determine the extent to which the better outcome achieved with the enhanced intervention was due to the additional attention that the CBI-E group received. Third, instead of asking participants to retrospectively recall their drinking during each week of the preceding three months, a more accurate record of their drinking might be achieved by asking participants to keep a prospective daily diary of their drinking. Fourth, this study was conducted in the United Kingdom, and it is not known how generalizable the findings are to other countries and other cultures with different drinking practices. Finally, it would be worthwhile in future to explore different combinations of the brief computerized interventions. For instance, how would the enhanced components of CBI-E alone fare as a brief intervention for university students when used after a comprehensive assessment of participants' drinking behavior? Also, would the enhanced components used alone be more effective for certain types of students (e.g., males and females who use protective behavioral strategies) than others?

Author Contributions: Conceptualization, methodology, and software writing were undertaken by L.M.H. under the PhD supervision of W.M.C.; data analysis and original draft preparation were undertaken by L.M.H. with manuscript writing jointly undertaken with L.M.H. and W.M.C. All authors have read and agreed to the published version of the manuscript.

Funding: The research reported in this article was supported by a Postgraduate Training Award (R42200134252) to Lee M. Hogan from the Economic Social and Research Council.

Institutional Review Board Statement: The study was conducted in accordance with the Declaration of Helsinki, and approved by the Institutional Review Ethical Board from Bangor University, School of Psychology Ethics Committee, originally awarded in 2003.

Informed Consent Statement: Informed consent was obtained from all participants involved in the study.

Data Availability Statement: Data supporting the results can be obtained by contacting L.M.H. at lee.hogan@bangor.ac.uk.

Acknowledgments: The Computerized Brief Intervention (CBI) was developed by the first author in collaboration with members of the counseling staff at Cygnor Alcohol Information Services (CAIS), Llandudno, North Wales, UK. The assistance of MSc. students Sarita Cooper and Laura Purdy in conducting a portion of the interviews is gratefully acknowledged.

Conflicts of Interest: The authors declare no conflict of interest.

References

1. Bagheri, M.; Cox, W.M. Self-regulation, adaptive motivation, and alcohol consumption: Understanding university students' motivation for drinking. *J. Subst. Use* **2024**, *29*, 389–392. [CrossRef]
2. Cox, W.M.; Hosier, S.G.; Crossley, S.; Kendall, B.; Roberts, K.L. Motives for drinking, alcohol consumption, and alcohol-related problems among British secondary-school and university students. *Addict. Behav.* **2006**, *31*, 2147–2157. [CrossRef] [PubMed]
3. Helle, A.C.; Boness, C.L.; Sher, K.J. College students' receptiveness to intervention approaches for alcohol and cannabis use. *Psychol. Addict. Behav.* **2022**, *36*, 157–176. [CrossRef]
4. Moagi, M.M.; van der Wath, A.E. Demand for alcohol use among students at higher education institutions: An integrative literature review. *J. Subst. Use* **2023**, *28*, 9–19. [CrossRef]
5. Richards, D.K.; Pearson, M.R.; Field, C.A. A comprehensive examination of alcohol-related motivations among college students: Unique relations of drinking motives and motivations for drinking responsibly. *Exp. Clin. Psychopharmacol.* **2022**, *30*, 809–819. [CrossRef]
6. Cox, W.M.; Klinger, E. Alcohol and its effects on the body. In *Why People Drink*; How People Change: A Guide to Alcohol and People's Motivation for Drinking It; Cox, W.M., Klinger, E., Eds.; Springer Nature: Berlin/Heidelberg, Germany, 2022.
7. Gajda, M.; Sedlaczek, K.; Szemik, S.; Kowalska, M. Determinants of Alcohol Consumption among Medical Students: Results from POLLEK Cohort Study. *Int. J. Environ. Res. Public Health* **2021**, *18*, 5872. [CrossRef]
8. DiClemente, C.C.; Corno, C.M.; Graydon, M.M.; Wiprovnick, A.E.; Knoblach, D.J. Motivational interviewing, enhancement, and brief interventions over the last decade: A review of reviews of efficacy and effectiveness. *Psychol. Addict. Behav.* **2017**, *31*, 862–887. [CrossRef]
9. Larimer, M.E.; Kilmer, J.R.; Cronce, J.M.; Hultgren, B.A.; Gilson, M.S.; Lee, C.M. Thirty years of BASICS: Dissemination and implementation progress and challenges. *Psychol. Addict. Behav.* **2022**, *36*, 664–677. [CrossRef]
10. Blume, A.W.; Marlatt, G.A. Motivational enhancement as a brief intervention for college student drinkers. In *Handbook of Motivational Counseling: Goal-Based Approaches to Assessment and Intervention with Addiction and Other Problems*, 2nd ed.; Cox, W.M., Klinger, E., Eds.; Wiley-Blackwell: Hoboken, NJ, USA, 2011; pp. 531–547.
11. Miller, W.R.; Rollnick, S. *Motivational Interviewing: Preparing People to Change Addictive Behavior*; Guilford: New York, NY, USA, 1991.
12. Miller, W.R.; Rollnick, S. *Motivational Interviewing: Preparing People for Change*, 2nd ed.; Guilford: New York, NY, USA, 2002.
13. Miller, W.R.; Rollnick, S. *Motivational Interviewing: Helping People Change*, 3rd ed.; Guilford: New York, NY, USA, 2013.
14. Resnicow, K.; Rollnick, S. Motivational interviewing in health promotion and behavioral medicine. In *Handbook of Motivational Counseling: Goal-Based Approaches to Assessment and Intervention with Addiction and Other Problems*, 2nd ed.; Cox, W.M., Klinger, E., Eds.; Wiley-Blackwell: Hoboken, NJ, USA, 2011; pp. 591–605.
15. Demmel, R. Motivational Interviewing: A Review. *Addict. J. Sci. Pract.* **2001**, *47*, 171–188.
16. Burke, B.L.; Arkowitz, H.; Menchola, M. The efficacy of motivational interviewing: A meta-analysis of controlled clinical trials. *J. Consult. Clin. Psychol.* **2003**, *71*, 843–861. [CrossRef]
17. Frost, H.; Campbell, P.; Maxwell, M.; O'Carroll, R.E.; Dombrowski, S.U.; Williams, B.; Cheyne, H.; Coles, E.; Pollock, A. Effectiveness of Motivational Interviewing on adult behaviour change in health and social care settings: A systematic review of reviews. *PLoS ONE* **2018**, *13*, 39. [CrossRef] [PubMed]
18. Lundahl, B.; Burke, B.L. The effectiveness and applicability of motivational interviewing: A practice-friendly review of four meta-analyses. *J. Clin. Psychol.* **2009**, *65*, 1232–1245. [CrossRef] [PubMed]
19. Magill, M.; Gaume, J.; Apodaca, T.R.; Walthers, J.; Mastroleo, N.R.; Borsari, B.; Longabaugh, R. The technical hypothesis of motivational interviewing: A meta-analysis of MI's key causal model. *J. Consult. Clin. Psychol.* **2014**, *82*, 973–983. [CrossRef] [PubMed]
20. Vasilaki, E.I.; Hosier, S.G.; Cox, W.M. The efficacy of motivational interviewing as a brief intervention for excessive drinking: A meta-analytic review. *Alcohol Alcohol.* **2006**, *41*, 328–335. [CrossRef] [PubMed]
21. Lenz, A.S.; Rosenbaum, L.; Sheperis, D. Meta-analysis of randomized controlled trials of motivational enhancement therapy for reducing substance use. *J. Addict. Offender Couns.* **2016**, *37*, 66–86. [CrossRef]

22. Miller, M.B.; Leffingwell, T.; Claborn, K.; Meier, E.; Walters, S.; Neighbors, C. Personalized feedback interventions for college alcohol misuse: An update of Walters & Neighbors (2005). *Psychol. Addict. Behav.* **2013**, *27*, 909–920.
23. Cox, W.M.; Klinger, E. Systematic Motivational Counseling: From motivational assessment to motivational change. In *Handbook of Motivational Counseling: Goal-Based Approaches to Assessment and Intervention with Addiction and Other Problems*, 2nd ed.; Cox, W.M., Klinger, E., Eds.; Wiley-Blackwell: Hoboken, NJ, USA, 2011; pp. 275–302.
24. Cox, W.M.; Klinger, E. A motivational model of alcohol use. *J. Abnorm. Psychol.* **1988**, *97*, 168–180. [CrossRef]
25. Cox, W.M.; Klinger, E. Incentive motivation, affective change, and alcohol use: A model. In *Why People Drink: Parameters of Alcohol as a Reinforcer*; Cox, W.M., Ed.; Psychology Press: Gardner, MA, USA, 1990.
26. Cox, W.M.; Klinger, E. A motivational model of alcohol use: Determinants of use and change. In *Handbook of Motivational Counseling: Concepts, Approaches, and Assessment*; Cox, W.M., Klinger, E., Eds.; Wiley: Hoboken, NJ, USA, 2004; pp. 121–138.
27. Cox, W.M.; Klinger, E. A motivational model of alcohol use: Determinants of use and change. In *Handbook of Motivational Counselling. Goal-Based Approaches to Assessment and Intervention with Addiction and Other Problems*; Cox, W.M., Klinger, E., Eds.; Wiley-Blackwell: Hoboken, NJ, USA, 2011; pp. 131–158.
28. Cox, W.M.; Klinger, E. *Why People Drink*; How People Change: A Guide to Alcohol and People's Motivation for Drinking It; Springer Nature: Berlin/Heidelberg, Germany, 2022.
29. Cox, W.M.; Fadardi, J.S.; Hosier, S.G.; Pothos, E.M. Differential effects and temporal course of attentional and motivational training on excessive drinking. *Exp. Clin. Psychopharmacol.* **2015**, *23*, 445–454. [CrossRef]
30. Jahan, Z.V.; Shamloo, Z.S.; Fadardi, J.S. Comparing the effectiveness of the Life Enhancement and Advancement Program and reality therapy on improving in-treatment substance abusers' recovery indices. *Res. Clin. Psychol. Couns.* **2013**, *3*, 99–118.
31. Cox, W.M.; Klinger, E. Measuring motivation: The Motivational Structure Questionnaire, Personal Concerns Inventory, and their variants. In *Handbook of Motivational Counseling: Goal-Based Approaches to Assessment and Intervention with Addiction and Other Problems*; Cox, W.M., Klinger, E., Eds.; Wiley-Blackwell: Hoboken, NJ, USA, 2011; pp. 161–204.
32. Cox, W.M.; Klinger, E. Motivational structure: Relationships with substance use and processes of change. *Addict. Behav.* **2002**, *27*, 925–940. [CrossRef]
33. Cox, W.M.; Schippers, G.M.; Klinger, E.; Skutle, A.; Stuchlíková, I.; Man, F.; King, A.L.; Inderhaug, I. Motivational structure and alcohol use of university students with consistency across four nations. *J. Stud. Alcohol* **2002**, *63*, 280–285. [CrossRef] [PubMed]
34. Walters, S.T.; Neighbors, C. Feedback interventions for college alcohol misuse: What, why and for whom? *Addict. Behav.* **2005**, *30*, 1168–1182. [CrossRef] [PubMed]
35. Hogan, L.; Patterson, C.W.; Cox, M. Accurately estimating alcohol consumption: A comparison of self-administrated and interview methods. *Subst. Use Misuse* **2020**, *55*, 1184–1188. [CrossRef] [PubMed]
36. Patterson, C.; Hogan, L.; Cox, M. A comparison between two retrospective alcohol consumption measures and the daily drinking diary method with university students. *Am. J. Drug Alcohol Abus.* **2019**, *45*, 248–253. [CrossRef] [PubMed]
37. Sobell, L.C.; Sobell, M.B. Timeline Follow-Back: A technique for assessing self-reported alcohol consumption. In *Measuring Alcohol Consumption: Psychosocial and Biochemical Methods*; Litten, R.Z., Allen, J.P., Eds.; Humana Press: Totowa, NJ, USA, 1992; pp. 41–72.
38. Miller, W.R.; Tonigan, J.S.; Longabaugh, R. *The Drinker Inventory of Consequences (DrInC): An Instrument for Assessing Adverse Consequences of Alcohol Abuse*; Project MATCH Monograph Series, Vol. 4. DHHS Publication No. 95-3911; National Institute on Alcohol Abuse and Alcoholism: Rockville, MD, USA, 1995.
39. Davidson, R.; Raitrick, D. The validity of the Short Alcohol Dependence Data (SADD) questionnaire: A short self-report questionnaire for the assessment of alcohol dependence. *Br. J. Addict.* **1986**, *81*, 217–222. [CrossRef] [PubMed]
40. Davidson, R.; Bunting, B.; Raitrick, D. The homogeneity of the alcohol dependence syndrome: A factor analysis of the SADD questionnaire. *Br. J. Addict.* **1989**, *84*, 907–915. [CrossRef] [PubMed]
41. Heather, N.; Gold, R.; Rollnick, S. *Readiness to Change Questionnaire: User's Manual. Technical Report 15*; National Drug and Alcohol Research Centre, University of New South Wales: Kensington, Australia, 1991.
42. Heather, N.; Rollnick, S.; Bell, A. Predictive validity of the Readiness to Change Questionnaire. *Addiction* **1993**, *88*, 1667–1677. [CrossRef] [PubMed]
43. Rollnick, S.; Heather, N.; Gold, R.; Hall, W. Development of a short 'readiness to change' questionnaire for use in brief, opportunistic interventions among excessive drinkers. *Addiction* **1992**, *87*, 743–754. [CrossRef] [PubMed]
44. Sher, K.J.; Wood, P.K.; Crews, T.M.; Vandiver, P.A. The Tridimensional Personality Questionnaire: Reliability and validity studies and short derivation of a short form. *Psychol. Assess.* **1995**, *7*, 195–208. [CrossRef]
45. Microsoft Corporation. Microsoft Excel. 2018. Available online: https://office.microsoft.com/excel (accessed on 23 March 2023).
46. Klinger, E.; Cox, W.M. The Motivational Structure Questionnaire, Personal Concerns Inventory, and their variants: Psychometric properties. In *Handbook of Motivational Counseling: Goal-Based Approaches to Assessment and Intervention with Addiction and Other Problems*; Cox, W.M., Klinger, E., Eds.; Wiley-Blackwell: Hoboken, NJ, USA, 2011; pp. 204–232.
47. House of Commons Health Committee. Alcohol. 2010. Available online: https://www.ias.org.uk/uploads/pdf/News%20stories/hchc-report-080110.pdf (accessed on 23 March 2023).
48. Feather, N.T.; Newton, J.W. Values, expectations, and the prediction of social action: An expectancy-valence analysis. *Motiv. Emot.* **1982**, *6*, 217–244. [CrossRef]

49. Klinger, E.; Cox, W.M. Motivation and the goal theory of current concerns. In *Handbook of Motivational Counseling: Goal-Based Approaches to Assessment and Intervention with Addiction and Other Problems*; Cox, W.M., Klinger, E., Eds.; Wiley-Blackwell: Hoboken, NJ, USA, 2011; pp. 3–47.
50. van Eerde, W.; Thierry, H. Vroom's expectancy models and work-related criteria: A meta-analysis. *J. Appl. Psychol.* **1996**, *81*, 575–586. [CrossRef]
51. Braitman, A.L.; Linden-Carmichael, A.; Henson, J.M. Protective behavioral strategies as a context-specific mediator: A multilevel examination of within- and between-person associations of daily drinking. *Exp. Clin. Psychopharmacol.* **2017**, *25*, 141–155. [CrossRef] [PubMed]
52. Gierski, F.; Benzerouk, F.; De Wever, E.; Duka, T.; Kaladjian, A.; Quaglino, V.; Naassila, M. Cloninger's temperament and character dimensions of personality and binge drinking among college students. *Alcohol. Clin. Exp. Res.* **2017**, *41*, 1970–1979. [CrossRef] [PubMed]
53. Carey, K.B.; DiBello, A.M.; Orazio, E.E.; Hatch, M.R.; Mastroleo, N.R. Predictors of receptivity to an alcohol intervention among mandated students. *Addict. Behav.* **2021**, *112*, 106605. [CrossRef] [PubMed]
54. Dunn, M.E.; Fried-Somerstein, A.; Flori, J.N.; Hall, T.V.; Dvorak, R.D. Reducing alcohol use in mandated college students: A comparison of a Brief Motivational Intervention (BMI) and the Expectancy Challenge Alcohol Literacy Curriculum (ECALC). *Exp. Clin. Psychopharmacol.* **2020**, *28*, 87–98. [CrossRef] [PubMed]
55. Babor, T.; Grant, M. (Eds.) *Project on Identification and Management of Alcohol-Related Problems. Report on Phase II: A Randomized Clinical Trial of Brief Interventions in Primary Health Care*; World Health Organization: Geneva, Switzerland, 1992.
56. Chang, G. Brief interventions for problem drinking and women. *J. Subst. Abus. Treat.* **2002**, *23*, 1–7. [CrossRef] [PubMed]
57. Collins, S.E.; Carey, K.B.; Sliwinski, M.J. Mailed personalized normative feedback as a brief interention for at-risk college drinkers. *J. Stud. Alcohol* **2002**, *63*, 559–567. [CrossRef]
58. Murphy, J.G.; Benson, T.A.; Vuchinich, R.E.; Deskins, M.M.; Eakin, D.; Flood, A.M.; McDevitt-Murphy, M.; Torrealday, O. A Comparison of Personalized Feedback for College Student Drinkers Delivered with and without a Motivational Interview. *J. Stud. Alcohol* **2004**, *65*, 200–203. [CrossRef]

behavioral sciences

MDPI

Article

Closing the Gap: How Psychological Distance Influences Willingness to Engage in Risky COVID Behavior

Ceridwen Williams [1], Paul Rauwolf [1], Matt Boulter [2] and John A. Parkinson [1,*]

[1] Wales Centre for Behaviour Change, Department of Psychology, Bangor University, Bangor LL57 2AS, UK; crw20zqf@bangor.ac.uk (C.W.); p.rauwolf@bangor.ac.uk (P.R.)
[2] School of Health and Life Sciences, University of the West of Scotland, Glasgow G72 0LH, UK; matt.boulter@uws.ac.uk
* Correspondence: j.parkinson@bangor.ac.uk

Abstract: Pandemics, and other risk-related contexts, require dynamic changes in behavior as situations develop. Human behavior is influenced by both explicit (cognitive) and implicit (intuitive) factors. In this study, we used psychological distance as a lens to understand what influences our decision-making with regard to risk in the context of COVID-19. This study was based on the rationale that our relational needs are more concrete to us than the risk of the virus. First, we explored the impact of social–psychological distance on participants' risk perceptions and behavioral willingness. As hypothesized, we found that close social relationships of agents promoted willingness to engage in risky behavior. In the second phase, we tested an intervention designed to increase the concreteness of information about virus transmission as a mechanism to mitigate the bias of social influence. We found that the concreteness intervention resulted in significantly reduced willingness to engage in risky behavior. As such, communications aimed at changing the behavior of citizens during times of increased risk or danger should consider conceptually concrete messaging when communicating complex risk, and hence may provide a valuable tool in promoting health-related behavior.

Keywords: psychological distance; construal level; behavior change; COVID-19

1. Introduction

In response to the SARS-CoV-2 COVID-19 (henceforth 'COVID') pandemic, a core response across the world was to introduce measures to reduce human contact through social distancing [1]. For example, such measures included mandating individuals to maintain a minimum distance (often between 1 and 2 m) in public and community situations, with the aim of protecting people from exposure to viral particles contained within exhaled respiratory droplets or in the air from infected individuals [2]. Such an approach acknowledges that a critical driving force behind viral pandemics is human social interaction [3]. Humans evolved as social animals and much of our behavior revolves around the development and maintenance of relationships. Indeed, there is evidence at behavioral and neuroscientific levels that we both consciously and unconsciously follow the behavior of others [4] and derive a deep-rooted comfort and sense of security in group settings and group coherence [5,6]. More specifically, socializing is known to help maintain a sense of identity [7] and fulfilment [8]. Furthermore, social pain due to rejection has been shown to activate similar areas of the brain to physical pain [9,10] and lacking social support has been linked to an increased risk of mortality [11]. As such, understanding the key drivers of human social behavior in pandemic contexts provides an important key for a successful response and risk mitigation [3,12].

The challenge is not inconsiderable: restrictions placed on individual freedoms pose the risk of triggering psychological reactance [13,14], whereby the desire to protect personal autonomy could potentially drive people to act in ways which could be harmful to themselves, or others. This is further compounded by the political climate, including a lack of trust, contradictory messaging and a lack of observable and consistent norms for desired behaviors [15]. In a survey, conducted in the UK by Imperial College, one of many across the pandemic period, 94% of respondents said that they did not meet up with friends or family beyond their immediate household, and 95% reported that they did not have visitors to their own home [16]. However, the authors noted that these results may be vulnerable to social desirability bias, and indeed, other data suggest that adherence to government regulations was poor. When asked to report on their actual behavior over a two-week time period, only 7.2% of 681 participants reported successful compliance. Almost half of these participants (48.6%) reported intentionally breaking the rules, and this was associated with normative pressure from family and friends [17]. Furthermore, a UK study found that compliance was more closely associated with people's practical abilities and intrinsic motivation to comply than by fear or deterrence [18]. Lower intention to socially distance has been associated with having higher self-interest, lower perceived susceptibility and being less socially responsible [17]. Taken together, these findings indicate that our decision making as it relates to minimizing the impact of COVID on our communities is heavily influenced by social and personal factors, and may be driven more by our relationship to others and our social goals than by rational evaluation of risk. Indeed, research has found that the risk of transmission appeared to be higher for interactions with friends and family than those with strangers [19] along with some evidence to suggest social norms were an important driver of social distancing behavior [20].

Social influence is argued to be strongest in situations of uncertainty, where social cues can help make decisions [21], and likewise, social norms often develop amongst an in-group to help shape appropriate behaviors for interactions and in- and out-group preferences [22]. Dual-process theory [23–26] considers social norms to have an unconscious and automatic influence over behavior that might undermine conscious and rational attempts to maintain a safe distance from others. Loewenstein and colleagues have developed a dual-process theory to account for the effects of emotion in decision-making and risk-based judgements [26]. They argue that immediate emotions, such as those triggered by the anticipation of spending time with family and friends, might bias risk judgements away from objectively more rational judgments, making decisions less sensitive to probabilities and more focused on the intensity of potential social gains. The closer the relationship, the stronger the affect, and the stronger the unconscious influence. This has been formalized in the concept of psychological distance, which offers a framework for exploring how social relationships might mediate risk behavior. Our perceived psychological distance from a person is influenced by how similar we are to them [27], how close our relationship is [28], and whether we perceive them to be part of our in-group or our out-group [27]. As such, friends and family are closer to us in psychological distance relative to strangers. Additionally, we are influenced more strongly as psychological distance reduces (i.e., proximity increases); for example, hotel guests were more likely to reuse their towels when they were told about a 're-use' norm of guests at the hotel in general, but this effect increased when the norm described the prior occupants of the very room they were staying in [15,29].

In the current context, deciding whether or not to engage in an activity that would involve some degree of risk of COVID transmission requires us to balance two conflicting goals: first, our desire to sustain our relationships with others; second, to avoid virus transmission, therefore risking our own health as well as perpetuating the difficulties created by the pandemic, including restrictions on activity. In this situation, the relationship goal is likely to be more concrete, both because our friends and family are more familiar to us (psychologically proximal) and because of the emotional connection we have with them. Virus transmission, on the other hand, is likely to be more abstract, because it is something we are less familiar with and is hence more of an abstract concept.

In the first part of this study, we explored whether social psychological distance influences perceived risk and willingness to engage in behaviors considered risky for COVID transmission. Risk perception and behavioral willingness are argued to sit within the sequence of decision-making such that perceptions around outcomes and their risks comes first, and then willingness to engage in potential behaviors follows, the latter being closer in processing to actual behavior [30,31]. Additionally, we included risk perception primarily to validate our design that the differing risk levels would be perceived as such by participants. Our hypothesis was that participants will perceive the risks of interactions with friends and family members as lower compared to activities that involve strangers, and additionally be more willing to engage in behaviors with them.

2. Materials and Methods: Study Phase 1

Participants. The study ran from April to May 2021, during which 182 participants (63% female, with the majority 69% from UK, then 14% from US, and included responses from 16 different countries in total) were recruited to participate in the study, which was hosted on qualtrics.com and distributed via web link (on Instagram, LinkedIn, Facebook, and through email distribution via the authors' and School's networks). No specific participant targeting strategy was employed (i.e., a convenience sample). Participants who completed at least half of the scenarios were included in this analysis (N = 153). The study was conducted in accordance with the Declaration of Helsinki, and approved by the School of Psychology Local Ethics Committee, Bangor University (Ethics reference 16893 approved February 2021).

Design. This study used a within-subjects design. There were two independent variables: psychological distance (with two levels: proximal or distal) and risk level (with three levels: low risk, ambiguous risk, or high risk). In this study, we defined proximal scenarios as those that described engaging in an activity with well-known others, specifically, friends or family members. A distal scenario would be an activity involving someone or some people who are unknown, such as a taxi driver or a shop assistant. To define the three levels of risk, a conscious decision was made not to rely on current policy (e.g., the 2 meter rule), as these policies vary by country and at different time periods. Instead, we sought a more objective evaluation of risk, and leveraged the helpful gradings of risk described by Jones et al. [2] which takes into consideration multiple factors that combine to determine risk level. This allowed us to codify a range of scenarios as either low, ambiguous (medium) or high risk, and to match scenarios across levels of distance/proximity by describing the same combination of factors and only changing the agents involved.

The dependent variables were risk perception and behavioral willingness. Risk perception is defined as the subjective judgement of risk, and was measured using a 7-point Likert scale (not at all risky–very risky), in line with previous research (e.g., [32]). Behavioral willingness was chosen because it has been found to be a better predictor of future behavior than behavioral intention or behavioral expectation [31].

Procedure. An initial pilot study involving ten volunteers examined the variance in responses to the scenarios in order to avoid ceiling and floor effects in either the ratings for risk and willingness. From the pilot, we were able to identify 16 scenarios in total, to be divided equally across two blocks (before and after the intervention—see study phase 2). Block 1 was used for study phase 1. Participants were invited to complete the questionnaire and task online, in their own time, on their own computer or smartphone. Participants were told that this study would be examining trade-off decisions we have all had to make during the COVID pandemic, and that we were interested in understanding what people think about the relative risk of some of these scenarios. To reduce social desirability bias, we reminded participants that their responses were strictly anonymous, and that there were no right or wrong answers—each scenario representing a genuinely complex trade-off decision, and each person may have their own personal or practical reasons for the responses they choose. Participants were also told that the research would involve evaluating the risk of COVID transmission in a range of scenarios, and were asked to assume that none of the agents described in each scenario were vaccinated at this point in time. This was felt to be necessary as the vaccine roll-out in various countries across the world had begun by the time the survey was launched, and this could have influenced how people perceived their relative risk of known others vs. unknown others.

Participants reviewed the first block of eight scenarios. At the end of each scenario, the participants responded to (1) risk and (2) willingness, an example of which can be seen in Box 1.

Box 1. Example survey item. For each of the 16 scenarios, participants were asked two questions to evaluate their risk perception and behavioral willingness.

Imagine the following scenario:

The gyms have re-opened, and you decide to go for a workout. As soon as you arrive at the gym, you run into a friend, and they suggest working out together as you haven't seen one another in a long time.

Assume that there are no lockdown restrictions in place, so none of the behaviors described are illegal, and to simplify it further please assume that no-one in the scenario has had the vaccine yet.

(1) How would you describe the risk of virus transmission in this scenario? (1 = Not at all risky, 7 = Very risky)

(2) How willing would you be to take on the risk in this scenario? (1 = Not at all willing, 7 = Very willing)

3. Results

Risk perception. To explore the effect of social distance on risk perceptions for different levels of risk, a two-way repeated measures ANOVA was conducted. We conducted analyses to understand how risk perception scores differed across different scenarios. The independent variables were risk, which had three levels (low, ambiguous, high) and proximity with two levels (proximal, distal).

A boxplot of risk perception revealed two outliers, and so these were removed before proceeding with the analysis. The number of data points included in the analysis was therefore $N = 151$. Mauchly's test of sphericity indicated that the assumption of sphericity had been violated for both risk ($\chi^2(2) = 13.92$, $p = 0.001$) and for the proximity $\times$ risk interaction ($\chi^2(2) = 15.10$, $p = 0.001$). The Greenhouse–Geisser estimate of the departure from sphericity for risk was $\varepsilon = 0.91$ and for proximity $\times$ risk was also $\varepsilon = 0.91$. The results were therefore considered only after correcting the degrees of freedom based on the Greenhouse–Geisser correction.

The repeated measures ANOVA found a significant main effect of proximity, $F(1, 141) = 9.20$, $p = 0.003$, $\eta^2 = 0.06$. On average, participants rated proximal scenarios ($M = 4.50$, $SE = 0.08$) as less risky than distal scenarios ($M = 4.68$, $SE = 0.07$). The main effect of risk was also significant ($F(1.83, 257.61) = 571.60$, $p < 0.001$, $\eta^2 = 0.80$), indicating that participants interpreted the high risk scenarios as the most risky ($M = 5.86$, $SE = 0.09$) followed by the ambiguous scenarios ($M = 4.85$, $SE = 0.08$), followed by the low risk scenarios ($M = 3.06$, $SE = 0.09$), as we expected.

The proximity x risk interaction was significant, $F(1.8, 255.84) = 9.40$, $p < 0.001$, $\eta^2 = 0.06$. This indicated that risk perceptions differed according to the social psychological distance to the person or people described in the scenario (see Figure 1).

A paired sample t-test was conducted to understand this interaction further. The rating of risk for objectively low-risk scenarios was lower when they were socially proximal (M = 2.92) as opposed to socially distal ($M = 3.18$). This difference was found to be significant (t (149) = −2.21, $p = 0.03$, $d = -0.18$). Similarly, for high-risk scenarios, risk perceptions were on average lower when they were socially proximal ($M = 5.59$) compared to when they were socially distal (M = 6.01) (t (144) = −5.19, $p < 0.001$, $d = -0.43$). The reverse was found for ambiguous scenarios; when they involved socially proximal individuals, risk perceptions were marginally higher (M = 4.90) than for socially distal individuals (M = 4.73), and this difference was also significant (t (150) = 2.14, $p = 0.03$, $d = 0.17$). However, the effect sizes indicate that only the effect seen in the high-risk condition exceeded Cohen's [33] convention for a small effect size, indicating that the differences in the other two conditions is negligible, even though they appear to be statistically significant. Therefore, we conclude that the only difference of note is for risk perceptions between proximal and distal scenarios in the high-risk condition.

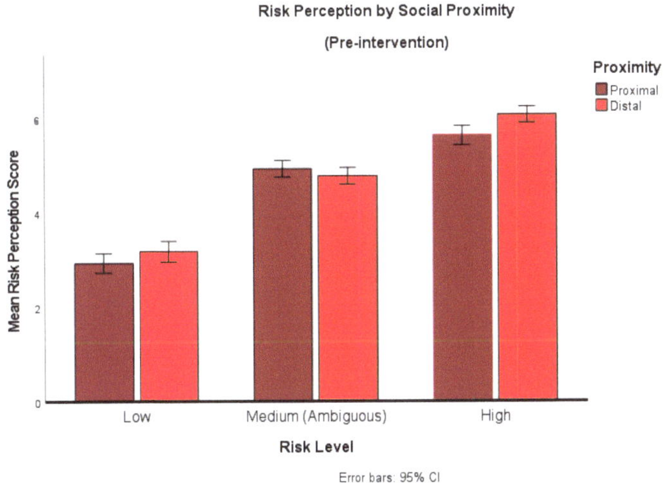

Figure 1. Risk perception by social distance. This graph compares risk perception for proximal vs. distal groups across scenarios that described different degrees of inherent risk (low, ambiguous, high).

Willingness. The differences in Willingness across low, ambiguous or high-risk scenarios involving either proximal or distal others were analyzed using a repeated measures ANOVA. A boxplot of willingness revealed no outliers. Mauchly's test of sphericity again indicated that the assumption was violated for both risk ($\chi^2(2) = 28.49$, $p < 0.001$) and for the proximity x risk interaction $\chi^2(2) = 13.63$, $p = 0.001$), and so results were again only considered after Greenhouse–Geisser correction.

The repeated-measures ANOVA revealed a significant main effect of proximity ($F(1, 137) = 81.79$, $p < 0.001$, $\eta^2 = 0.37$) and risk ($F(1.68, 230.45) = 215.73$, $p < 0.001$, $\eta^2 = 0.61$). The ANOVA also revealed a significant interaction effect of proximity $\times$ risk ($F(1.83, 250.15) = 6.07$, $p = 0.004$, $\eta^2 = 0.042$) (see Figure 2).

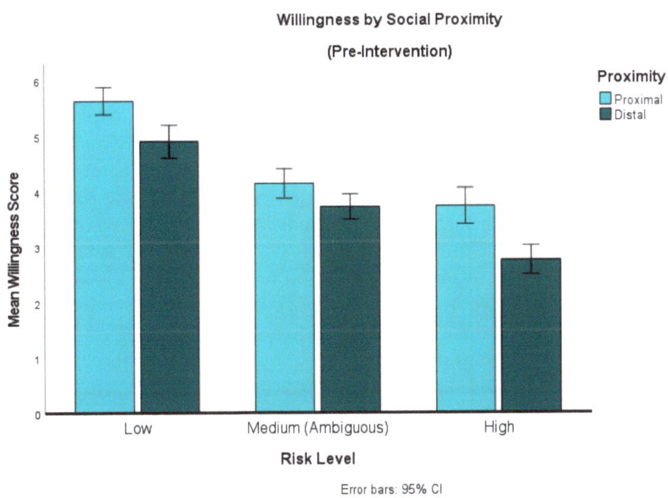

Figure 2. Behavioral willingness by social distance. This graph compares willingness to engage in behaviors involving socially proximal vs. distal others across scenarios (low, ambiguous or high risk).

To explore these effects further, we conducted post hoc *t*-tests, and found that mean willingness was higher for proximal than for distal scenarios across all three levels of Risk, and these differences were significant at the 0.05 level. The differences in willingness between proximal and distal scenarios was greatest in the high-risk condition (mean difference = 0.94; t (143) = 7.78, $p < 0.001$, $d = 0.65$), followed by low risk (mean difference = 0.78; t (146) = 5.92, $p < 0.001$, d = 0.49). For each of these the effect size would be considered medium according to Cohen's [33] criteria. The difference was smallest for the ambiguous scenarios (mean difference = 0.34; t (151) = 3.21, $p = 0.002$, $d = 0.26$), a significant but small effect.

Risk and willingness were found to be significantly negatively correlated ($r = -0.63$, $p < 0.001$), which served to validate our assumption (Figure 3).

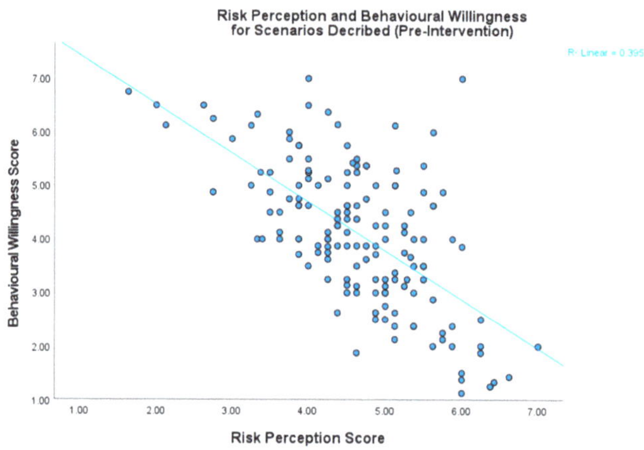

Figure 3. The relationship between risk perception and behavioral willingness. These two scores were negatively correlated, which validates our assumption that participants generally want to avoid engaging in situations they perceive to be risky.

4. Discussion of Study Phase 1 and Introduction to Study Phase 2

Participants viewed scenarios involving friends and family as less risky and showed a greater behavioral willingness to engage. The effects were greater with the behavioral willingness measure, and we observed the largest effects in the high-risk scenarios. Whilst the study successfully reflected observations in the real world, as outlined in the introduction, the study does not give a clear picture as to what is driving the effects, and hence how one might intervene to influence them. On the one hand, we have a lifetime of experience of safely interacting with our friends and family members, and familiarity is considered to be a form of close psychological proximity, whereas paucity of knowledge, for example with regard to the virus, indicates increased psychological distance [27], and processing of more abstract information has been shown to lead participants to rate events as less likely [34]. Individuals might, therefore, be making an unconscious evaluation of risk based on either past history of positive time with family, or on the likely more abstract representation of viral risk and its negative outcomes. As such, judgements might reflect the core representational nature of the events and not just their psychological distance. Psychological distance is argued to influence the 'level of construal', meaning the way individuals mentally represent events. Higher levels of psychological distance (e.g., future events, distant relationships) lead to more abstract and global construals, while lower levels (e.g., immediate events, close relationships) result in more concrete and detailed construals. The level of construal then acts to influence decisions in different ways. For example, concrete construals are more likely to influence immediate decisions, whereas abstract construals will have a stronger influence on future events [35]. Furthermore, if an event is perceived as being less probable we tend to view it more abstractly, and if it is perceived as expected, we view it more concretely [34].

Although our intentions tend to be aligned to our higher-order goals, we often underestimate how our behavior in the moment will be affected by low-level factors, such as how we feel [36,37]. As such, while our cognitive appraisal of the probability of an outcome tends to remain stable over time, our emotional anticipation increases as the event draws nearer and the outcome becomes more concrete [37]. When making decisions about interactions with family, the close and concrete nature of the representations may have a significant impact of our intentions. Additionally, as information about COVID is often presented in abstract terms, such as schematics of the molecular structure of a virus alongside population case numbers, we might also view it as less probable, more psychologically distant, and certainly less concrete or emotionally engaging. Therefore, by making the concept of the virus more concrete, one might increase its impact on immediate decision-making. Indeed, some recent research suggests that anthropomorphizing diseases makes them feel more proximal [38]. Therefore, we developed a brief intervention manipulating the level of construal of the virus to see if it could promote better social distancing intentions, i.e., behavioral willingness. In the study phase 2, we wanted to explore the impact of this intervention designed to increase the level of concreteness with which participants conceptualize how the virus transmits to see whether this would impact their willingness to engage in risky behaviors. As such, our hypothesis for phase 2 was that increasing the level of concreteness for transmission of the virus, through an intervention, would reduce willingness to engage in risky behavior.

5. Materials and Methods of Study Phase 2

Participants. The same participants proceeded to the second stage of the research. Participants who completed at least half of the scenarios in the second block were included in this analysis ($N = 136$).

Design. Initially, participants were randomly assigned to one of three groups: a control ($N = 48$), and then also two interventions groups (verbal, $N = 41$, and visual + verbal $N = 47$). The rationale behind the two intervention groups was to test two levels of 'concreteness' by including vivid imagery in one intervention condition, and text only in the other. However, preliminary analysis showed there was no difference between the behavior of the two groups following these interventions (all $t < 2$), and so, given that both forms of intervention were designed to increase concreteness, we combined these two groups into a single "intervention" group ($N = 88$), resulting in a $2 \times 2 \times 2$ design with time having two levels (pre-intervention, post-intervention), psychological distance having two levels (proximal, distal), and another group having two levels (control group, intervention group). The dependent variable was behavioral willingness, for which part one of the study served as our baseline.

Procedure. Following directly on from part one, participants were now asked to complete a short task. In the verbal condition, participants were asked to read a short paragraph of text about COVID-19 transmission (see Appendix A—*Intervention*). They were then asked to answer some simple questions about the article. This served to ensure participants had engaged with the content of the intervention. In the visual + verbal condition, the same information and task was given, but this time supported by visuals. In the control condition, participants saw a neutral message ("You're halfway through. Thank you for making it this far! When you're ready, click to continue on to the remaining scenarios"). They then completed their second block of eight scenarios, different in content to the first set but matched in terms of the factors that determined the level of risk (e.g., masks, ventilation, number of people, and amount of time).

6. Results of Study Phase 2

The independent variables were time with two levels (pre- and post- intervention), proximity with two levels (proximal, distal) and group with two levels (intervention group, control group). The dependent variable was behavioral willingness. Levene's test was not significant. A boxplot analysis revealed no outliers. As none of the independent variables exceeded three levels, sphericity could also be assumed, so we proceeded with a three-way repeated measures ANOVA.

The results show that there was a small but significant main effect of time (F (1, 134) = 8.158, $p = 0.005$, $\eta^2 = 0.06$). However, qualifying this effect was a significant interaction effect for time × group (F (1, 134 = 7.18, $p = 0.008$, $\eta^2 = 0.05$); see Figure 4.

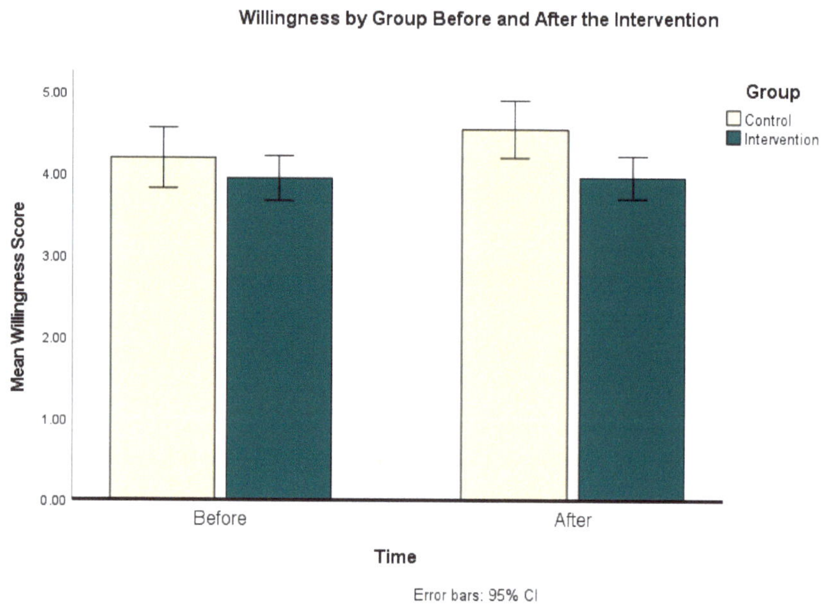

Figure 4. Behavioral willingness by group before the intervention (Time 1) and after (Time 2).

Finally, there was also a main effect of proximity, F(1, 134) = 84.26, $p < 0.001$, $\eta^2 = 0.39$. None of the other main effects or interactions were significant.

To explore the time x group interaction effect further, a paired sample *t*-test was used to see whether the difference in willingness from before the intervention and after the intervention was significant for each of the groups. The results showed that the control group were significantly more willing to engage in the behaviors described in the scenarios in the second block ($M = 4.55$, $SD = 1.31$) than in the first block ($M = 4.20$, $SD = 1.39$), t(47) = −3.41, $p = .001$, $d = -0.43$), an intermediate effect size. For the intervention group, the difference in willingness pre- and post- was not significant (t(87) = 0.230, $p = 0.82$).

An independent samples *t*-test was used to examine the difference between the control group and the intervention group pre- and post- intervention. The results showed that these groups were not significantly different before the intervention (t(134) = 1.091, $p = 0.277$, $d = 0.20$), but that after the intervention willingness was higher in the control group ($M = 4.5$, $SD = 1.30$) than in the intervention group ($M = 3.96$, $SD = 1.20$), t(134) = 2.67, $p = 0.008$, $d = 0.48$), with a medium effect size.

However, because there was a difference pre-intervention and a 27.7% chance that this difference was by chance, a second analysis was conducted to remove the potential confound of differences within the groups. A new variable was created for each individual's change in willingness pre- and post-intervention, and an independent samples *t*-test was run to see whether the change in willingness was different between the two groups. The results were t(134) = 2.65, $p = 0.009$, $d = 0.48$, 95% CI [0.09, 0.59]. This indicates that the change in Willingness for each group was significantly different, and the effect size for this was small to moderate.

7. Discussion

Within the context of COVID and the risk to health, this study asked participants to rate how willing they were to engage in social behaviors in a variety of real-world scenarios. The key difference in the scenarios was that half were involved agents who were psychologically distant (e.g., strangers), and the other half were psychologically proximal (e.g., friends or family). While relationships to others did have a small and significant effect on perceptions of how risky a behavior was, it had a larger effect on self-reported willingness to engage in that behavior. This effect was greatest in the high-risk scenarios condition. In a second phase of the study, we manipulated construal level as part of an intervention, specifically to make representations of the COVID virus more concrete and hence psychologically proximal. Participants in the experimental group read a script (which, in some cases, included a representation; see Appendix A) that presented COVID in concrete, literal, and operational terms—as defined by construal level theory [27,34,35]. This was expected to lower the construal level of representation for information about the virus because it introduced specific details about how the virus transmits, as well as concrete examples about how wearing a mask or ventilating a space would affect this. Subsequently, participants who read the script were significantly less willing to engage in risky scenarios relative to controls, and this effect was observed across all scenarios, i.e., not restricted to either proximal or distal groups. As such, the intervention appeared to successfully influence participants such that they become less willing to engage in COVID-related risk behaviors in all scenarios.

Traditional risk-value models struggle to explain the findings from Block 1, i.e., differences in judgement for social groups, as, for example, the expected value of the goal should be the same, but decisions often systematically vary according to factors such as psychological distance [39]. Indeed, research has demonstrated how social influence can introduce an element of bias to judgements and evaluations [21]. Such biases are pervasive and form very early in our lives. For example, studies have demonstrated in-group preference in children as young as five years old [40]. A recent review [15] highlighted in-group norms as being particularly influential for adherence to COVID-19 prevention and control guidelines. In this study, it is possible that the scenarios describing proximal others conveyed information about an in-group norm and hence produced a systematic social influence towards engaging. For example, if a friend is offering you a lift in their car, the implication is that the friend does not see anything wrong with this behavior, and if you view this behavior as exemplary for the group, you could be motivated to behave in accordance with the rest of the group.

A nuanced finding was the observation that risk perception scores were lower for proximal scenarios when the level of risk was clear, but when the level of risk was ambiguous, this finding was reversed. Furthermore, differences in willingness for proximal groups were smaller for the ambiguous scenarios. Dual-process models of information processing, such as the Elaboration Likelihood Model [41], highlight the influence that our degree of engagement with information has on how it is processed. These models distinguish between central and peripheral routes of processing, and demonstrate that outcomes may differ depending on which route is activated. It is possible that, when the level of risk was obvious, participants were not required to process the information deeply; this allowed heuristics such as in-group bias to exert more influence on the subsequent ratings for risk and willingness. However, when the scenario was ambiguous, they needed to pay more attention to the detail, which may have brought the level of construal for this information down (e.g., made it more concrete), making this form of influence more powerful.

Social relationships are considered to have special psychological importance across many different aspects of psychology, and so they could be considered a form of super-ordinate goal. For example, most theories of fundamental human needs include an element of "social connection" (Maslow's hierarchy: [42]; self-determination theory: [43]; core social motives theory: [44]), and the belief that our behavior is motivated by achieving need satisfaction or avoiding need frustration. Furthermore, we ran this study between April and May 2021, when many participants had endured months of social distancing and numerous local and nationwide lockdowns. Therefore, connectedness goals may have been particularly salient for these participants. In line with this interpretation, participants' informal comments during the study revealed that they felt their responses were influenced by how much they valued the activity described.

Our membership to particular sub-groups such as the political party one supports has been shown to mediate our response to an energy conservation nudge [45]. In group exercise settings, where exercise is likely to be a group norm, the degree to which one identifies with the group predicts participation in the activity [46]. These are both examples of how group membership, group identity and other social or situational factors [21,47,48] may exert an influence on the efficacy of a social norm, but by what mechanism is less clear. As an example, picture an image of a crowded beach. The impact that this has on you may vary drastically depending on your interpretation of the scene. While some may decide it must be safe to go to the beach, given that many other people are going, others may conclude that the beach is no longer safe, given that so many people decided to go. It could also depend on who is on the beach, and whether they are people you know, or strangers, and whether or not you identify with the group that they belong to. The importance of how norm information is processed was highlighted in a recent study. Jiang et al. [49] investigated the impact of social norms on the relationship between news attention and social-distancing behavior, and reported that—contrary to their hypothesis—norms exerted a negative interaction effect. That is, if an individual perceived a strong norm to practice social distancing in their in-group, they may be less likely to engage in this behavior themselves, despite believing it to be effective and the consequences to be severe. On the other hand, if they did not believe that others in their inner circle were social distancing, they compensated by being more diligent themselves. While authors did not offer an interpretation as to why this effect was observed, it serves to reinforce that norms can have unexpected consequences, and also further highlights the gap in our understanding of the underlying mechanisms by which norms may influence behavior.

An explanation for our current findings based on construal level theory suggests that reducing psychological distance influences the nature of outcome evaluations. Decisions viewed as distant are typically judged by outcome desirability, whereas those seen as close are assessed by feasibility [32,35]. For example, when considering whether to attend a guest lecture, when the guest lecturer's name was similar to their own, participants were swayed more by feasibility (how convenient it is to get there), and when the name sounded different, they were more swayed by outcome (how interesting the lecture is). By having a similar name, the psychological distance was reduced, and this shifted their preferences [50]. In this study, pre-intervention scenarios were likely considered abstractly, emphasizing outcome desirability, such as the appeal of social interactions. Post-intervention, awareness of transmission risks rendered these decisions more concrete, prioritizing feasibility over desirability and possibly reducing willingness to take risks.

Alternatively, as the concreteness intervention reduced willingness to engage across all scenarios (not just those psychologically proximal), it may have more generally been the effect of generating more intense immediate emotions that influenced all decision-making [26,37], in this case, by increasing fear of the virus and hence suppressing all behavioral intentions. Such an influence has also been described as the "immediacy bias" in that people focus on current and affectively arousing information when making immediate decisions about behavior. There are two assumptions here. The first is that the information in the intervention produced an affective response, and second, that when making the decisions, the participants were conceptualizing their responses in terms of an immediate behavior, i.e., they were making a decision about something they were going to do now, and not at some future date. It would be valuable, in future work, to explore both these assumptions. For example, whether the power of the concreteness intervention rests on increasing the affective influence on decision-making in the moment [26]. Likewise, exploring decisions for immediate behavior versus ones that will take place in the future. This would also test a further prediction of construal-level theory, which is that that whilst concrete construals impact immediate decision-making, abstract construals should have a stronger impact on future decision events [39,51]

Our study had several limitations, partially due to the rapid changes in context while it was being conducted. At the time of the study, the rollout of the COVID-19 vaccine was just beginning, meaning that we had to clarify in the instructions that participants should assume no-one in the scenarios described had been vaccinated yet. Otherwise, knowledge of friends or family's vaccine status compared with lack of knowledge about strangers' vaccine status could have confounded our findings. However, there is still a chance that this influenced the results. Willingness to engage in behaviors associated with the risk of virus transmission was significantly lower for the intervention group relative to the controls. Visually exploring this data, we saw that the willingness of the control group was higher for the second block of scenarios than for the first block. This may indicate that, although the scenarios were developed with a rubric to ensure they were mapped to the first block of scenarios in terms of risk variability, there may still have been some other variables that influenced the baseline level of willingness for these scenarios. This indicated that the between-group comparison may be more reliable than within groups. Importantly, there were no differences between the control group and the intervention group at baseline, meaning that the between-groups comparison was meaningful. Furthermore, we conducted a within-group analysis to control for any between-group confounds, and confirmed that willingness increased more for the control group than for the intervention group. An additional consideration with the intervention was that we originally designed two configurations, one purely written, and one with a supporting visual representation (Appendix A). The impact of the two did not differ even though we expected that the visual form might have been more impactful. The differences in presentation format warrant future exploration to determine the most impactful way to present an important message. Finally, some of our results may have been artefacts of the study design rather than a true replication of how these decisions are processed in a real world setting. For example, we opted for a simple Likert scale of not at all willing to very willing, which implies that the decision being made is binary (to engage or not to engage in the behavior). In reality, these decisions are rarely binary as there are often many different options for how to respond: for example, taking an at-home COVID test before attending a social gathering, opening a window or choosing to wear a mask, as means of adjusting the relative risk of the situation. Presenting different options at once, known as choice bracketing, has been shown to influence choice independently of construal level [32]. A final avenue for further work is that the results in the current study intervention might have reflected a general suppression of behavior (a fear response), rather than an impact specifically on COVID protective behaviors.

8. Conclusions

This study has shown that people are influenced in decisions about behavioral willingness by their relationships to those around them, and that concretizing representations of the COVID virus can go some way to mitigating risky behaviors. Concrete representations of the negative consequences of behavior have been widely used in attempts to reduce addictive behaviors, e.g., cigarette packaging, but the approach has been criticized as it can generate anxiety and also does not directly promote the desired behavior [52] though see [53]. However, in certain circumstances, such as during immediate decisions in uncertain circumstances, such interventions may serve to bias behavior in a safer direction [12,53]. In contrast, a natural tendency for communicating risk to groups is to use higher-level abstract construals (such as public communications) [54]. For immediate behaviors, concreteness interventions could be particularly effective in situations where there is a conflict between the desired behavior and competing super-ordinate goals such as our desire for social connectedness. There is a need here to provide a clear indication of what the 'safe' or desired behavior would be. Communicating risk in health messages is increasingly important for sustainability of both people and the planet. Dual-process approaches help to reveal the myriad ways human behavior is influenced, and this work demonstrates the importance of understanding behavioral drivers, in this case construal level, in designing communications. Ultimately, it serves to emphasize the importance of building capability and capacity in behavioral science in building an effective and coherent response to threats to society in an increasingly uncertain world.

Author Contributions: Conceptualization, C.W. and J.A.P.; methodology, C.W., J.A.P. and P.R.; software, C.W. and P.R.; formal analysis, C.W. and P.R.; investigation, C.W.; writing—original draft preparation, C.W. and J.A.P.; writing—review and editing, C.W., P.R., M.B. and J.A.P.; project administration, J.A.P. All authors have read and agreed to the published version of the manuscript.

Funding: This research received no external funding.

Institutional Review Board Statement: The study was conducted in accordance with the Declaration of Helsinki, and approved by the School of Psychology Local Ethics Committee, Bangor University (Ethics reference 16893 approved February 2021).

Informed Consent Statement: Informed consent was obtained from all participants involved in the study.

Data Availability Statement: Where relevant, all anonymized primary data is available via the corresponding author.

Conflicts of Interest: The authors declare no conflicts of interest.

Appendix A

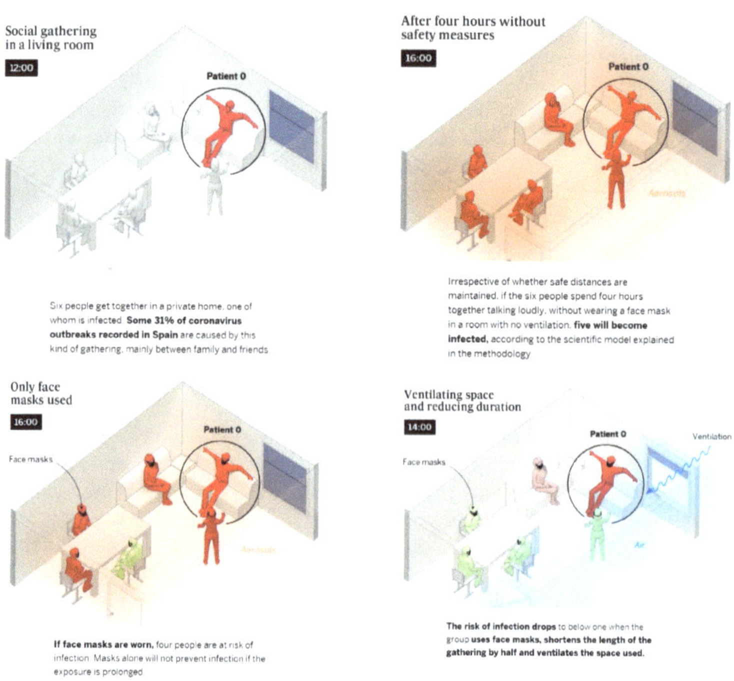

Figure A1. Intervention Materials.

References

1. Murphy, C.; Lim, W.W.; Mills, C.; Wong, J.Y.; Chen, D.X.; Xie, Y.; Li, M.W.; Gould, S.; Xin, H.L.; Cheung, J.K.; et al. Effectiveness of social distancing measures and lockdowns for reducing transmission of COVID-19 in non-healthcare, community-based settings. *Philos. Trans. R. Soc. A* **2023**, *381*, 20230132. [CrossRef] [PubMed]
2. Jones, N.R.; Qureshi, Z.U.; Temple, R.J.; Larwood, J.P.J.; Greenhalgh, T.; Bourouiba, L. Two metres or one: What is the evidence for physical distancing in COVID-19? *Bmj-Brit. Med. J.* **2020**, *370*, m3223. [CrossRef] [PubMed]
3. Bavel, J.J.V.; Baicker, K.; Boggio, P.S.; Capraro, V.; Cichocka, A.; Cikara, M.; Crockett, M.J.; Crum, A.J.; Douglas, K.M.; Druckman, J.N.; et al. Using social and behavioural science to support COVID-19 pandemic response. *Nat. Hum. Behav.* **2020**, *4*, 460–471. [CrossRef] [PubMed]
4. Kameda, T.H.R. Herd Behavior. In *Emerging Trends in the Social and Behavioral Sciences*; Kosslyn, R., Ed.; Wiley: Hoboken, NJ, USA, 2015; pp. 1–14.
5. Ryan, R.M.; Deci, E.L. Intrinsic and extrinsic motivation from a self-determination theory perspective: Definitions, theory, practices, and future directions. *Contemp. Educ. Psychol.* **2020**, *61*, 101860. [CrossRef]
6. Raafat, R.M.; Chater, N.; Frith, C. Herding in humans (vol 13, pg 420, 2009). *Trends Cogn. Sci.* **2009**, *13*, 504. [CrossRef]
7. Tajfel, H.; Turner, J.C.; Austin, W.G.; Worchel, S. An integrative theory of intergroup conflict. *Organ. Identity* **1979**, *56*, 65.
8. Eisenberger, N.I.; Cole, S.W. Social neuroscience and health: Neurophysiological mechanisms linking social ties with physical health. *Nat. Neurosci.* **2012**, *15*, 669–674. [CrossRef]
9. Eisenberger, N.I.; Jarcho, J.M.; Lieberman, M.D.; Naliboff, B.D. An experimental study of shared sensitivity to physical pain and social rejection. *Pain* **2006**, *126*, 132–138. [CrossRef] [PubMed]
10. Eisenberger, N.I.; Lieberman, M.D.; Williams, K.D. Does rejection hurt? An fMRI study of social exclusion. *Science* **2003**, *302*, 290–292. [CrossRef]
11. Holt-Lunstad, J.; Smith, T.B.; Layton, J.B. Social Relationships and Mortality Risk: A Meta-analytic Review. *PLoS Med.* **2010**, *7*, e1000316. [CrossRef]
12. Gould, A.; Lewis, L.; Evans, L.; Greening, L.; Howe-Davies, H.; West, J.; Roberts, C.; Parkinson, J.A. COVID-19 Personal Protective Behaviors during Large Social Events: The Value of Behavioral Observations. *Behav. Sci.* **2024**, *14*, 63. [CrossRef] [PubMed]
13. Fogarty, J.S. Reactance theory and patient noncompliance. *Soc. Sci. Med.* **1997**, *45*, 1277–1288. [CrossRef] [PubMed]
14. Taylor, S.; Asmundson, G.J.G. Negative attitudes about facemasks during the COVID-19 pandemic: The dual importance of perceived ineffectiveness and psychological reactance. *PLoS ONE* **2021**, *16*, e0246317. [CrossRef] [PubMed]
15. Young, S.D.; Goldstein, N.J. Applying social norms interventions to increase adherence to COVID-19 prevention and control guidelines. *Prev. Med.* **2021**, *145*, 106424. [CrossRef] [PubMed]
16. Smith, L.E.; Amlôt, R.; Lambert, H.; Oliver, I.; Robin, C.; Yardley, L.; Rubin, G.J. Factors associated with adherence to self-isolation and lockdown measures in the UK: A cross-sectional survey. *Public Health* **2020**, *187*, 41–52. [CrossRef] [PubMed]
17. Hills, S.; Eraso, Y. Factors associated with non-adherence to social distancing rules during the COVID-19 pandemic: A logistic regression analysis. *Bmc Public Health* **2021**, *21*, 352. [CrossRef] [PubMed]
18. Kooistra, E.B.; Reinders Folmer, C.; Kuiper, M.E.; Olthuis, E.; Brownlee, M.; Fine, A.; Van Rooij, B. *Mitigating COVID-19 in a Nationally Representative uk Sample: Personal Abilities and Obligation to Obey the Law Shape Compliance with Mitigation Measures*; Soscial Science Research Network: Amsterdam, The Netherlands, 2020. [CrossRef]
19. Thompson, H.A.; Mousa, A.; Dighe, A.; Fu, H.; Arnedo-Pena, A.; Barrett, P.; Bellido-Blasco, J.; Bi, Q.F.; Caputi, A.; Chaw, L.; et al. Severe Acute Respiratory Syndrome Coronavirus 2 (SARS-CoV-2) Setting-Specific Transmission Rates: A Systematic Review and Meta-analysis. *Clin. Infect. Dis.* **2021**, *73*, E754–E764. [CrossRef] [PubMed]
20. Martínez, D.; Parilli, C.; Scartascini, C.; Simpser, A. Let's (not) get together! The role of social norms on social distancing during COVID-19. *PLoS ONE* **2021**, *16*, e0247454. [CrossRef] [PubMed]
21. Spears, R. Social Influence and Group Identity. *Annu. Rev. Psychol.* **2021**, *72*, 367–390. [CrossRef]
22. McDonald, R.I.; Crandall, C.S. Social norms and social influence. *Curr. Opin. Behav. Sci.* **2015**, *3*, 147–151. [CrossRef]
23. Evans, J.S.T. In two minds: Dual-process accounts of reasoning. *Trends Cogn. Sci.* **2003**, *7*, 454–459. [CrossRef] [PubMed]
24. Evans, J.S.T.; Stanovich, K.E. Dual-Process Theories of Higher Cognition: Advancing the Debate. *Perspect. Psychol. Sci.* **2013**, *8*, 223–241. [CrossRef] [PubMed]
25. Kahneman, D. *Thinking, Fast and Slow*, 1st ed.; Farrar, Straus and Giroux: New York, NY, USA, 2013; 499p.
26. Loewenstein, G.; O'Donoghue, T.; Bhatia, S. Modeling the interplay between affect and deliberation. *Decision* **2015**, *2*, 55–81. [CrossRef]
27. Trope, Y.; Liberman, N.; Wakslak, C. Construal levels and psychological distance: Effects on representation, prediction, evaluation, and behavior. *J. Consum. Psychol.* **2007**, *17*, 83–95. [CrossRef] [PubMed]
28. Aron, A.; Aron, E.N.; Smollan, D. Inclusion of Other in the Self Scale and the Structure of Interpersonal Closeness. *J. Pers. Soc. Psychol.* **1992**, *63*, 596–612. [CrossRef]
29. Goldstein, N.J.; Cialdini, R.B.; Griskevicius, V. A room with a viewpoint: Using social norms to motivate environmental conservation in hotels. *J. Consum. Res.* **2008**, *35*, 472–482. [CrossRef]
30. Maartensson, H.; Loi, N.M. Exploring the relationships between risk perception, behavioural willingness, and constructive hope in pro-environmental behaviour. *Environ. Educ. Res.* **2022**, *28*, 600–613. [CrossRef]

31. Pomery, E.A.; Gibbons, F.X.; Reis-Bergan, M.; Gerrard, M. From Willingness to Intention: Experience Moderates the Shift From Reactive to Reasoned Behavior. *Pers. Soc. Psychol. B* **2009**, *35*, 894–908. [CrossRef]
32. Webb, E.C.; Shu, S.B. The Effect of Perceived Similarity on Sequential Risk Taking. *J. Mark. Res.* **2018**, *55*, 916–933. [CrossRef]
33. Cohen, J. Statistical Power Analysis for the Behavioral-Sciences. *Percept. Mot. Ski.* **1988**, *67*, 1007.
34. Wakslak, C.; Trope, Y. The Effect of Construal Level on Subjective Probability Estimates. *Psychol. Sci.* **2009**, *20*, 52–58. [CrossRef]
35. Trope, Y.; Liberman, N. Temporal construal and time-dependent changes in preference. *J. Pers. Soc. Psychol.* **2000**, *79*, 876–889. [CrossRef]
36. Gerrard, M.; Gibbons, F.X.; Houlihan, A.E.; Stock, M.L.; Pomery, E.A. A dual-process approach to health risk decision making: The prototype willingness model. *Dev. Rev.* **2008**, *28*, 29–61. [CrossRef]
37. Loewenstein, G. Emotions in economic theory and economic behavior. *Am. Econ. Rev.* **2000**, *90*, 426–432. [CrossRef]
38. Wan, J.; Kulow, K.; Cowan, K. It's Alive! Increasing Protective Action against the Coronavirus through Anthropomorphism and Construal. *J. Assoc. Consum. Res.* **2022**, *7*, 81–88. [CrossRef]
39. Liberman, N.; Trope, Y. Traversing psychological distance. *Trends Cogn. Sci.* **2014**, *18*, 364–369. [CrossRef]
40. Buttelmann, D.; Böhm, R. The Ontogeny of the Motivation That Underlies In-Group Bias. *Psychol. Sci.* **2014**, *25*, 921–927. [CrossRef]
41. Petty, R.E.; Cacioppo, J.T.; Petty, R.E.; Cacioppo, J.T. *The Elaboration Likelihood Model of Persuasion*; Springer: New York, NY, USA, 1986.
42. Maslow, A.H. *Motivation and Personality*, 2nd ed.; Harper & Row: New York, NY, USA, 1970; 369p.
43. Deci, E.L.; Ryan, R.M. The "what" and "why" of goal pursuits: Human needs and the self-determination of behavior. *Psychol. Inq.* **2000**, *11*, 227–268. [CrossRef]
44. Stevens, L.E.; Fiske, S.T. Motivation and cognition in social life: A social survival perspective. *Soc. Cogn.* **1995**, *13*, 189–214. [CrossRef]
45. Costa, D.L.; Kahn, M.E. Energy Conservation "Nudges" and Environmentalist Ideology: Evidence from a Randomized Residential Electricity Field Experiment. *J. Eur. Econ. Assoc.* **2013**, *11*, 680–702. [CrossRef]
46. Stevens, M.; Rees, T.; Polman, R. Social identification, exercise participation, and positive exercise experiences: Evidence from parkrun. *J. Sport Sci.* **2019**, *37*, 221–228. [CrossRef]
47. Cialdini, R.B. Crafting normative messages to protect the environment. *Curr. Dir. Psychol. Sci.* **2003**, *12*, 105–109. [CrossRef]
48. Allcott, H. Social norms and energy conservation. *J. Public Econ.* **2011**, *95*, 1082–1095. [CrossRef]
49. Jiang, X.Y.; Hwang, J.; Shah, D.V.; Ghosh, S.; Brauer, M. News Attention and Social-Distancing Behavior Amid COVID-19: How Media Trust and Social Norms Moderate a Mediated Relationship. *Health Commun.* **2022**, *37*, 768–777. [CrossRef]
50. Liviatan, I.; Trope, Y.; Liberman, N. Interpersonal similarity as a social distance dimension: Implications for perception of others' actions. *J. Exp. Soc. Psychol.* **2008**, *44*, 1256–1269. [CrossRef]
51. Liberman, N.; Sagristano, M.D.; Trope, Y. The effect of temporal distance on level of mental construal. *J. Exp. Soc. Psychol.* **2002**, *38*, 523–534. [CrossRef]
52. Stolow, J.A.; Moses, L.M.; Lederer, A.M.; Carter, R. How Fear Appeal Approaches in COVID-19 Health Communication May Be Harming the Global Community. *Health Educ. Behav.* **2020**, *47*, 531–535. [CrossRef]
53. Harper, C.A.; Satchell, L.P.; Fido, D.; Latzman, R.D. Functional Fear Predicts Public Health Compliance in the COVID-19 Pandemic. *Int. J. Ment. Health Addict.* **2021**, *19*, 1875–1888. [CrossRef]
54. Joshi, P.D.; Wakslak, C.J. Communicating with the Crowd: Speakers Use Abstract Messages When Addressing Larger Audiences. *J. Exp. Psychol. Gen.* **2014**, *143*, 351–362. [CrossRef]

behavioral sciences

MDPI

Article

Milking the Alternatives: Understanding Coffee Consumers' Preferences for Non-Dairy Milk

Nibal Halabi [1], Velina Hristova [2,3,*] and Ivo Vlaev [1,*]

[1] Warwick Business School, University of Warwick, Scarman Rd., Coventry CV4 7 AL, UK; nibal.halabi@warwick.ac.uk
[2] Psychology Department, Sofia University "St. Kliment Ohridski", bul. "Tsar Osvoboditel" 15, 1504 Sofia, Bulgaria
[3] Institute for Population and Human Studies, Bulgarian Academy of Sciences, Acad. G. Bonchev Str. 6, 1113 Sofia, Bulgaria
* Correspondence: velina.hristova@iphs.bas.bg (V.H.); ivo.vlaev@wbs.ac.uk (I.V.)

Abstract: Consumer interest in plant-based milk alternatives is growing, despite extra charges in coffeehouses. While much research exists on non-dairy alternatives, plant-based milks in coffee drinks remain understudied. This study examines consumer preferences and behaviors regarding milk alternatives in coffee, using the Theoretical Domains Framework (TDF) and the Behavior Change Wheel (BCW). A survey of 200 participants from 19 countries explored demographics, coffee habits, attitudes towards non-dairy milk charges, and marketing awareness. Market insights showed taste as the main reason for coffee choice, with a preference for cow's milk and local cafes for quality. Many opposed the extra charges for non-dairy options, citing lactose intolerance or allergies, especially among Gen Z and Millennials. Regional variations included stronger opposition in the UK and Germany compared to the UAE and USA. The marketing for non-dairy milk was less memorable than general coffee advertisements. Regression analysis confirmed that viewing non-dairy milk as a dietary staple increased consumption, aligning with the TDF's "Beliefs about Consequences" domain. Finally, within the BCW framework, the intervention strategies centered on training and coercion were discussed. Implementing these approaches could encourage the wider adoption of non-dairy milk options in coffee shops, fostering inclusivity, health awareness, and supporting environmental sustainability efforts.

Keywords: consumer behavior; Theoretical Domains Framework; Behavior Change Wheel; non-dairy industry; plant-based dairy alternatives

1. Introduction

Increasing interest in sustainability, along with concerns for the environment and animal welfare, is motivating more consumers to choose plant-based milks. The marketing of plant-based dairy alternatives (PBDA) often emphasizes their commitment to sustainability, environmental protection, natural ingredients, and humane animal treatment, which gives them a competitive edge over traditional dairy products.

Across key environmental metrics—such as land use, greenhouse gas emissions, water use, and eutrophication—cow's milk has a much greater impact, producing about three times more greenhouse gases [1]. In comparison, research indicates that plant-based drinks have significantly lower greenhouse gas emissions, reduced by 59–71% per 250 mL [2]. Dairy production also uses around ten times more land, consumes two to twenty times more freshwater, and contributes significantly more to eutrophication [1]. Among plant-based options, almond milk has lower greenhouse gas emissions and land use than soy milk but requires more water and results in more eutrophication. While all plant-based alternatives are more environmentally friendly than dairy, none is the clear winner across all sustainability metrics. Oat and soy drinks, for instance, use considerably less water than dairy milk, yet rice drinks do not share this advantage. However, consumers must navigate these nuances to make informed and sustainable choices, as each type of plant-based milk presents its own set of environmental trade-offs.

Additionally, reducing our reliance on animal-based foods aligns with several United Nations Sustainable Development Goals (UN SDGs), particularly those focused on sustainable consumption and production, the sustainable management of natural resources, and urgent climate action [3]. By adopting planetary diets, which prioritize plant-based foods, individuals can significantly decrease their environmental footprint, helping to mitigate climate change, preserve biodiversity, and promote the sustainable use of resources. Research shows that substituting the 250 mL serving of dairy milk allowed within the EAT Lancet Planetary Health Diet with a fortified plant-based alternative maintains nutritional adequacy while substantially lowering environmental impact [4,5].

1.1. The Individuals' Health Factor

The most common adverse reactions associated with milk consumption are cow's milk protein allergies (CMPAs) and lactose intolerance (LI). These conditions arise from the body's inability to properly digest, absorb, and metabolize specific components of milk. In the case of CMPA, the immune system reacts abnormally to proteins found in cow's milk, leading to allergic reactions. Lactose intolerance, on the other hand, is due to the malabsorption of lactose, the sugar in milk, caused by a deficiency of the enzyme lactase. This deficiency is particularly prevalent, with about two-thirds of the world's population affected, though the prevalence varies significantly across different regions [6].

Digestibility issues and lactose intolerance are the primary reasons for consumers to turn to plant-based milks [7–9]. For those with LI, consuming dairy can lead to symptoms like bloating, diarrhea, and stomach cramps, making dairy alternatives a more comfortable choice. Similarly, individuals with CMPA must avoid cow's milk altogether, necessitating alternatives that do not trigger allergic reactions.

These issues have compelled specific populations to seek out milk alternatives that are nutritionally similar to conventional milk.

1.2. Nutritional Content of Dairy versus Plant-Based Beverages

Studies from different parts of the world have analyzed the nutritional content of non-dairy milk compared to plant-based alternatives [2,10–15]. Plant-based milk alternatives (PBMAs) have distinct nutritional profiles compared to bovine milk, influenced by their plant sources, processing methods, and fortification with additional ingredients.

Cow and goat milks are naturally rich in essential minerals such as calcium, potassium, magnesium, sodium, and phosphorus, as well as trace elements like selenium and zinc [10]. Conversely, PBMAs require fortification to reach similar nutritional levels. Furthermore, PBMAs contain antinutrients like phytic acid, trypsin inhibitors, and inositol phosphates, which can interfere with mineral absorption and reduce protein digestibility but also provide beneficial components that are not present in cow's milk, such as isoflavones (especially in soy-based alternatives) and dietary fibers [9].

Regarding macronutrients, PBMAs typically have a lower protein content than cow's milk, with animal proteins being superior in nutritional quality and digestibility, due to their varied amino acids [16]. Only soy-based milk has a protein content comparable to that of cow's milk [13].

Unlike cow's milk, PBMAs are free from lactose and cholesterol and have higher levels of unsaturated fatty acids. Additionally, PBMAs have very low levels of saturated fats, minimal sodium [4], and have no cholesterol, all of which contribute positively to a healthier diet. Additionally, dairy consumption is related to some dermatological conditions [9,17].

1.3. Pricing Strategies in the Dairy versus Alternative Milk Industry

Shareholders and common ownership significantly influence the dynamics of the dairy and alternative milk industry. Institutional investors often hold stakes in multiple companies within these sectors, driving pricing decisions to maximize portfolio returns. When non-dairy milk producers are commonly owned by the same institutional investors, competitive pricing incentives may diminish, potentially leading to higher prices for non-dairy milks.

An OECD document from 2017 notes the rise in common ownership, with institutional investors holding stakes in multiple-sector companies [18]. Alex Edmans discussed, in a 2009 article, how shareholder activities impact market dynamics and corporate governance, including pricing strategies [19]. Aghion et al. [20] also explored how liquidity impacts shareholder incentives, noting that easily tradable shares can lead to short-term profit strategies at the expense of long-term company health. In the context of pricing, this managerial myopia might result in higher prices and underinvestment in necessary innovations, explaining the high cost of non-dairy products. While coordinated pricing among commonly owned firms can lead to stable prices, it might also reduce the competitive pressure, keeping prices high, which negatively impacts price-sensitive consumers or those dependent on non-dairy milks due to dietary restrictions. The OECD suggests that common ownership may encourage unilateral pricing behaviors that favor institutional investor portfolios, potentially facilitating collusive outcomes [18]. This can lead to pricing strategies, such as charging extra for non-dairy milks, that prioritize short-term profits over consumer interests and market sustainability.

Unless someone has a health issue or concern, such as diet consciousness, lactose intolerance, or a dairy allergy, there is one large barrier to entry for the adoption and proliferation of plant-based milks: cost. One of the primary challenges facing PBMAs is their elevated production costs, which impact every stage of the plant-based milk supply chain [9]. The higher production costs of plant milk (due to expensive processes, packaging, marketing, and logistics) compared to dairy milk provide plant milk suppliers with significant bargaining power when negotiating with retailers like large coffee shops [21]. While retailers face a medium level of buyer bargaining power and some flexibility in choosing suppliers, partnering with suppliers can reduce costs through larger purchase quantities and optimized supply chain management.

Once retailers acquire soy milk and offer it to customers, their bargaining power remains constrained—they cannot provide the product for free, yet customers can choose alternative suppliers where costs are lower or the product is free. This complex market landscape, including various dairy milk alternatives and consumer preferences like drinking espresso or coffee without milk, illustrates the intricate dynamics described by Porter's Five Forces model, as depicted in Figure 1.

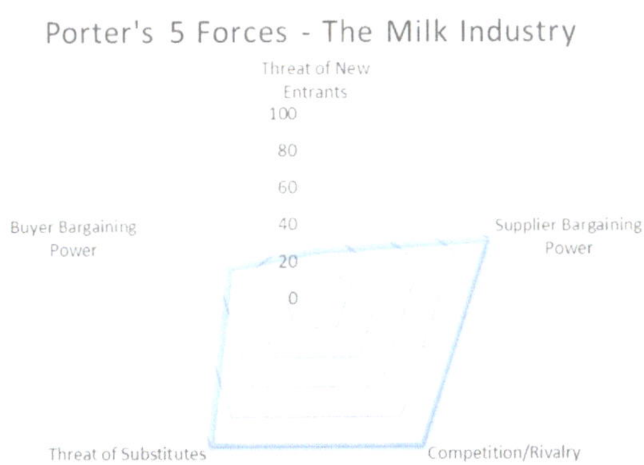

Figure 1. Porter's Five Forces—dairy and plant-based milks.

While there is substantial research on non-dairy alternatives, there is a notable lack of studies specifically focusing on the use of plant-based milks in coffee drinks. This study aims to fill this gap by examining consumer preferences and behaviors related to non-dairy milk alternatives in the context of coffee consumption.

1.4. Theoretical Domains Framework (TDF) Model

To achieve its goal, the present study employed the Theoretical Domains Framework (TDF) [22] within the Behavior Change Wheel (BCW) [23] approach. The TDF was chosen because it offers a comprehensive framework that integrates 128 constructs from 33 behavior change theories into 14 domains, providing a thorough understanding of the factors influencing behavior, including the following: knowledge, skill, beliefs about capabilities, beliefs about consequences, behavioral regulation, optimism, emotion, environmental context and resources, social/professional role and identity, intention, goal, reinforcement, social influence, and memory, attention, and decisional processes. Secondly, the BCW complements the TDF by offering a structured approach to designing and evaluating behavior change interventions, ensuring that this study's findings can be effectively translated into practical strategies for promoting non-dairy milk consumption. By combining these frameworks, this study can uncover a nuanced picture of consumer behaviors and preferences, identify key barriers and facilitators, and develop targeted interventions to encourage the adoption of non-dairy milk alternatives in coffee shops.

The TDF has demonstrated its effectiveness and utility within public health and healthcare contexts, dietary behaviors [22,24,25], the promotion of children's milk consumption [26], and the adoption of sustainable agri-environmental practices [27].

However, the utilization of this behavior change methodology is not widely embraced within the domain of coffee consumer choice behavior, especially dairy alternatives. Therefore, to our knowledge, this is the first study to use the TDF and other components of the BCW to explore the barriers and facilitators in the context of non-dairy and plant-based milks in coffee drinks. Previous research has investigated barriers to the consumption of plant-based beverages among US consumers using a multi-response method (emotional, conceptual, situational, and conative) [28]. It was found that fitting expectations and negative associations were dominant among consumers who had never consumed plant-based beverages, with these associations varying by product type. For instance, negative perceptions were the strongest for oat milk, followed by fruit smoothies with soy milk, and iced coffee with almond milk. Food neophobia also negatively influenced the perceptions of less familiar products, including plant-based beverages. However, this research was limited to a small number of beverages and plant-based alternatives. Another systematic review investigated the determinants of real-life behavioral interventions to promote more plant-based and less animal-based diets, finding that targeting individual or environmental determinants is most effective [29]. None of these studies used the TDF and BCW, nor did they investigate plant-based alternatives to dairy specifically for coffee drinks.

2. Materials and Methods

2.1. Subjects and Design

This study employed a cross-sectional design. A total of 215 participants from 19 countries, including prominent regions such as the UAE, USA, UK, Germany, and Canada, participated in this study. However, 15 participants were excluded due to incomplete survey submissions, ensuring the integrity of our results. The final sample size consisted of 200 respondents. Of these 200 participants, approximately 56% identified as male, 42% as female, and 4 participants (2%) identified as transgender, non-binary, or another not-listed gender. According to the Beresford Research classification of age groups, Millennials (aged 26–41) constituted the largest demographic in this study, comprising 53% (106 participants) of the sample [30]. Generation X (aged 42–57) accounted for 26% of respondents, while Generation Z (aged 18–25) made up 16%. Geographically, roughly one quarter of the respondents (23%) resided in the USA, followed by 22% in the United

Arab Emirates. The UK and Germany each accounted for around 11% of participants, and Canada represented 9%. The participants were also asked about food allergies, with 81% indicating they do not have any, while about 10% of those with an allergy reported having a milk allergy.

2.2. Instruments

The survey utilized in this study consisted of 31 questions, including a 10-item TDF-based scale. The survey began with a series of 7 questions to capture the demographic information about the participants. Following the inquiry about coffee consumption, the participants who reported being coffee drinkers proceeded to respond to nine more questions related to coffee, whereas non-coffee drinkers moved directly to the next section of the survey. Following the coffee-related questions, all 200 participants answered 3 questions related to their attitudes towards non-dairy milk charges at coffee shops. After this, the participants responded to two questions about their awareness of marketing campaigns for coffee or coffee shops in general, as well as specific promotions for non-dairy milk coffee beverages.

The final section of the survey asked the participants to evaluate 10 statements developed using the Theoretical Domains Framework (TDF). The survey instrument was developed specifically for this research by the authors and had not been previously validated. It was constructed based on elements and recommendations from the Theoretical Domains Framework (TDF) [23], informed by previous TDF surveys and interview guides [31–33], as well as a validated TDF scale [34]. The full questionnaire is provided in Appendix A.

2.3. Procedure

Primary data were collected online through a survey featuring both closed and open-ended questions. The survey was administered using a Computer-Assisted Web Interviewing (CAWI) platform, with data collection occurring from May to July 2023.

The survey was reviewed and approved by Warwick Business School (WBS), following the guidelines of the University of Warwick's Humanities and Social Science Research Ethics Committee (HSSREC) on 15 July 2022. All participants provided informed consent before participating. The survey was conducted anonymously, adhering to GDPR compliance, as per the University of Warwick's data protection policies. Detailed information on data management practices is available in the University of Warwick Research Privacy Notice.

2.4. Data Analysis

To comprehensively explore the participants' coffee-related behaviors and preferences and gain market research insights, a series of analytical methods were employed in this study. A frequency analysis was conducted to identify patterns and distributions in the participants' coffee-related behaviors, attitudes, and preferences. This analysis involved examining the frequencies of responses to questions regarding coffee consumption habits, preferences for types of milk, and locations where coffee is typically consumed. The results of this analysis provided valuable insights into the prevalence of various behaviors and preferences among the study participants, offering a picture of their coffee consumption patterns. In addition to exploring the behaviors and preferences, this study conducted market research comparisons based on geographical location, age group, attitudes towards charges for non-dairy milks, and awareness of marketing campaigns. Multiple regression analysis was performed to investigate the relationship between the Theoretical Domains Framework (TDF) questions (independent variables) and the consumption of non-dairy milk (dependent variable). This analysis provided a deeper understanding of which TDF domains significantly influenced the participants' likelihood of adopting or rejecting non-dairy milk. Finally, based on the BCW, practical suggestions for intervention strategies were discussed.

3. Results

3.1. Coffee-Related Behavior

Of the 200 participants, 177 (approximately 89%) were coffee drinkers and responded to the coffee-related questions. The first question inquired why the participants drink coffee, offering four predefined options and an "other" category, with the participants being allowed to select multiple reasons. The most common reason was taste, selected by about 85% of the respondents, followed by caffeine or energy at 64%. Social reasons accounted for 47%, stress relief for 26%, and 10% chose "other."

Understanding why consumers drink coffee is essential for grasping their preferences for different types of coffee, such as milk-based or black. The subsequent five questions explored the participants' coffee drinking habits, including the time of day and preferred locations, providing insights into their consumption patterns. The data revealed that 92% of the respondents primarily drink coffee at home, followed by 64% at coffee shops, and 58% at the office. These insights highlight the various factors influencing coffee drinkers' preferences. For instance, those drinking coffee at the office might face challenges with dairy-alternative milks due to limited company provisions, whereas coffee shops offer a wider range of options.

The participants were then asked about their milk preferences in coffee. The responses indicated that 61% preferred cow's milk, 53% chose no milk or espresso, and 51% opted for plant-based or other milks. This question is significant for understanding the milk preferences of coffee drinkers and serves as a key reference point for our later analysis.

The final two questions asked the coffee drinkers about their preferred coffee shop or brand and the reasons for their preference. Among the 177 respondents, approximately 40% (69 individuals) preferred local cafes or small businesses, 15% favored Starbucks, 10% chose another large coffee chain or brand, and 30% selected home or other options. The most frequently cited reasons for their preferences were the quality or taste of the coffee (83%), followed by the ambiance (37%), and the location or availability (36%).

3.2. Attitudes towards Non-Dairy Milk Charges at Coffee Shops

After completing the coffee section of the survey, all 200 participants were asked three questions about dairy milk alternatives and their preferences. The first question assessed their awareness of the additional charges for non-dairy milks at coffee shops. More than half (54%) indicated that their coffee shop charges extra, 14% said that it does not, and 32% were unsure or unaware of the policy.

The second question explored the participants' beliefs on whether customers should pay extra for non-dairy milks (Figure 2). Among the "yes" responses, the most common reason was that non-dairy milk costs more to produce (34%). The highest response overall was "No, because customers should not have to pay due to an allergy/intolerance" (43%).

When analyzed by age group, Gen Z (18–25) most strongly believed that non-dairy milk should not be chargeable due to allergies (53%), followed by Millennials (26–41) at 43%, Gen X (42–57) at 39%, and Boomer I (58–67) at 13%. The youngest and eldest groups, each with one respondent, both scored 100%, which were considered statistical anomalies.

The final question related to non-dairy milk charges asked the participants if they would visit a coffee shop or brand more often if it did not charge extra for non-dairy milks. Nearly 43% stated that this would not change their behavior, with about 22% more saying that they do not drink dairy milk, so it does not affect them. The remaining responses were affirmative, with 15% saying they would always visit or order from such a coffee shop more often, and 21% mentioning they would do so only if the shop was close by or convenient.

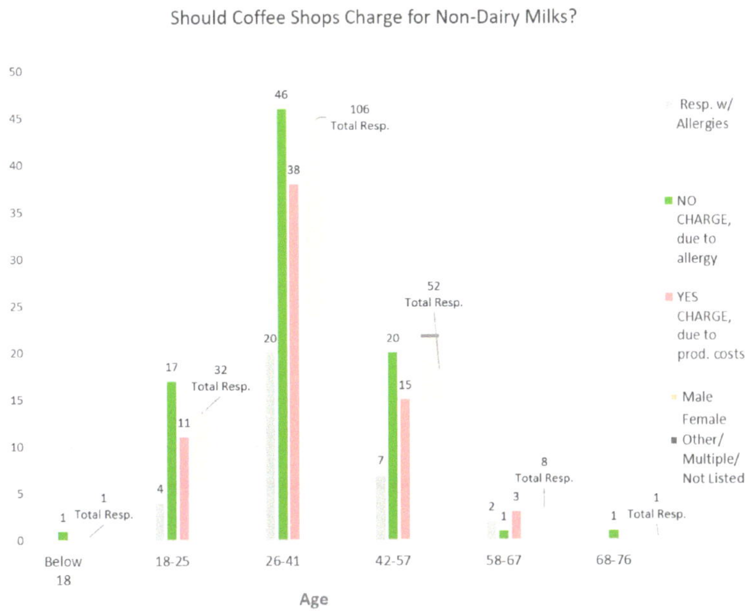

Figure 2. Distribution of data by participants' beliefs on whether customers should pay extra for non-dairy milks.

3.3. Marketing Campaigns Awareness

After completing the survey section on dairy milk alternatives, the participants were asked about their awareness of marketing campaigns for coffee and specifically for non-dairy milk coffee beverages. Notably, 61% of the respondents recalled seeing advertisements for a coffee shop or brand, while 35% remembered campaigns promoting non-dairy milk beverages.

3.4. TDF Framework Results

The participants' perceptions regarding dairy and non-dairy milk were further assessed through 10 TDF-based items. The ten TDF statements, along with their scores, means, standard deviations, and variances, are detailed in the table below (Table 1).

The statement regarding taste yielded a mean response of 2.65, indicating a slight negativity towards non-dairy milk taste, although the high standard deviation (1.28) highlighted diverse opinions. Social influences were explored in the statement about peers and family members not consuming non-dairy milk, which had a mean of 2.59, indicating variability. The wording may have influenced the responses, necessitating cautious interpretation. Concerns about the cost showed a mean response of 3.35, suggesting a generally affirmative perception with a narrower range of opinions. The participants strongly agreed (mean 4.47) with the statements related to dairy consumption in upbringing, indicating a widespread consensus. Statements on health considerations generally reflected positive inclinations towards incorporating non-dairy milk into diets, with means of around 3.16 and relatively consistent responses, underscoring growing health awareness and dietary flexibility among the participants.

Table 1. TDF statement descriptions.

	TDF Items	Min	Max	Mean	SD	Var
1	I drink non-dairy milk. (Beliefs about Capabilities)	1.00	5.00	3.07	1.61	2.61
2	Non-dairy milk tastes bad. (Beliefs about Consequences)	1.00	5.00	2.65	1.28	1.64
3	Non-dairy milk is too expensive. (Environmental Context and Resources)	1.00	5.00	3.35	1.03	1.07
4	Non-dairy milk is not available to me. (Environmental Context and Resources)	1.00	5.00	1.76	1.07	1.15
5	My friends/colleagues/family do not drink non-dairy milk. (Social Influences)	1.00	5.00	2.59	1.31	1.73
6	Dairy milk (cow's milk) should be part of a normal diet. (Beliefs about Consequences)	1.00	5.00	2.91	1.07	1.15
7	I grew up drinking dairy (cow's milk). (Social Role and Identity)	1.00	5.00	4.47	0.98	0.95
8	Non-dairy milk should be part of a normal diet. (Beliefs about Consequences)	1.00	5.00	3.16	0.96	0.92
9	I am conscious about the amount of calories I consume. (Behavioral Regulation)	1.00	5.00	3.40	1.24	1.54
10	I am conscious about the amount of calories in different types of milk. (Knowledge, Behavioral Regulation)	1.00	5.00	2.68	1.38	1.91

3.5. Regression Analysis Results

The regression analysis explored how the TDF questions (independent variables) relate to non-dairy milk consumption (dependent variable) (Table 2). The results showed a moderate positive correlation (Multiple R = 0.5969), indicating that higher agreement with the TDF questions was associated with increased non-dairy milk consumption About 35.63% of consumption variance was explained by TDF question variations (R Square = 0.356). The model was statistically significant (F = 10.46, $p < 0.001$), confirming that TDF questions collectively influenced consumption. Notably, questions on dairy and non-dairy milk in diets had the lowest *p*-values, indicating a significant impact on consumption.

Table 2. Regression analysis results.

Consumption of Plant-Based Milk Alternatives in the Coffee Drink				
F (10, 189)	10.462, $p < 0.001$			
Multiple R	0.5969			
R^2	0.356			
Independent Variable	***ß***	***SE***	***t***	***p*-Value ***
I drink non-dairy milk.	0.124	0.020	6.121	0.000
Non-dairy milk tastes bad.	−0.023	0.028	−0.822	0.412
Non-dairy milk is too expensive.	−0.030	0.028	−1.041	0.299
Non-dairy milk is not available to me.	−0.023	0.027	−0.836	0.404
My friends/colleagues/family do not drink non-dairy milk.	0.005	0.022	0.244	0.807
Dairy milk (cow's milk) should be part of a normal diet.	−0.072	0.031	−2.338	0.020 *
I grew up drinking dairy (cow's milk).	−0.017	0.030	−0.572	0.568
Non-dairy milk should be part of a normal diet.	0.066	0.031	2.177	0.036 *
I am conscious about the amount of calories I consume.	0.015	0.029	0.518	0.605
I am conscious about the amount of calories in different types of milk.	−0.007	0.026	−0.256	0.798

* $p < 0.05$.

The coefficient for "Dairy milk as part of a normal diet" was −0.072, indicating a negative association with non-dairy milk consumption (Table 2). In contrast, "Non-dairy milk as part of a normal diet" had a coefficient of 0.066, signifying a positive association—suggesting that those who view non-dairy milk as a dietary staple are more inclined to consume it. Conversely, other factors such as taste, price, availability, social influence, and calorie consciousness did not exhibit statistically significant correlations with non-dairy milk consumption based on our analyses.

3.6. Geographical Location

Of particular interest is the high representation of participants from the United States and the United Arab Emirates, where Starbucks imposes a "plant-based tax" by charging extra for non-dairy milk. In contrast, the survey also identified the United Kingdom and Germany as the third and fourth most represented countries, respectively, where Starbucks does not charge for non-dairy milks [35]. The strong representation from these four countries suggests that their perspectives, behaviors, and opinions may have a significant influence on the overall findings, as visualized in Figures 3 and 4 below.

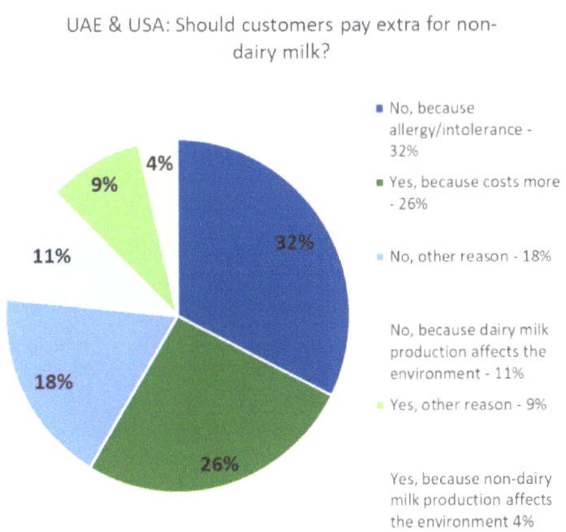

Figure 3. Distribution of data by participants' beliefs on whether customers should pay extra for non-dairy milks based on geographical location: UAE & USA.

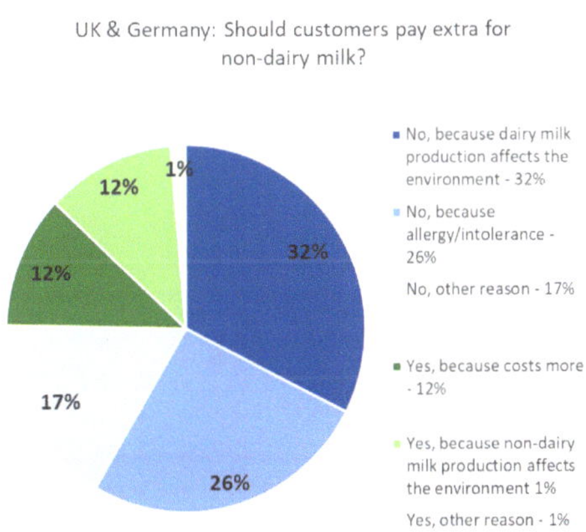

Figure 4. Distribution of data by participants' beliefs on whether customers should pay extra for non-dairy milks based on geographical location: UK & Germany.

A significant majority of respondents from the UK and Germany across all age groups believe that no one should pay additional charges for non-dairy milk, regardless of the circumstances, compared to respondents from the UAE and USA. Although the younger respondents from the UAE and USA also prioritize inclusivity similarly to their counterparts in the UK and Germany, their consideration appears to be balanced with economic considerations favoring the USA and UAE respondents.

Based on awareness of marketing campaigns (Table 3), Canada had the highest visibility for coffee advertisements (82%) but the lowest for non-dairy milk coffee beverage advertisements (7%). Conversely, while the USA had the second-highest visibility for coffee advertisements (74%), it scored the highest for non-dairy milk advertisements at 65%.

Table 3. Marketing campaigns awareness frequencies based on location.

Have You Seen a Coffee Advertisement in the Last 6 Months?				
	N	**Yes**	**No**	**I Do Not Remember**
USA	46	74%	15%	11%
UAE	43	49%	23%	28%
UK	22	55%	9%	36%
Germany	21	67%	10%	24%
Canada	17	82%	12%	6%
Have You Seen a Non-Dairy Milk Coffee Beverage Advertisement in the Last 6 Months?				
USA	39	65%	14%	21%
UAE	33	23%	39%	38%
UK	20	40%	15%	45%
Germany	19	42%	32%	26%
Canada	15	7%	67%	27%

Furthermore, the regions of the UAE and USA appeared to be more conscious of overall calorie intake and the calories in milk, as indicated by higher means on the relevant TDF statements (Table 4). The UK and Germany demonstrated a stronger upbringing on dairy and the belief that it should be part of a diet.

Table 4. TDF statement means based on location.

Respondents' Country	**Grew Up Drinking Milk**		**Non-Dairy Should Be Part of a Diet**		**Dairy Should Be Part of a Diet**		**Conscious about Overall Calories**		**Conscious about Milk Calories**	
	Mean	**Var**	**Mean**	**Var**	**Mean**	**Var**	**Mean**	**Var**	**Mean**	**Var**
UAE and USA	4.4	0.8	3.4	0.8	3.1	1.0	3.9	1.0	3.3	1.9
UK and Germany	4.8	0.2	2.4	0.8	3.7	2.3	3.2	1.7	2.0	1.8

4. Discussion

The findings from this study provide a nuanced understanding of consumer behavior and preferences surrounding the use of non-dairy milks in coffee consumption. Taste emerged as one of the primary drivers influencing participants' coffee choices, highlighting the significance of sensory satisfaction in beverage selection. Many participants indicated a preference for adding cow's milk to their coffee, highlighting a strong preference for dairy taste, established dietary habits, and potential cultural influences.

Sensory properties are crucial in plant-based drinks, as highlighted by prior research [4,36]. Established consumers of plant-based alternatives generally perceive the taste positively, whereas taste perception remains a significant barrier for non-consumers [37]. Previous studies have shown that expectations and negative associations are common among those who have never tried plant-based beverages, with these associations varying by product type [28]. Additionally, food neophobia—a fear of trying unfamiliar foods—negatively affects the perceptions of plant-based beverages.

A significant aspect of this study was the awareness among the participants regarding extra charges for non-dairy milks at coffee shops. This issue generated diverse opinions, with some arguing against such charges on the grounds of fairness, particularly for individuals with allergies or intolerances for whom plant-based alternatives are the only option. Conversely, supporters of the surcharges cited higher production costs for plant-based alternatives. In reality, one of the primary challenges facing PBMAs is their elevated production costs, which impact every stage of the plant-based milk supply chain [9].

Notably, younger generations like Gen Z and Millennials exhibited stronger opposition to these fees. This inclination could stem from their upbringing in an era marked by extensive access to information and heightened awareness of social and environmental issues, such as the importance of planetary health and the United Nations Sustainable Development Goals. Conversely, older age groups may demonstrate a more nuanced perspective, possibly influenced by evolving societal norms and personal experiences over time. The middle age group, in particular, seems to weigh economic sustainability alongside inclusivity, reflecting a stage of life where financial responsibilities and stability become more prominent concerns. Understanding these generational dynamics is crucial for businesses aiming to align with the values and preferences of their evolving consumer base, ensuring that their practices resonate with both economic realities and social aspirations across different age demographics.

Regional disparities were also evident, with the respondents from the UK and Germany being more inclined to oppose the extra charges for non-dairy milks compared to those from the UAE and USA, where economic factors often tempered inclusivity concerns. This outcome may be influenced by Starbucks' pricing strategy, which, since 2023, does not impose additional charges for non-dairy milk in the UK and Germany, whereas, in the UAE and USA, there is an extra charge for non-dairy milk in their coffees. Interestingly, despite this inclusive pricing, individuals from the UK and Germany were raised with a stronger emphasis on dairy consumption, often viewing it as a dietary staple more so than their counterparts from the UAE and USA. This difference could be attributed to robust marketing campaigns, the perceived nutritional benefits of dairy milk, or traditional dietary habits and education. It is important to note that a preference for dairy does not undermine the belief in inclusivity, but rather reflects personal choices or perceptions of dairy's benefits.

This study also revealed nuances in consumer awareness and preferences regarding calorie consciousness in general and in milk products, particularly evident in regions like the USA and UAE. This heightened awareness may explain why coffee shops or brands in these regions target their customers with advertisements for non-dairy milk options, which generally contain fewer calories, based on the respondents' feedback.

Moreover, while the participants widely recalled advertisements for coffee shops or brands, campaigns specifically promoting non-dairy milk beverages were notably less memorable. This discrepancy suggests that there is significant room for improvement in marketing strategies aimed at increasing the visibility and appeal of plant-based alternatives. Targeted marketing efforts could effectively address this gap by highlighting the benefits of non-dairy milks, such as their environmental sustainability [1,2], health advantages [4,9], and suitability for those with dietary restrictions [7–9]. By focusing on these unique selling points, companies could not only enhance consumer awareness but also foster a stronger connection with the growing demographic that values inclusivity and sustainability in their dietary choices.

Behavior Change Suggestions

The results from the regression analysis showed that the participants who viewed non-dairy milk as a dietary staple were more likely to consume it. This finding aligns with the "Beliefs about Consequences" domain from the Theoretical Domains Framework (TDF) (refer to Table 1 and Appendix A for details).

The Belief about Consequences domain refers to an individual's perception of the positive or negative outcomes and the effects associated with specific behaviors or actions [22]. The participants who see non-dairy milk as a dietary staple likely believe in its positive outcomes, such as health benefits [4,9], environmental sustainability [1,2], or alignment with dietary restrictions [7–9]. These anticipated positive consequences potentially reinforce their choice to consume non-dairy milk. Their consumption behavior is influenced by their belief in the favorable results of integrating non-dairy milk into their diet.

The Behavior Change Wheel (BCW) [23] can be used to transition from identifying behavioral patterns to designing interventions. Ojo et al. [38] have adapted the BCW, as shown in Figure 5, to illustrate how the Theoretical Domains Framework (TDF) domains align with the BCW. This mapping facilitates the selection of appropriate intervention functions and policy categories that can effectively address the behavioral determinants identified in our study. In the BCW, the intervention functions corresponding to the Beliefs about Consequences domain are Training and Coercion.

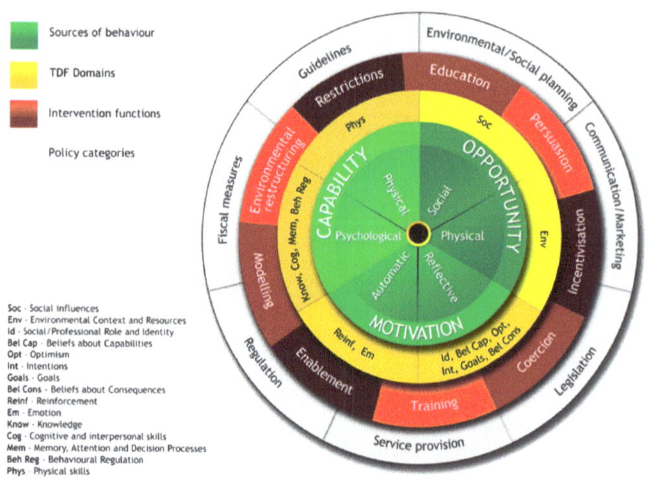

Figure 5. Behavior Change Wheel with TDF Domains mapped [23,38].

To align with the Training function of the Behavior Change Wheel (BCW), coffee shops can implement comprehensive training programs for baristas that extend beyond the basics of non-dairy milk preparation. These programs can include advanced preparation techniques, where baristas are trained in how to steam and froth various non-dairy milks to achieve the perfect texture and consistency for different coffee beverages. Sensory training is also essential, as educating staff on the taste, mouthfeel, and aroma profiles of different non-dairy milks will allow them to make informed recommendations to customers based on individual taste preferences. This approach can help to address food neophobia and challenge the negative expectations and associations commonly held by those unfamiliar with plant-based beverages [28]. Our survey results indicate that taste is a significant factor in coffee consumption decisions. Additionally, providing baristas with knowledge about the nutritional benefits and potential allergens associated with different non-dairy milks will help them to address customer inquiries more accurately and confidently. Educating staff in the coffee shops on the positive consequences of drinking plant-based alternatives for both individuals and the planet's health, as well as informing them about sustainability and ethical issues, can further enhance customer engagement and satisfaction.

In terms of Coercion, which involves the expectation of costs or punishment [23], it can be implemented in a more positive and strategic manner to promote non-dairy milk consumption. Offering time-limited discounts or promotions on beverages made with non-dairy milk can be an effective approach. For instance, implementing "Non-Dairy

Mondays" where all non-dairy milk beverages are discounted encourages customers to try them out. Developing loyalty programs that reward customers for choosing non-dairy milk is another strategy (similar to the Starbucks "Gold" program). For example, a point system where customers earn extra points for each non-dairy milk purchase, which can be redeemed for free beverages or other rewards, can enhance customer loyalty.

Environmental incentives can also be tied to non-dairy milk consumption. Implementing eco-friendly initiatives where customers who bring reusable cups and choose non-dairy milk receive a discount or a small reward promotes not only non-dairy milk but also sustainable practices. Subscription plans can be introduced for frequent customers, offering benefits such as free non-dairy milk options or reduced surcharges for non-dairy milk over a set period. Special events and campaigns can further promote non-dairy milk. Hosting events like a "Non-Dairy Milk Week" with special offers, tastings, and informational sessions can raise awareness and encourage more customers to try non-dairy milk options.

By incorporating these strategies, both training and coercion can be effectively used to promote the adoption and acceptance of non-dairy milk options in coffee shops. This comprehensive approach will ultimately lead to a more inclusive and health-conscious customer base, while also supporting environmental sustainability.

5. Conclusions

The present study examined consumer preferences and behaviors related to non-dairy milk alternatives in the context of coffee consumption. Based on the results of the survey, we gained valuable insights into the demographics, coffee-related responses, dairy milk alternative preferences, marketing, and beliefs that influence consumer choices. This study revealed that taste was the primary reason participants drank coffee. Most participants consumed coffee at home, followed by coffee shops and the office. Cow's milk was the preferred additive in coffee for the majority of the respondents. Many favored local cafes or small businesses, citing coffee quality or taste as reasons why. A significant number of participants were aware of extra charges for non-dairy milks at coffee shops, with a majority reporting that their coffee shop applied such charges. Arguments against extra charges included concerns that they should not be due to allergies or intolerances, while those in favor argued that production costs for plant-based alternatives were higher. Gen Z and Millennials were particularly likely to oppose charges for non-dairy milks due to lactose intolerance or allergies. The respondents from the UK and Germany were more inclined to believe that no one should pay extra for non-dairy milk compared to those from the UAE and USA, where economic considerations balanced inclusivity concerns. The majority of participants remembered encountering advertisements for coffee shops or brands, while only approximately one-third recalled seeing campaigns promoting non-dairy milk beverages. Finally, the results from the regression analysis indicated that the participants who viewed non-dairy milk as a dietary staple were more likely to consume it. This finding aligns with the "Beliefs about Consequences" domain from the Theoretical Domains Framework (TDF), as these individuals likely associate non-dairy milk with positive outcomes, such as health benefits and environmental sustainability. Finally, based on the BCW, practical suggestions for intervention strategies based on Training and Coercion were discussed.

As with any survey, there are limitations to consider. Although the findings were statistically significant, the sample size of 200 participants does not comprehensively represent the diverse perspectives and preferences of all coffee consumers. A larger sample size would enhance the reliability and generalizability of the results. Conducting more extensive surveys in each of the top five countries, which provided particularly interesting insights, could yield stronger and more nuanced findings. Additionally, future studies should delve deeper into the impact of cultural factors on milk preferences. Cultural norms, dietary habits, and traditional beliefs can significantly influence consumer behavior and attitudes towards dairy and non-dairy milk. Understanding these cultural influences would provide a more holistic view of consumer preferences and could inform more targeted marketing and policy-making efforts. This expanded approach would help us to create a comprehensive understanding of the global market for dairy and non-dairy milk in coffee consumption.

Author Contributions: Conceptualization, I.V. and N.H.; Data curation, V.H.; Writing—original draft, N.H. and V.H.; Writing—review & editing, V.H.; Supervision, I.V.; Project administration, I.V. All authors have read and agreed to the published version of the manuscript.

Funding: This work was supported by the National Recovery and Resilience Plan of the Republic of Bulgaria under contract SUMMIT BG-RRP-2.004-0008-C01.

Institutional Review Board Statement: The study was conducted in accordance with the University of Warwick's Humanities and Social Science Research Ethics Committee (HSSREC) Program: DMBA; student number: 2068044; on 15 July 2022.

Informed Consent Statement: Informed consent was obtained from all subjects involved in the study.

Data Availability Statement: Data are contained within the article.

Conflicts of Interest: The authors declare no conflict of interest.

Appendix A. Survey Questions

Demographics:	
1	What is your age?
2	What gender do you identify as?
3	What country do you live in (spend most of your days in a year)?
4	What is your employment status?
5	If employed, do you work from home, office, or hybrid?
6	Do you have any food allergies?
7	Do you drink coffee?
Coffee-related behavior:	
1	Why do you drink coffee?
2	How often do you drink coffee?
3	If daily, how many coffee beverages do you consume a day on average?
4	What time of the day do you drink coffee?
5	Do you drink your coffee hot or cold?
6	Where do you drink your coffee?
7	What kind of milk do you take with your coffee, if any?
8	Which coffee shop or brand do you prefer the most to drink from?
9	Why do you prefer to drink from the coffee shop/brand you selected in the previous answer?
Attitudes towards non-dairy milk charges at coffee shops:	
1	Your opinion on dairy milk alternatives: does the coffee shop you visit or are aware of charge for non-dairy milks (i.e., soy, almond, oats, other)?
2	Should customers pay extra for non-dairy milks (i.e., soy, almond, oats, other)?
3	If the coffee shop did not charge extra for non-dairy milks, would you visit it/order from it more often?
Marketing campaigns awareness:	
1	In the last 6 months, have you seen any advertisement for coffee/coffee shop (either in public or online/mobile or other)?
2	Have you seen any advertisement for non-dairy milk coffee beverages in the same period?

Theoretical-Domains-Framework-based questions:
How much do you agree with the following statements about non-dairy milk (i.e., soy, almond, oats, other)? (5-point Likert scale)

	TDF Statement	TDF Domain
1	I drink non-dairy milk.	Beliefs about Capabilities
2	Non-dairy milk tastes bad.	Beliefs about Consequences
3	Non-dairy milk is too expensive.	Environmental Context and Resources
4	Non-dairy milk is not available to me.	Environmental Context and Resources
5	My friends/colleagues/family do not drink non-dairy milk.	Social Influences
6	Dairy milk (cow's milk) should be part of a normal diet.	Beliefs about Consequences
7	I grew up drinking dairy milk (cow's milk).	Social Role and Identity
8	Non-dairy milk should be part of a normal diet.	Beliefs about Consequences
9	I am conscious of the number of calories I consume.	Behavioral Regulation
10	I am conscious of the number of calories in different types of milk.	Knowledge, Behavioral Regulation

References

1. Ritchie, H. Dairy vs. Plant-Based Milk: What Are the Environmental Impacts? Published Online at OurWorldInData.org. 2022. Available online: https://ourworldindata.org/environmental-impact-milks (accessed on 20 June 2024).
2. Craig, W.; Messina, V.; Rowland, I.; Frankowska, A.; Bradbury, J.; Smetana, S.; Medici, E. Plant-Based Dairy Alternatives Contribute to a Healthy and Sustainable Diet. *Nutrients* **2023**, *15*, 3393. [CrossRef]
3. United Nations (UN). Transforming Our World: The 2030 Agenda for Sustainable Development. United Nations. Available online: https://sdgs.un.org/2030agenda (accessed on 17 June 2024).
4. Craig, W.; Fresán, U. International Analysis of the Nutritional Content and a Review of Health Benefits of Non-Dairy Plant-Based Beverages. *Nutrients* **2021**, *13*, 842. [CrossRef]
5. EAT. The EAT-Lancet Commission on Food, Planet and Health: The Planetary Health Diet. EAT. Available online: https://eatforum.org/eat-lancet-commission/the-planetary-health-diet-and-you/ (accessed on 20 June 2024).
6. Storhaug, C.; Fosse, S.; Fadnes, L. Country, regional, and global estimates for lactose malabsorption in adults: A systematic review and meta-analysis. *Lancet Gastroenterol. Hepatol.* **2017**, *2*, 10. [CrossRef]
7. Ramsing, R.; Santo, R.; Kim, B.; Altema-Johnson, D.; Wooden, A.; Chang, K.; Semba, R.; Love, D. Dairy and Plant-Based Milks: Implications for Nutrition and Planetary Health. *Curr. Environ. Health Rep.* **2023**, *10*, 291–302. [CrossRef]
8. Ammann, J.; Grande, A.; Inderbitzin, J.; Guggenbühl, B. Understanding Swiss consumption of plant-based alternatives to dairy products. *Food Qual. Prefer.* **2023**, *110*, 104947. [CrossRef]
9. Plamada, D.; Teleky, B.-E.; Nemes, S.A.; Mitrea, L.; Szabo, K.; Călinoiu, L.-F.; Pascuta, M.S.; Varvara, R.-A.; Ciont, C.; Martău, G.A.; et al. Plant-Based Dairy Alternatives—A Future Direction to the Milky Way. *Foods* **2023**, *12*, 1883. [CrossRef]
10. Astolfi, M.; Marconi, E.; Protano, C.; Canepari, S. Comparative elemental analysis of dairy milk and plant-based milk alternatives. *Food Control.* **2020**, *116*, 107327. [CrossRef]
11. Clegg, M.; Ribes, A.; Reynolds, R.; Kliem, K.; Stergiadis, S. A comparative assessment of the nutritional composition of dairy and plant-based dairy alternatives available for sale in the UK and the implications for consumers' dietary intakes. *Food Res. Int.* **2021**, *148*, 110586. [CrossRef]
12. D'Andrea, A.; Kinchla, A.; Nolden, A. A comparison of the nutritional profile and nutrient density of commercially available plant-based and dairy yogurts in the United States. *Front. Nutr.* **2023**, *10*, 1195045. [CrossRef]
13. Glover, A.; Hayes, H.E.; Ni, H.; Raikos, V. A comparison of the nutritional content and price between dairy and non-dairy milks and cheeses in UK supermarkets: A cross-sectional analysis. *Nutr. Health* **2024**, *30*, 157–165. [CrossRef]
14. Moshtaghian, H.; Hallström, E.; Bianchi, M.; Bryngelsson, S. Nutritional profile of plant-based dairy alternatives in the Swedish market. *Curr. Res. Food Sci.* **2024**, *8*, 100712. [CrossRef] [PubMed]
15. Marchese, L.; Hendrie, G.; McNaughton, S.; Brooker, P.; Dickinson, K.; Livingstone, K. Comparison of the nutritional composition of supermarket plant-based meat and dairy alternatives with the Australian Food Composition Database. *J. Food Compos. Anal.* **2024**, *129*, 106017. [CrossRef]
16. Silva, A.; Silva, M.; Ribeiro, B. Health issues and technological aspects of plant-based alternative milk. *Food Res. Int.* **2020**, *131*, 108972. [CrossRef]
17. Baldwin, H.; Tan, J. Effects of Diet on Acne and Its Response to Treatment. *Am. J. Clin. Dermatol.* **2021**, *22*, 55–65. [CrossRef] [PubMed]
18. OECD. Common Ownership by Institutional Investors and Its Impact on Competition. Organisation for Economic Co-Operation and Development. 2017. Available online: https://one.oecd.org/document/daf/comp(2017)10/en/pdf (accessed on 21 June 2023).
19. Edmans, A. Blockholder trading, market efficiency, and managerial myopia. *J. Financ.* **2009**, *64*, 2481–2513. [CrossRef]
20. Aghion, P.; Bolton, P.; Tirole, J. Exit options in Corporate Finance: Liquidity versus incentives. *Rev. Financ.* **2004**, *8*, 327–353. [CrossRef]
21. Goldenberg, M.; Frost, S. Mintec Insight Series: Are Plant-Based Products Sold at (un)-Justified Premiums? Mintec Insight Series. Available online: https://mintecglobal.pagetiger.com/whitepaper/plant-based-foods (accessed on 10 June 2024).

22. Cane, J.; O'Connor, D.; Michie, S. Validation of the theoretical domains framework for use in behavior change and Implementation Research. *Implement. Sci.* **2012**, *7*, 37. [CrossRef]
23. Michie, S.; Atkins, L.; West, R. *The Behaviour Change Wheel: A Guide to Designing Interventions*; Silverback Publishing: London, UK, 2014.
24. Grady, A.; Seward, K.; Finch, M.; Fielding, A.; Stacey, F.; Jones, J.; Wolfenden, L.; Yoong, S. Barriers and Enablers to Implementation of Dietary Guidelines in Early Childhood Education Centers in Australia: Application of the Theoretical Domains Framework. *J. Nutr. Educ. Behav.* **2018**, *50*, 3. [CrossRef] [PubMed]
25. Timlin, D.; Giannantoni, B.; McCormack, J.; Polito, A.; Ciarapica, D.; Azzini, E.; Giles, M.; Simpson, E. Comparison of barriers and facilitators of MIND diet uptake among adults from Northern Ireland and Italy. *BMC Public Health* **2021**, *21*, 265. [CrossRef]
26. Greene, E.; Hunt, E.; Kilduff, O.; Murrin, C. Factors influencing the implementation of the EU School Milk Scheme in Irish primary schools. *Eur. J. Public Health* **2024**, *33*, 2. [CrossRef]
27. Baaken, M.; Bartkowski, B.; Rode, J. Exploring farmers'support needs for the adoption of agrienvironmental practices: An application of the theoretical domains framework. *Environ. Res. Commun.* **2023**, *5*, 111004. [CrossRef]
28. Jaeger, S.; Giacalone, D. Barriers to consumption of plant-based beverages: A comparison of product users and non-users on emotional, conceptual, situational, conative and psychographic variables. *Food Res. Int.* **2021**, *144*, 110363. [CrossRef] [PubMed]
29. Taufik, D.; Verain, M.; Bouwman, E.; Reinders, M. Determinants of real-life behavioural interventions to stimulate more plant-based and less animal-based diets: A systematic review. *Trends Food Sci. Technol.* **2019**, *93*, 281–303. [CrossRef]
30. Beresford Research. Age Range by Generation. Beresford Research. 2023. Available online: https://www.beresfordresearch.com/age-range-by-generation/ (accessed on 17 March 2023).
31. Amemori, M.; Michie, S.; Korhonen, T.; Murtomaa, H.; Kinnunen, T.H. Assessing implementation difficulties in tobacco use prevention and cessation counselling among dental providers. *Implement. Sci.* **2011**, *6*, 1–10. [CrossRef] [PubMed]
32. Gainforth, H.; Sheals, K.; Atkins, L.; Jackson, R.; Michie, S. Developing interventions to change recycling behaviors: A case study of applying behavioral science. *Appl. Environ. Educ. Commun.* **2016**, *15*, 325–339. [CrossRef]
33. Smith, J.; Corace, K.; MacDonald, T.; Fabrigar, L.; Saedi, A.; Chaplin, A.; MacFarlane, S.; Valickis, D.; Garber, G. Application of the Theoretical Domains Framework to identify factors that influence hand hygiene compliance in long-term care. *J. Hosp. Infect.* **2019**, *101*, 393–398. [CrossRef] [PubMed]
34. Huijg, J.M.; Gebhardt, W.A.; Crone, M.R.; Dusseldorp, E.; Presseau, J. Discriminant content validity of a theoretical domains framework questionnaire for use in implementation research. *Implement. Sci.* **2014**, *9*, 1–16. [CrossRef] [PubMed]
35. Valko, A. Customers Are Upset Starbucks Is 'Unfairly' Overcharging for Non-Dairy Milks. Yahoo! 2023. Available online: https://www.yahoo.com/lifestyle/customers-upset-starbucks-unfairly-overcharging-210028672.html (accessed on 21 June 2023).
36. Cardello, A.; Llobell, F.; Giacalone, D.; Roigard, C.; Jaeger, S. Plant-based alternatives vs. dairy milk: Consumer segments and their sensory, emotional, cognitive and situational use responses to tasted products. *Food Qual. Prefer.* **2022**, *100*, 104599. [CrossRef]
37. Laila, A.; Topakas, N.; Farr, E.; Haines, J.; Ma, D.; Newton, G.; Buchholz, A. Barriers and facilitators of household provision of dairy and plant-based dairy alternatives in families with preschool-age children. *Public Health Nutr.* **2021**, *24*, 5673–5685. [CrossRef]
38. Ojo, S.O.; Bailey, D.P.; Brierley, M.L.; Hewson, D.J.; Chater, A.M. Breaking barriers: Using the behavior change wheel to develop a tailored intervention to overcome workplace inhibitors to breaking up sitting time. *BMC Public Health* **2019**, *19*, 7468. [CrossRef]

behavioral sciences

MDPI

Article

Effectiveness of the Life Enhancement and Advancement Program for Weight Management in Overweight and Obese Females

Raheleh Maddah Shourche [1], Mohsen Nematy [2], W. Miles Cox [3] and Javad S. Fadardi [1,3,4,*]

[1] Faculty of Education and Psychology, Ferdowsi University of Mashhad, Mashhad 9177948991, Iran; ra_ma889@mail.um.ac.ir
[2] Department of Nutrition, Mashhad Medical Sciences University, Mashhad 9177899191, Iran; nematym@mums.ac.ir
[3] School of Psychology and Sport Science, Bangor University, Bangor LL57 2DG, UK; m.cox@bangor.ac.uk
[4] School of Community and Global Health, Claremont Graduate University, Claremont, CA 91711, USA
* Correspondence: javad.fadardi@cgu.edu

Abstract: Background: Obesity has been shown to have many deleterious physical and psychological consequences. Objective: This study examined the effectiveness of adding the Life Enhancement and Advancement Program (LEAP) to a weight management program. Design: To evaluate the different components of a weight loss program, this study included four groups: (1) dieting, exercise, and LEAP; (2) dieting, exercise, and sham training; (3) dieting and exercise; and (4) exercise only. An assessment was administered at baseline, post-intervention, and a three-month follow-up. Participants: Forty female participants with a body mass index (BMI) $\geq$ 25 were recruited from a local sports center. They provided informed consent and were randomly assigned to one of the four groups. Measures: Participants' heights were recorded at baseline, and their weight, waist circumference (WC), and BMI were measured at each of the three assessments. Participants completed the Personal Concerns Inventory (PCI) to assess their adaptive motivation at all three assessments. Results: A MANCOVA indicated that participants who received LEAP along with dieting and exercise had a greater reduction in BMI and WC and improved more in adaptive motivation than the other groups. Conclusions: The results suggest that adding LEAP to a weight management program enhanced participants' ability to achieve and maintain weight loss. LEAP enabled participants to pursue and achieve their important goals successfully.

Keywords: exercise; dieting; adaptive motivational structure; personal concerns inventory

1. Introduction

Overweight and obesity are defined as excessive or abnormal fat accumulation, which may cause health-related problems and reduce a person's lifespan. Obesity represents an increasing global epidemic [1,2]. It is the fifth leading cause of death worldwide. Each year, at least 2.8 million adults die because of problems associated with being overweight or obese. Overweight and obesity result from complex interactions among various genetic, physiological, psychological, and environmental factors, which have many psychological and physical consequences [3]. It has also been shown that women are more likely than men to suffer from obesity [4,5].

Interventions for being overweight or obese require a combination of approaches to improve the person's diet and physical activity and address various psychological factors. Customary weight loss programs include dieting and exercise [6]. Successful weight loss programs should, however, also promote healthy lifestyles so that overweight individuals can lose weight safely and maintain weight loss. There is ample evidence that losing weight is difficult for most individuals. Collectively, these studies support the potential of motivational interventions, particularly when combined with exercise and dietary modifications, for promoting weight loss and improving psychological well-being. Jacob et al.'s [7] meta-analysis underscores the broader effectiveness of cognitive–behavioral interventions for weight management and psychological health. Weinreich et al.'s [8] research demonstrates the potential of integrating psychological components into lifestyle interventions, while Butryn et al.'s [9] review emphasizes the value of behavioral treatments in addressing obesity. These findings highlight the importance of incorporating motivational strategies to enhance the effectiveness of exercise-based weight loss programs and improve long-term outcomes for individuals seeking to manage their weight. Moreover, there is a strong likelihood that lost weight will be regained [10]; therefore, the effects of weight loss programs may not persist over the long term [11]. More than 50% of the people who start an exercise program seem to lose their motivation and usually drop out within three to six months [12,13]. Similarly, most dieters abandon their program after weight loss, causing them to regain the lost weight [14–16]

Overweight individuals cite various factors that hinder their weight management, including both psychological (e.g., negative emotions, depression, stress, lack of motivation, and inconsistency in adhering to their exercise routine) and situational (e.g., tempting food commercials and the easy availability of unhealthy food and drinks) barriers [17]. There are other reasons, such as a lack of information about effective methods for losing weight or the calorie content of various foods [18–20]. Therefore, a psychological intervention should be a major component of an effective weight management program [21]. It is very important, moreover, for treatment gains to be maintained over the long term. Considering the multi-dimensional nature of being overweight or obese [3] and the high failure rates of obesity treatments (dieting, exercise), multidisciplinary programs would be expected to improve the success of weight loss programs [22–25].

To better help overweight people, dieting, exercise, and psychoeducational interventions must be combined. An important addition to such an intervention would be a motivational intervention focusing on people's goal choices and how they pursue their goals. Different people have diverse ways of choosing and pursuing their goals. One factor that affects people's success or failure at achieving their goals is their motivational structure [26–29], which can be adaptive or maladaptive [30,31] and is assessed with the Personal Concerns Inventory (PCI) [32–34]. An adaptive motivation structure is characterized by expected happiness from goal attainments, choosing goals that have realistic chances of being achieved, and commitment to the pursuits. People's motivational structure predicts their ability to alleviate problematic behaviors [35]. Therefore, overweight people who can lose weight and maintain the loss in the long term would be expected to have a more adaptive motivational structure.

Cox and Klinger developed Systematic Motivational Counseling (SMC) to assess and change maladaptive motivational patterns into adaptive ones [36,37]. SMC aims to help people lead happier and more fulfilling lives by identifying better ways to resolve their current concerns. SMC has been used for individuals with alcohol and other substance abuse disorders, and evaluations have been consistently favorable [36–38].

Similarly, the Life Enhancement and Advancement Program (LEAP) was designed as a motivational restructuring technique for helping individuals to find emotional satisfaction without using chemical substances [35,39]. LEAP includes four major components: First, participants are shown how their lack of satisfaction in other areas of their lives can affect their motivation to engage in unhealthy behaviors. Second, they are asked to discuss the goals they named on the PCI, which they completed at the beginning of the program. Third, they complete a goal matrix to assess how each goal facilitates or hinders the achievement of other goals. In turn, they select valued and realistic goals that will not interfere with achieving other goals. Fourth, they specify actions to be taken that will help them reach their chosen goals, and then they develop a plan for achieving each action. In the case of people who use alcohol excessively, LEAP is effective in changing maladaptive behavioral patterns, thereby enabling people to moderate their drinking [35].

Overweight and obesity are multifaceted conditions that place people at risk of developing multiple health problems [40]. There is ample evidence that being overweight is not simply a problem of self-control or a lack of willpower; rather, it is linked to various comorbid conditions [21]. An effective weight loss program requires combining exercise and dietary intervention with a psychological intervention [22,25,41]. Thus, the major goal of the current study was to assess the effectiveness of adding LEAP to a weight management program for overweight and obese females. This goal was achieved by evaluating the different components of the program separately and in combination. Accordingly, there were four groups whose intervention consisted of (a) dieting, exercise, and LEAP; (b) dieting, exercise, and sham training; (c) dieting and exercise; or (d) exercise only. We hypothesized that the group that received the combined dieting, exercise, and LEAP training would show a greater reduction in BMI and WC and greater improvement in adaptive motivation than any of the other three groups.

2. Methods

2.1. Design

We adopted a 4 (groups: (a) exercise, dieting, and LEAP; (b) exercise, dieting, and sham training; (c) exercise and dieting; (d) exercise only) × 3 (time: pre vs. post vs. follow-up) design. The Ethics Committee of the Department of Psychology, Ferdowsi University of Mashhad, approved the study protocol and the data collection procedures on 24 June 2019 (IR.UM.REC.1398.043).

2.2. Sampling, Setting, and Procedure

The convenience sampling method was utilized due to limited resources and time; however, future studies should consider random sampling for greater generalizability. Participants were recruited from one of the local sports centers in the city of Mashhad, Iran. This study was completed within one year after the study adverts were distributed, upon which the follow-up assessment was completed. After announcing this study at a local sports center, potential participants interested in this study contacted the first author (R.M.S., a psychologist with an M.A. degree and sports coaching credentials). She then made the initial contact with the volunteers. To each participant, the goals and method of the research were carefully explained, and she was assured of the confidentiality and anonymity of the data and that participants would be provided with the study results. Each participant then provided written information consent before participation. Next, she conducted the initial eligibility screening using self-reported information and targeted questions. Each participant was randomly assigned to one of the four groups: Group 1: exercise, dieting, and LEAP; Group 2: exercise, dieting, and sham training; Group 3: exercise and dieting; Group 4: (d) exercise only. All four groups attended six of the 45-to-55 min sessions of an exercise program with three sessions per week, each supervised by the same coach and with a target heart rate of 40% to 60% of maximum heart rate. The three groups trained in dieting were referred to a physician nutrition specialist (PNS) in Mashhad, Iran to participate in a dieting program supervised by the second author (M.N.). The group that received the LEAP intervention [39] (see Table 1) had six 2 h sessions conducted by the first author. She was supervised by the fourth author (J.S.F., Full Professor of Psychology with extensive clinical experience). The group that received sham training attended six weekly 2 h classes in learning English.

The participants' height was recorded at baseline, and their weight, waist circumference, and BMI were measured at baseline, post-intervention, and three-month follow-up. All participants completed the PCI at all three assessments. Participants' demographic characteristics, such as age, education level, history of dieting failures, and weight changes during the past three months, were recorded at baseline.

Table 1. Steps in the Life Enhancement and Advancement Program (LEAP) used in this study.

Session	Goal	Topics	Task
1	Introduction to LEAP	Established rapport. Explained the rationale and method of LEAP; the importance of goals and their successful pursuit for emotional satisfaction; how LEAP can improve people's quality of life and happiness. Discussed the nature of people's goals and goal-seeking activities and adaptive and maladaptive motivational structures. Introduced the Personal Concerns Inventory (PCI) and how it should be completed.	Administered the PCI
2	How to score and interpret the PCI	Helped participants complete and score the PCI and interpret the results. Discussed adaptive vs. maladaptive motivation, different motivational profiles, and how to achieve adaptive motivation, e.g., by taking a more active role in goal pursuits, examining sources of control, and planning how to pursue specific goals, such as weight control. Identified new incentives and goals for participants to pursue and helped them to disengage from inappropriate goals.	Worked on enhancing participants motivation. Completed the Satisfaction with Life Scale (SWLS) and Dutch Eating Behavior Questionnaire (DEBQ).
3	Helped to improve participants' knowledge about and sense of control over their eating behavior	Discussed general and personal causes of overeating and consuming too many high-calorie foods. Compiled a list of false beliefs vs. facts about eating high-calorie foods. Identified situations that motivate the consumption of high-calorie foods (why, when, where, how, with whom).	Provided a list of personal advantages and disadvantages of weight control.
4	Promoted goal commitment by clarifying the link between lifestyle, weight control, and resulting gratification	Explained different eating styles (emotional, external, inhibited) and how they are related to food consumption. Discussed realistic weight control targets and the relationship between weight control and having a happier lifestyle. Explained three general methods for achieving a happier lifestyle. Identified individual sources of happiness and stress and ways to reduce daily life stresses. Explored alternative activities to the consumption of high-calorie foods.	Identified the sources of daily feelings related to overeating; focused on activities that can reduce food intake.
5	Reviewed participants' goals and ways to achieve appropriate goals	Reviewed participants' personal goals that might increase their happiness. Focused on both the quantity (using a goal matrix) and quality of participants' goals and the nature of people's satisfaction upon achieving their goals. Discussed how other goals impact the goal of losing weight; the importance of goal planning based on each participant's PCI results.	Completed a list of things that are important to me; completed a goal matrix and a sample goal ladder.
6	Learned how to design a goal ladder	Developed a plan for achieving the goal of losing weight. Introduced SMART (specific, measurable, attainable, relevant, time-bound) goals and the prioritization of goals. Designed a goal ladder and prioritized steps for losing weight (eating less, changing bad eating habits, reducing the size of meals, increasing the number of meals, increasing physical activity). Discussed specific steps for achieving these goals. Identified potential obstacles and ways to overcome them. Designed a target ladder for reading a specific weight loss goal. Obtained feedback from other participants.	Reviewed the sessions and drew conclusions. Identified dates for the follow-up assessments.

Note. At the beginning of each session, participants' homework from the previous session was checked and discussed.

The group that received sham training was instructed in basic reading skills according to the International English Language Testing System (IELTS). The course involved identifying the main components of texts and paragraphs, such as introduction, conclusions, and keywords. This group was also informed that the sessions were designed to assess their reading skills and that no oral or written exams would be required.

Following completion of this study, participants in the three groups that had not had the LEAP intervention could participate in LEAP sessions if they wished.

2.3. Participants

Only females were recruited because the incidence of obesity is higher among females than males [42]. Inclusion criteria were as follows: female gender, 18-to-45 years old (because BMI cannot be assessed in people younger than 18), BMI $\geq$ 25, willingness to lose 5-to-7% in body weight, ability to understand and communicate in Persian, having given written informed consent. Exclusion criteria were as follows: body weight greater than 150 kg, pregnant or planned pregnancy within three months, currently seeing a dietitian or participating in a weight loss program, weight loss or gain of more than 3% of body weight within the previous month, physical or psychological condition within the past year that would interfere with the ability to undergo the intervention (e.g., backache or knee pain, eating disorder, depression). Ultimately, no participants were excluded from this study.

2.4. Outcome Measures

Personal Concerns Inventory. The PCI measures participants' motivational structure [32,34]. Respondents are encouraged to consider their major concerns, wishes, and goals. They then rank each goal (from 0 to 10) on various scales that depict the important dimensions of the goal pursuit (e.g., appetitive or aversive valence, commitment, control, realistic plans) and their expectation from goal achievement (e.g., optimism, emotional satisfaction). In turn, PCI indices are derived from the ratings that indicate the degree to which the motivational structure is adaptive versus maladaptive. An adaptive motivational structure is characterized by having appetitive goals to which the person feels committed to pursue and from which they expect to derive emotional satisfaction and have realistic chances of success. The reliability and validity of the PCI have been confirmed [34,43]. Fadardi et al. developed a summary score that measures adaptive motivation and showed that the summary scores are highly correlated (r = 0.98) with PCI adaptive motivation derived from factor analysis or principal component analysis [44].

Body weight. While dressed in light clothing, each participant's body weight was measured to a precision of 100 g using a Seca digital scale.

Height. While standing barefoot against a wall, each participant's height was measured using a portable stadiometer (OTM; Tehran, Iran) to a precision of 0.10 cm.

Body mass index. Body mass index (BMI) is a commonly used index of height and weight. It is calculated by dividing weight (in kg) by height (m^2) [45].

2.5. Bias Control

This study followed a single-anonymized design because the first author responsible for data collection was aware of participants' group allocation; therefore, the outcomes should be interpreted cautiously. We took a few steps to control other potential sources of bias. The reason for the absence of a diet-only group is that all participants were recruited from a sports center whose aim was to lose weight through exercise. It could cause resistance to participation if they were invited to follow a diet-only routine, which could bias the study outcomes. Dietary compliance was monitored using a multifaceted approach based on PNS protocol, including self-reported dietary logs, validated food frequency questionnaires, and regular consultations. These measures allowed for ongoing assessment of adherence to the prescribed dietary guidelines, providing feedback and support to participants throughout the intervention period. Although non-compliance was an exclusion criterion, all participants maintained satisfactory adherence levels. The goal of having sham training was to control for the effects of attention and social interaction. A flow diagram of this study is shown in Figure 1. While initial weight loss may be evident within two weeks, a three-month follow-up is essential to assess the long-term sustainability of weight loss results and their impact on overall lifestyle behaviors. A three-month follow-up aligns with established research practices, such as the Diabetes Prevention Program (DPP), demonstrating the importance of sustained weight loss at three months for long-term diabetes prevention [46]. Additionally, research in obesity highlights that weight regain is common within the first few months after initial weight loss, making the 3-month mark a critical point for evaluating the efficacy of interventions and identifying factors that predict long-term success [9].

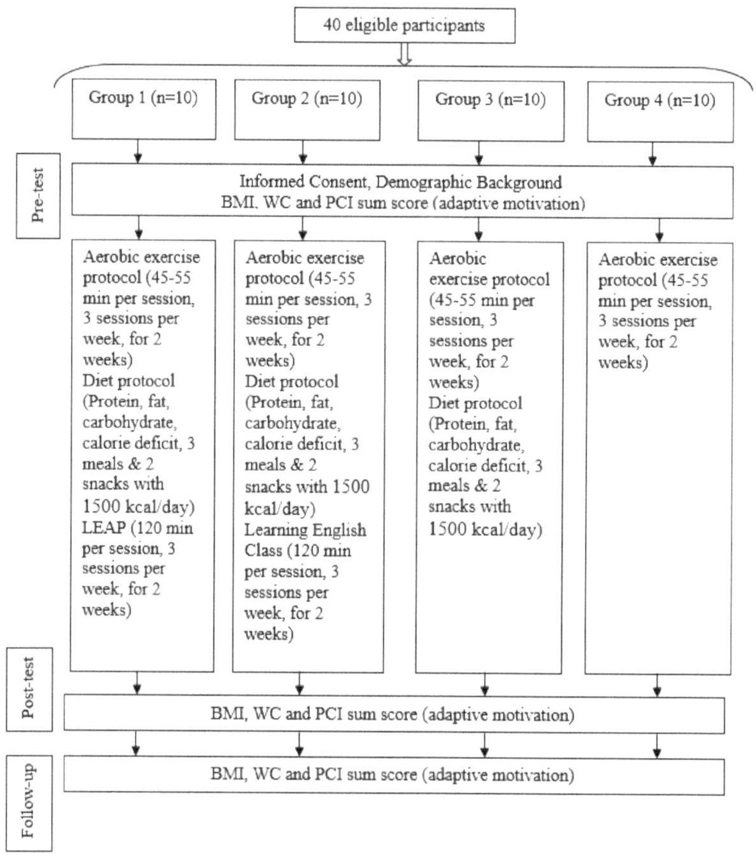

Figure 1. Flow diagram of this study's procedure. Note. Group 1: exercise, dieting, LEAP; Group 2: exercise, dieting, English class; Group 3: exercise, dieting; Group 4: exercise. BMI: body mass index; WC: waist circumference; PCI: Personal Concerns Inventory; posttest assessment was conducted after a two-week intervention; follow-up assessment was conducted three months post-intervention.

2.6. Sample Size

Although convenience sampling was used due to practical constraints, estimating the required sample size through a power analysis is recommended to ensure sufficient statistical power. Using G*Power 3.0.3 software and considering effect size estimates ($f^2 = 0.28$) from similar studies [47–49], with $\alpha = 0.05$, power = 0.80, number of groups = 4, number of predictors = 6 (four groups and two covariates), and number of response variables = 2, a minimum sample size of 37 was calculated. To account for potential attrition, we aimed to recruit 40 obese or overweight females (BMI $\geq$ 25 kg/m^2) from a pool of 60 volunteers at a local sports center.

2.7. Analysis

Analyses included descriptive statistics (e.g., means and standard deviations) and inferential statistics. MANCOVA and Bonferroni post-hoc and paired t-tests were used to compare the four groups on the various dependent variables. All data were checked for normality using Q-Q plots [50]. A p-value of ≤ 0.05 was set for all analyses.

3. Results

Participants' demographic characteristics, including their education, age, body weight, BMI, WC, history of dieting failures, and weight changes during the previous six months are shown separately for the four groups in Table 2.

Table 2. Participants' demographic characteristics.

	Group							
	Group 1 (n = 10)		Group 2 (n = 10)		Group 3 (n = 10)		Group 4 (n = 10)	
	%		%		%		%	
Education								
<High school	18.2%		9.1%		45.5%		27.3%	
High school	27.3%		27.3%		0.00%		0.00%	
Associate's degree	27.3%		0.00%		0.00%		36.4%	
Bachelor's degree	27.3%		54.5%		45.5%		18.2%	
Master's degree	0.00%		0.00%		0.00%		9.1%	
	M	sd	M	sd	M	sd	M	sd
Age	30.00	7.94	27.80	9.72	32.30	9.09	29.90	7.62
Weight (kg.)	81.27	11.59	72.20	6.86	77.10	12.11	76.7	9.49
Height (cm.)	1.64	7.00	1.57	7.10	1.61	6.15	1.59	5.40
BMI	29.68	3.31	29.30	3.06	29.28	3.07	30.28	3.30
WC (cm.)	101.95	4.07	102.56	4.35	100.89	5.15	101.62	4.20
No. of dieting failures	2.90	2.94	2.50	2.32	1.80	2.04	3.10	2.33
Weight changes during last 6 months (kg.)	−0.27	2.28	−0.10	3.21	−0.20	3.58	1.00	5.33

Note. Group 1: exercise, dieting, LEAP; Group 2: exercise, dieting, English class; Group 3: exercise, dieting; Group 4: exercise.

The means and standard deviations of participants' BMI, WC, and PCI adaptive motivation summary scores at baseline, post-intervention, and three-month follow-up are shown in Table 3. Three separate MANCOVAs were conducted to test the hypothesis that the group receiving exercise, dieting, and LEAP would show a greater reduction in BMI and WC and a greater improvement in PCI adaptive motivation than any of the other three groups. In each MANCOVA, BMI, WC, or PCI adaptive motivation for the post-intervention and the three-month follow-up was entered as the dependent variable, with as the predictor variable. The covariates were participants' age and education and their baseline BMI, WC, and PCI adaptive motivation scores.

As Table 4 shows, the results of the first MANCOVA showed a significant overall effect for Group 1 on participants' BMI with a large effect size, $d = 0.95$ (eta squared effect sizes were converted to Cohen's d, whose values are 0.20, 0.50, and 0.80, for small, medium, and large effects, respectively). Group 1 was not significant at post-intervention, but it was significant at the three-month follow-up. Bonferroni tests indicated that Group 1 (exercise, dieting, and LEAP) was significantly lower on BMI than Group 2 ($p = 0.005$), Group 3 ($p < 0.001$), and Group 4 ($p < 0.001$) at the follow-up; no other group differences were found.

Table 3. Means and standard deviations of participants' BMI, WC, PCI adaptive motivation scores.

		BMI		WC		PCI	
		M	sd	M	sd	M	sd
Group 1	Pretest	29.68	3.31	101.95	4.07	54.71	2.37
	Posttest	28.52	3.53	97.13	5.03	62.30	1.83
	Follow-up	26.50	2.34	88.95	3.97	62.63	1.88
Group 2	Pretest	29.30	3.06	102.56	4.35	55.72	2.07
	Posttest	28.001	2.58	101.88	4.77	55.26	2.33
	Follow-up	27.99	2.52	101.19	4.83	54.76	2.401
Group 3	Pretest	28.93	3.31	100.89	5.15	54.83	2.63
	Posttest	28.00	3.05	100.00	5.35	55.007	2.11
	Follow-up	28.68	3.09	99.16	5.19	54.66	2.17
Group 4	Pretest	29.01	3.62	101.62	4.20	54.89	2.82
	Posttest	29.10	3.37	100.56	3.81	54.34	2.11
	Follow-up	29.08	3.52	100.90	6.84	54.26	2.17

Note. Group 1: exercise, dieting, LEAP; Group 2: exercise, dieting, English class; Group 3: exercise, dieting; Group 4: exercise.

Table 4. MANCOVA results for the effects of group on BMI, WC, and PCI adaptive motivation.

Outcome Variable	Overall Effect $F(6, 56)$ [d]	Post-Intervention $F(3, 36)$ [d]	Follow-Up $F(3, 36)$ [d]	Post-Hoc Comparisons (Bonferroni)
BMI	7.05 ** [0.95]	0.72 [0.31]	17.79 ** [1.52]	Group 1 < Group 2, 3, 4
Waist circumference (WC)	45.40 ** [2.43]	14.72 ** [1.38]	31.20 ** [2.01]	Group 1 < Group 2, 3, 4
PCI adaptive motivation	21.57 * [1.67]	3.69 * [0.69]	17.79 ** [1.52]	Group 1 > Group 2, 3, 4

Note. Group 1: exercise, dieting, LEAP; Group 2: exercise, dieting, English class; Group 3: exercise, dieting; Group 4: exercise; d = Cohen's d, calculated from eta squared effect sizes. p-values = ** $p < 0.01$; * $p < 0.05$.

The results of the second MANCOVA showed a significant overall effect for Group 1 on participants' WC with a large effect size, $d = 2.43$. The Group 1 effect was significant at both post-intervention and the three-month follow-up. A Bonferroni test indicated that Group 1 had significantly lower WC measurements than Group 2 ($p < 0.001$), Group 3 ($p < 0.001$), and Group 4 ($p < 0.001$) at the follow-up; no other group differences were found.

Finally, the third MANCOVA showed a significant overall effect for Group 1 on participants' PCI adaptive motivation scores with a large effect size, $d = 1.67$. There was also a significant effect for Group 1 at both post-intervention and the three-month follow-up. A Bonferroni test indicated that the adaptive motivation of Group 1 had significantly improved at the follow-up compared to Group 2 ($p < 0.001$), Group 3 ($p = 0.01$), and Group 4 ($p < 0.001$); nonetheless, the difference between other groups was not significant.

Next, paired t-tests were calculated to identify the source of Group 1 X Time interactions on the PCI indices. The results showed improvements in the PCI indices in Group 1 (exercise, dieting, and LEAP), including moral rightness of goal pursuits, plans for goal pursuits, commitment to goal pursuits, and optimism about goal achievements (see Table 5). Participants' PCI indices in the other three groups did not change significantly from baseline to the other two assessment points. These results, therefore, supported this study's hypotheses.

At follow-up, participants in Group 1 (exercise, dieting, and LEAP) reported continuing to pursue their new healthy lifestyle, which included exercising and dieting. This further indicates the success of the intervention that Group 1 received.

Table 5. Results of paired t-tests of PCI scores at baseline, post-intervention, and follow-up in Group 1.

PCI Index	Time	p	$t_{(9)}$
Moral rightness	T_1–T_2	0.01	3.02
	T_1–T_3	0.01	3.11
Plans for goal pursuits	T_1–T_2	0.04	2.22
	T_1–T_3	0.04	2.20
Commitment to goal pursuits	T_1–T_2	0.001	4.45
	T_1–T_3	0.001	4.52
Optimism about goal achievements	T_1–T_2	0.04	2.31
	T_1–T_3	0.02	2.54

Notes. There was no significant change in the other PCI indices across the assessment points, including T_2–T_3. Group 1: exercise, dieting, and LEAP.

4. Discussion

This study aimed to assess the effectiveness of LEAP as an add-on intervention to exercise and dieting in a weight management program for overweight and obese females. It is important to acknowledge that this study utilized a convenience sampling method, which may limit the generalizability of the findings to the broader population. While convenience sampling offers practical advantages in feasibility and recruitment, it can introduce potential bias due to the non-random selection of participants. Therefore, caution should be exercised when extrapolating the results beyond the specific characteristics and context of the sampled population. The results supported the hypothesis that *Group 1* (exercise, dieting, and LEAP) would be more successful in helping participants to lose weight than would *Group 2* (exercise, dieting, and sham training to control for the attention that Group 1 received), *Group 3* (exercise and dieting), or *Group 4* (exercise only). Unlike any of the other three groups, the intervention in Group 1 enabled participants to reduce their BMI and WC to maintain the reductions for at least three months.

Previous studies have shown that interventions for weight management that include both exercise and dieting are more effective than only one of these components [51,52], and the inclusion of a psychological intervention can improve the results even further [3,53]. The results of the present study are also consistent with previous studies that have demonstrated the effectiveness of both *Systematic Motivational Counseling* and the related intervention *Life Enhancement and Advancement Program (LEAP)* for improving treatment outcomes [35,37,38].

In the current study, Group 1 (exercise, dieting, and LEAP) showed other positive outcomes that can be attributed to the effects of LEAP on improving participants' adaptive motivation. For example, Group 1 showed significant improvements from baseline to post-treatment and from baseline to the follow-up in participants' (a) willingness to seek information that would facilitate their goal attainments, (b) commitment to achieving their goals, (c) optimism about reaching their goals, and (d) expected chances of success in reaching their goals. Participants in Group 1 were instructed to take an appetitive approach to pursuing their goals, thereby focusing on positive things they would like to achieve instead of negative things they wanted to avoid or get rid of. This attitude, in turn, seemed to strengthen their commitment to goal pursuits [54]. The participants also appeared more likely to seek information to help them achieve their goals than participants in the other three groups. They seemed to become more adept at planning and scheduling their activities that would facilitate their goal attainments and more adept at asking for help when they needed it. As a result, they felt more in control, more committed to their goal pursuits, and more optimistic about reaching their goals. Because participants in Group 1 were instructed to adopt an adaptive motivational approach in their weight loss program, they seemed to derive greater satisfaction from their goal achievements than participants in the other three groups. Finally, participants in Group 1 seemed to believe in the importance of their own role in achieving their weight loss goals. These differences among the participants in the four intervention groups were confirmed by improvements only in Group 1's motivational structure, which became more adaptive during this study.

An adaptive motivational structure is characterized by having appetitive goals that the person wants to achieve, knowing the steps to take to reach one's goals, commitment to and a sense of control over goal pursuits, expectations of success in reaching one's goals, and expected emotional satisfaction upon reaching one's goals [32]. From the current study, we conclude that participants in Group 1 (exercise, dieting, and LEAP) achieved more adaptive motivation from having participated in LEAP. It is designed to replace participants' maladaptive motivational structure with a more adaptive one. The LEAP component of the intervention in Group 1 focused largely on participants' motivational structure, rather than solely on exercise or dieting. Using LEAP, we initially assessed the characteristics of the goals that the participants named (e.g., the degree to which they were appetitive or aversive) and then tried to shift them from aversive to appetitive goals. We did so by using strategies such as goals prioritization, enhancing commitment to realistic and achievable goals, finding solutions to conflicts among different goals, and identifying realistic steps to goal attainment.

The overarching goal of LEAP was to promote participants' happiness and satisfaction by maximizing their success in reaching attractive and achievable goals. Research has shown that life satisfaction is achieved by having positive outcomes in various life domains [55]. Life satisfaction derived from achieving small goals is key to motivating people to modify their life circumstances by working to achieve their personal goals. By the end of the LEAP sessions, the participants seemed to have more realistic beliefs about weight loss, and their motivation for weight loss appeared to be more internalized, whereby they sought to lose weight to promote their long-term health.

The current study utilized novel techniques to evaluate the cumulative effects of weight loss components (LEAP, dieting, and exercise) for overweight and obese females. The minimum and maximum weight loss was achieved, respectively, in Group 4 (exercise only) and in Group 1 (exercise, dieting, and LEAP), thereby confirming the greater effectiveness of the intervention that Group 1 received. We used the sham training in Group 2 (exercise, dieting, English class) to control for the additional attention that Group 1 (exercise, dieting, LEAP) received. As noted, the improvements in Group 1 can be attributed to the specific effects of LEAP rather than the supportive–expressive effects of being in the group. Moreover, the LEAP might fortify the effects of dieting and exercise by addressing motivational components, especially those significantly improved post-training (i.e., moral rightness, plans for goal pursuits, commitment to goal pursuits, and optimism about goal achievements).

While BMI is a widely used and convenient measure, it does not differentiate between fat and lean mass, potentially leading to misclassification in individuals with high muscle mass [45]. The lack of significant group differences between the exercise-only group and the exercise plus diet groups in this study, as indicated by BMI and WC, might be attributed to this limitation of BMI. It is plausible that participants in the exercise-only group experienced increased muscle mass that offset any potential fat loss, resulting in minimal change in BMI despite improvements in body composition.

Incorporating measures such as waist-to-hip ratio (WHR) and body fat percentage would provide a more comprehensive assessment of body composition and adiposity distribution, offering valuable insights into the health risks associated with obesity [42]. These measures could potentially reveal differences between groups not captured by BMI alone. For example, the exercise-only group might show decreased body fat percentage or a more favorable WHR than the exercise plus diet groups, even if their BMI remained relatively stable.

This study primarily focused on BMI and WC due to their established associations with cardiometabolic risk factors and their widespread use in clinical practice [3]. However, we recognize the value of including additional measures like WHR and body fat percentage in future research to enhance the understanding of the impact of lifestyle interventions on body composition and overall health. Notwithstanding the strengths of the present study, there were also some limitations. First, we selected participants from clients enrolling with a sports center in Mashhad, and the sampling method might limit the generalizability of the results. Second, the follow-up assessment (three months) was relatively short. Despite the favorable outcomes among participants in Group 1 (exercise, dieting, LEAP), caution should be exercised in drawing definitive conclusions from the results. Accordingly, larger studies with a more diverse sample (e.g., male and female participants) and a longer follow-up period (e.g., 12 months) are warranted. Finally, future research would benefit from comparing LEAP with other weight management interventions and psychological approaches to augment the effects of exercise and diet in achieving weight loss.

5. Conclusions

Although dieting and exercise can have short-term effects on weight loss, it is essential to focus on broader motivational issues to help participants achieve long-term effects. The present study confirmed that motivational training in addition to dieting and exercise improved female participants' ability to lose weight by enhancing their adaptive motivation. The results of this study point to the need for additional research on the use of dieting, exercise, and LEAP in weight management for overweight and obese females.

Author Contributions: R.M.S. contributed to the conceptualization, methodology, data collection, analysis, and writing the original draft of the manuscript. M.N. assisted with data collection and editing of the manuscript. W.M.C. edited the manuscript. J.S.F. contributed to conceptualization, methodology, analysis, student supervision, writing the original draft, and editing of the manuscript. All authors have read and agreed to the published version of the manuscript.

Funding: This study was supported by a small grant (46475) to the first and last authors from the Research Office of Ferdowsi University of Mashhad.

Institutional Review Board Statement: The study was conducted in accordance with the Declaration of Helsinki, and approved by the Ethics Committee of Department of Psychology, Ferdowsi University of Mashhad (protocol code IR.UM.REC.1398.043 and date of 24 June 2019).

Informed Consent Statement: All participants provided written informed consent prior to their participation in this study.

Data Availability Statement: Data are contained within the article. Additional data are unavailable due to privacy and ethical restrictions.

Acknowledgments: The authors would like to thank all participants who participated in this study.

Conflicts of Interest: The authors declare no conflicts of interest.

References

1. Apovian, C.M. The obesity epidemic—Understanding the disease and the treatment. *N. Engl. J. Med.* **2016**, *374*, 177–179. [CrossRef]
2. Castillo, F.; González, D.R.; Moore-Carrasco, R. Effects of Phaseolus vulgaris extract on lipolytic activity and differentiation of 3T3-L1 preadipocytes into mature adipocytes: A strategy to prevent obesity. *J. Nutr. Metab.* **2019**, *2019*, 5093654. [CrossRef] [PubMed]
3. Wharton, S.; Lau, D.C.; Vallis, M.; Sharma, A.M.; Biertho, L.; Campbell-Scherer, D.; Adamo, K.; Alberga, A.; Bell, R.; Boulé, N. Obesity in adults: A clinical practice guideline. *Can. Med. Assoc. J.* **2020**, *192*, E875–E891. [CrossRef]
4. World Health Organization. Obesity and Overweight. Available online: https://www.who.int/news-room/fact-sheets/detail/obesity-and-overweight (accessed on 10 July 2024).
5. Flegal, K.M.; Carroll, M.D.; Kit, B.K.; Ogden, C.L. Prevalence of obesity and trends in the distribution of body mass index among USs adults, 1999–2010. *JAMA* **2012**, *307*, 491–497. [CrossRef]
6. Obert, J.; Pearlman, M.; Obert, L.; Chapin, S. Popular weight loss strategies: A review of four weight loss techniques. *Curr. Gastroenterol. Rep.* **2017**, *19*, 61. [CrossRef]
7. Jacob, A.; Moullec, G.; Lavoie, K.L.; Laurin, C.; Cowan, T.; Tisshaw, C.; Kazazian, C.; Raddatz, C.; Bacon, S.L. Impact of cognitive-behavioral interventions on weight loss and psychological outcomes: A meta-analysis. *Health Psychol.* **2018**, *37*, 417–432. [CrossRef]

8. Weinreich, T.; Filz, H.P.; Gresser, U.; Richartz, B.M. Effectiveness of A Four-Week Diet Regimen, Exercise and Psychological Intervention for Weight Loss. *J. Clin. Diagn. Res.* **2017**, *11*, LC20–LC24. [CrossRef]
9. Butryn, M.L.; Webb, V.; Wadden, T.A. Behavioral treatment of obesity. *Psychiatr. Clin.* **2011**, *34*, 841–859. [CrossRef] [PubMed]
10. Hall, K.D.; Kahan, S. Maintenance of lost weight and long-term management of obesity. *Med. Clin.* **2018**, *102*, 183–197. [CrossRef] [PubMed]
11. Tronieri, J.S.; Wadden, T.A.; Chao, A.M.; Tsai, A.G. Primary care interventions for obesity: Review of the evidence. *Curr. Obes. Rep.* **2019**, *8*, 128–136. [CrossRef]
12. Elmer, P.J.; Obarzanek, E.; Vollmer, W.M.; Simons-Morton, D.; Stevens, V.J.; Young, D.R.; Lin, P.-H.; Champagne, C.; Harsha, D.W.; Svetkey, L.P. Effects of comprehensive lifestyle modification on diet, weight, physical fitness, and blood pressure control: 18-month results of a randomized trial. *Ann. Int. Med.* **2006**, *144*, 485–495. [CrossRef]
13. Linke, S.E.; Gallo, L.C.; Norman, G.J. Attrition and adherence rates of sustained vs. intermittent exercise interventions. *Ann. Behav. Med.* **2011**, *42*, 197–209. [CrossRef]
14. Papies, E.K.; Stroebe, W.; Aarts, H. Understanding dieting: A social cognitive analysis of hedonic processes in self-regulation. *Eur. Rev. Soc. Psychol.* **2008**, *19*, 339–383. [CrossRef]
15. Sares-Jäske, L.; Knekt, P.; Männistö, S.; Lindfors, O.; Heliövaara, M. Self-report dieting and long-term changes in body mass index and waist circumference. *Obes. Sci. Pract.* **2019**, *5*, 291–303. [CrossRef]
16. Werrij, M.Q.; Jansen, A.; Mulkens, S.; Elgersma, H.J.; Ament, A.J.; Hospers, H.J. Adding cognitive therapy to dietetic treatment is associated with less relapse in obesity. *J. Psychosom. Res.* **2009**, *67*, 315–324. [CrossRef] [PubMed]
17. Beck, A.L.; Iturralde, E.; Haya-Fisher, J.; Kim, S.; Keeton, V.; Fernandez, A. Barriers and facilitators to healthy eating among low-income Latino adolescents. *Appetite* **2019**, *138*, 215–222. [CrossRef]
18. Burke, L.E.; Steenkiste, A.; Music, E.; Styn, M.A. A descriptive study of past experiences with weight-loss treatment. *J. Am. Diet. Assoc.* **2008**, *108*, 640–647. [CrossRef] [PubMed]
19. Elfhag, K.; Morey, L.C. Personality traits and eating behavior in the obese: Poor self-control in emotional and external eating but personality assets in restrained eating. *Eat. Behav.* **2008**, *9*, 285–293. [CrossRef]
20. Govender, R.; Al-Shamsi, S.; Regmi, D. Weight bias and eating behaviours of persons with overweight and obesity attending a general medical practice in Durban, South Africa. *S. Afr. Fam. Pract.* **2019**, *61*, 85–90. [CrossRef]
21. Bean, M.K.; Stewart, K.; Olbrisch, M.E. Obesity in America: Implications for clinical and health psychologists. *J. Clin. Psychol. Med. Settings* **2008**, *15*, 214–224. [CrossRef]
22. Branco, B.H.M.; Valladares, D.; De Oliveira, F.M.; Carvalho, I.Z.; Marques, D.C.; Coelho, A.A.; De Oliveira, L.P.; Bertolini, S.M.M.G. Effects of the order of physical exercises on body composition, physical fitness, and cardiometabolic risk in adolescents participating in an interdisciplinary program focusing on the treatment of obesity. *Front. Physiol.* **2019**, *10*, 1013. [CrossRef]
23. Dicker, D.; Alfadda, A.A.; Coutinho, W.; Cuevas, A.; Halford, J.C.; Hughes, C.A.; Iwabu, M.; Kang, J.-H.; Nawar, R.; Reynoso, R. Patient motivation to lose weight: Importance of healthcare professional support, goals and self-efficacy. *Eur. J. Intern. Med.* **2021**, *91*, 10–16. [CrossRef]
24. Svetkey, L.P.; Stevens, V.J.; Brantley, P.J.; Appel, L.J.; Hollis, J.F.; Loria, C.M.; Vollmer, W.M.; Gullion, C.M.; Funk, K.; Smith, P. Comparison of strategies for sustaining weight loss: The weight loss maintenance randomized controlled trial. *JAMA* **2008**, *299*, 1139–1148. [CrossRef]
25. Zolotarjova, J.; Ten Velde, G.; Vreugdenhil, A. Effects of multidisciplinary interventions on weight loss and health outcomes in children and adolescents with morbid obesity. *Obes. Rev.* **2018**, *19*, 931–946. [CrossRef]
26. Cox, W.M.; Klinger, E. *Why People Drink; How People Change: A Guide to Alcohol and People's Motivation for Drinking It*; Springer: Berlin/Heidelberg, Germany, 2022.
27. Cox, W.M.; Klinger, E.; Fadardi, J.S. Nonconscious motivational influences on cognitive processes in addictive behaviors. In *Addiction and Choice: Rethinking the Relationship*; Oxford University Press: Oxford, UK, 2017.
28. Klinger, E. The goal theory of current concerns and its applications at year 45. In *Why People Do the Things They Do: Building on Julius Kuhl's Contributions to the Psychology of Motivation and Volition*; Hogrefe: Göttingen, Germany, 2018.
29. Klinger, E.; Cox, W.M. Motivation and the goal theory of current concerns. In *Handbook of Motivational Counseling: Goal-Based Approaches to Assessment and Intervention with Addiction and Other Problems*; Wiley Online Library: Hoboken, NJ, USA, 2011; pp. 1–47.
30. Cox, W.M.; Klinger, E. Motivational structure: Relationships with substance use and processes of change. *Addict. Behav.* **2002**, *27*, 925–940. [CrossRef] [PubMed]
31. Cox, W.M.; Schippers, G.M.; Klinger, E.; Skutle, A.; Stuchlíková, I.; Man, F.; King, A.L.; Inderhaug, R. Motivational structure and alcohol use of university students across four nations. *J. Stud. Alcohol* **2002**, *63*, 280–285. [CrossRef] [PubMed]
32. Cox, W.M.; Klinger, E. Measuring motivation: The motivational structure questionnaire and personal concerns inventory and their variants. In *Handbook of Motivational Counseling: Goal-Based Approaches to Assessment and Intervention with Addiction and Other Problems*; Wiley Online Library: Hoboken, NJ, USA, 2011; pp. 159–204.
33. Cox, W.M.; Klinger, E. Assessing current concerns and goals idiographically: A review of the Motivational Structure Questionnaire family of instruments. *J. Clin. Psychol.* **2023**, *79*, 667–682. [CrossRef]
34. Klinger, E.; Cox, W.M. The motivational structure questionnaire, personal concerns inventory, and their variants: Psychometric properties. In *Handbook of Motivational Counseling*; Wiley Online Library: Hoboken, NJ, USA, 2011; pp. 205–232.

35. Cox, W.M.; Fadardi, J.S.; Hosier, S.G.; Pothos, E.M. Differential effects and temporal course of attentional and motivational training on excessive drinking. *Exp. Clin. Psychopharmacol.* **2015**, *23*, 445. [CrossRef]
36. Cox, W.M.; Klinger, E. Systematic motivational counseling: The Motivational Structure Questionnaire in action. In *Handbook of Motivational Counseling: Concepts, Approaches, and Assessment*; Wiley Online Library: Hoboken, NJ, USA, 2004; pp. 217–237.
37. Cox, W.M.; Klinger, E. Systematic motivational counseling: From motivational assessment to motivational change. In *Handbook of Motivational Counseling: Goal-Based Approaches to Assessment and Intervention with Addiction and Other Problems*; Wiley Blackwell: Hoboken, NJ, USA, 2011.
38. Cox, W.M.; Klinger, E. A psychological-systems goal theory model of alcohol consumption and treatment. In *The Handbook of Alcohol Use*; Elsevier: Amsterdam, The Netherlands, 2021; pp. 237–260.
39. Fadardi, J.; Cox, W.; Klinger, E. *Life Enrichment and Advancement Program (LEAP): A Self-Help Manual for Reducing Your Need to Drink*; Bangor University: Bangor, UK, 2006; unpublished manual.
40. Robinson, E.; Hunger, J.; Daly, M. Perceived weight status and risk of weight gain across life in US and UK adults. *Int. J. Obes.* **2015**, *39*, 1721–1726. [CrossRef]
41. Lang, A.; Froelicher, E.S. Management of overweight and obesity in adults: Behavioral intervention for long-term weight loss and maintenance. *Eur. J. Cardiovasc. Nurs.* **2006**, *5*, 102–114. [CrossRef]
42. Tauqeer, Z.; Gomez, G.; Stanford, F.C. Obesity in women: Insights for the clinician. *J. Women's Health* **2018**, *27*, 444–457. [CrossRef] [PubMed]
43. Aghamohammadian Sharbaf, H.; Salehi Fadardi, J.; Cox, W. Validation of The Persian-Personal-Concerns Inventory. In Proceedings of the 12th Iranian of the Researchers Conference in Europe (IRCE), Manchester, UK, 3–4 July 2004.
44. Salehi, F.J.; Maddah, S.R.; Nemati, M. A comparison of motivational structure and eating behaviors between overweight and obese and normal weight women. *J. Fundam. Ment. Health* **2011**, *13*, 170–181.
45. Ghesmaty Sangachin, M.; Cavuoto, L.A.; Wang, Y. Use of various obesity measurement and classification methods in occupational safety and health research: A systematic review of the literature. *BMC Obes.* **2018**, *5*, 28. [CrossRef]
46. Knowler, W.C.; Barrett-Connor, E.; Fowler, S.E.; Hamman, R.F.; Lachin, J.M.; Walker, E.A.; Nathan, D.M.; Diabetes Prevention Program Research, G. Reduction in the incidence of type 2 diabetes with lifestyle intervention or metformin. *N. Engl. J. Med.* **2002**, *346*, 393–403. [CrossRef]
47. Abdolhosseini, F. The Effectiveness of Life Enhancement and Advancement Program and Rational Emotive Behavior Therapy on the Improvement of Addiction Treatment Indexes in Misuser Addicted Females. Master's Thesis, Ferdowsi University of Mashhad, Mashhad, Iran, 2010.
48. Faul, F.; Erdfelder, E.; Lang, A.-G.; Buchner, A. G* Power 3: A flexible statistical power analysis program for the social, behavioral, and biomedical sciences. *Behav. Res. Methods* **2007**, *39*, 175–191. [CrossRef]
49. Harlow, L.L. *The Essence of Multivariate Thinking: Basic Themes and Methods*; Routledge: Oxfordshire, UK, 2014.
50. Parrone, D.; Ghergo, S.; Preziosi, E. A multi-method approach for the assessment of natural background levels in groundwater. *Sci. Total Environ.* **2019**, *659*, 884–894. [CrossRef]
51. Morrow, A.; Walker, K.; Calder-MacPhee, N.; Ozakinci, G. The active ingredients of physical activity and/or dietary workplace-based interventions to achieve weight loss in overweight and obese healthcare staff: A systematic review. *J. Behav. Med.* **2022**, *45*, 331–349. [CrossRef]
52. Xie, C.; Wang, X.; Zhou, C.; Xu, C.; Chang, Y.-K. Exercise and dietary program-induced weight reduction is associated with cognitive function among obese adolescents: A longitudinal study. *PeerJ* **2017**, *5*, e3286. [CrossRef]
53. Carels, R.A.; Darby, L.; Cacciapaglia, H.M.; Konrad, K.; Coit, C.; Harper, J.; Kaplar, M.E.; Young, K.; Baylen, C.A.; Versland, A. Using motivational interviewing as a supplement to obesity treatment: A stepped-care approach. *Health Psychol.* **2007**, *26*, 369. [CrossRef]
54. Vakharia, J.D.; Thaweethai, T.; Licht, P.; Wexler, D.J.; Delahanty, L.M. Psychological and Behavioral Predictors of Weight Loss in the Reach Ahead for Lifestyle and Health-Diabetes Lifestyle Intervention Cohort. *J. Acad. Nutr. Diet.* **2023**, *123*, 1033–1043. e1031. [CrossRef]
55. Luhmann, M.; Hennecke, M. The motivational consequences of life satisfaction. *Motiv. Sci.* **2017**, *3*, 51. [CrossRef]

behavioral sciences

MDPI

Article

Factors Influencing Intentions of People with Hearing Impairments to Use Augmented Reality Glasses as Hearing Aids

Liyuan Deng [1], Jiangjie Chen [2] and Dongning Li [1,*]

[1] School of Design, Jiangnan University, Wuxi 214122, China; 7210306013@stu.jiangnan.edu.cn
[2] College of Fine Arts, Huaqiao University, Quanzhou 362021, China; chenjiangjie@hqu.edu.cn
* Correspondence: lidongning@jiangnan.edu.cn

Abstract: The advent and progression of AR (augmented reality) technology, coupled with the emergence of AR hearing aid glasses, offer a novel opportunity for people with hearing impairments (PHI). This study aims to explore the intention of this population to employ AR hearing aid glasses as their choice of hearing aid device and the specific factors influencing their preference. This study utilized the partial least squares SEM (PLS-SEM) analytical method to create structural equation model for intentions of PHI to use AR glasses as hearing aids. Data were gathered from on-site experiences across multiple locations; a total of 189 valid questionnaires from individuals with varying degrees of hearing disabilities were used for statistical analysis. According to the data analysis results, we discovered that functionality quality, perceived interaction speed, and perceived usability significantly influence communication effectiveness. Further, communication effectiveness positively influences confidence and societal perception, and the latter has a positive impact on information. Both of these factors positively influence behavioral intention. Based on these findings, this study offers design recommendations for AR hearing aid glasses to cater to the specific needs of PHI, aiming to enhance their quality of life. Furthermore, this study provides pivotal insights for the prospective growth of this emerging industry.

Keywords: hearing impairments; AR technology; AR hearing aid glasses; use intentions

1. Introduction

Hearing is one of the most important yet fragile functions in a person's life, susceptible to various factors that can lead to hearing loss at any time for anyone [1–3]. As a result, hearing impairment has become the third most common cause of disability [4,5]. According to the World Hearing Report published by the World Health Organization, by 2021, over 5% of the global population suffered from hearing loss, and by 2050, it is projected that nearly 2.5 billion individuals will have different degree of hearing loss [6]. Hence, hearing impairment has gravely threatened global public health [7–9].

Unlike individuals who are deaf, people with hearing impairments (PHI), despite facing various difficulties due to hearing loss [10,11], can address these issues with the help of hearing aid products [12]. However, the adoption rate of assistive devices in the real-world context remains low among PHI [13,14]. Among them, hearing aids are the primary choice for hearing impairment rehabilitation [15–17], yet their adoption rate is less than 20% [18]. One of the main reasons for this phenomenon is the stigma associated with them [19,20]. Because hearing impairment is an invisible disability, the use of such assistive devices may inadvertently highlight it, leading to the bearer being labeled or perceived as disabled or an outsider in society [21–26]

Consequently, many individuals, before seeking medical intervention and receiving a diagnosis of hearing impairment, may prefer to experiment with devices that appear "normal" in any public setting, such as smart glasses [27–29], mobile phones [30,31], and smart earbuds like AirPods and Samsung Galaxy Buds Pro [32]. However, mobile phones as hearing-assistive agents are not suitable for everyday face-to-face communication, and smart earbuds, which merely amplify sounds, might risk further deterioration in hearing. In contrast, smart glasses offer advantages such as a natural appearance, sensory compensation, comfortable wear, and a broad range of applicability. They emerge as a superior choice. As dos Santos, Ferrari [33] pointed out, both glasses and hearing aids can assist those with hearing difficulties, but the stigma associated with glasses is significantly less.

With the advancement and proliferation of augmented reality (AR) technology, AR glasses demonstrate greater potential as hearing aid devices [28,33]. With AR technology, hearing-assistive glasses have transcended their basic function of merely integrating sound amplifiers into their frames. Instead, they now incorporate AR tech into the lens interface and visual effects, amalgamating features like real-time voice-to-text captions, specialized word prompts, spatial sound indicators, etc., into the AR glasses display system, enabling users with hearing impairments to communicate normally through AR glasses [29,34]. It is evident that AR hearing glasses have unique advantages in terms of technological functionality, social acceptance, and interactive experience. As a hearing aid device, they possess immense growth potential and a vast market outlook, holding significant social and economic value.

Given the anticipated significant increase in the number of PHI over the next 30 years, understanding their attitudes towards adopting and intention to use hearing-assistive technology is crucial [6,35]. However, current research on the adoption and usage of hearing aid devices mainly focuses on traditional hearing aids [36–38], and studies on the emerging product of AR hearing glasses are relatively scarce. Existing research on AR hearing aid glasses primarily centers on technological development, functional innovation, experience design, and product development [14,27–29,34,39], with insufficient exploration of whether PHI can truly accept and use AR hearing aid glasses. Most studies approach the issue from a single perspective, either technological functionality or sociocultural aspects [40–44], with few studies comprehensively exploring the willingness of PHI to adopt AR hearing aid glasses from an integrated perspective.

Therefore, this study, based on sociotechnical systems theory (STS), explores the factors and mechanisms influencing the intention of PHI to use AR hearing aid glasses from a comprehensive perspective encompassing technical, social, and individual dimensions. This research aims to provide insights and references for optimizing the design and enhancing the acceptance of AR hearing aid glasses, offering a new practical direction to improve the communication experience and social integration of PHI.

2. Theoretical Framework and Research Hypotheses

Sociotechnical systems theory (STS) is an interdisciplinary theory that provides a comprehensive perspective for understanding and designing technological systems by considering the complex interactions between technical, social, and individual factors [45,46]. The core idea of this theory is that various subsystems (technical, social, and individual) are interdependent and mutually influential. The design and implementation of any new technology, product, or service system must simultaneously consider the potential impacts on these subsystems to achieve optimal results [47,48]. This paper adopts the three-dimensional framework of sociotechnical systems theory—technical subsystem, social subsystem, and individual subsystem—as the theoretical foundation for the following reasons: On one hand, sociotechnical systems theory provides a comprehensive analytical framework for emerging issues related to hearing impairment behavior, hearing aid technology, and AR hearing glasses. On the other hand, research on hearing impairment and hearing aid technology is not merely a technical or individual health issue; it is a complex phenomenon that encompasses personal physiology, product technical functions, and social life [33,49]. Through the integrated perspective of sociotechnical systems theory, we can gain a more comprehensive understanding of the motivations and behavioral impact mechanisms of PHI using AR hearing glasses.

Based on the three dimensions of sociotechnical systems theory, this study explores the technical features of AR hearing aid glasses, the personal physiological characteristics of PHI, and the relevant factors of social life. It ultimately identifies seven factors, namely: functional quality, perceived interaction speed, perceived ease of use, communication effectiveness, social image, confidence, and behavioral intention. The operational definitions for each construct are presented in Table 1.

Table 1. Operational definitions of constructs.

Construct	Operational Definition	Source
Function quality	The completeness and quality of functions of AR smart glasses.	Wang and Chuan-Chuan Lin [50]
Perceived interaction speed	The response speed of AR smart glasses as perceived by PHI.	Steuer, Biocca and Levy [51]
Perceived ease of use	The ease of use of AR smart glasses as perceived by PHI.	Davis [52]
Communication effectiveness	The effectiveness and quality of interactions and communication between PHI and others.	Sweeney, Morrison [53]
Social image	The views and respect that PHI receive from others.	Lin and Bhattacherjee [54]
Confidence	The confidence of PHI that AR glasses can assist them in communication.	Wilkes [55]
Behavioral intention	The intention of PHI to use AR smart glasses as hearing aids.	Taylor and Todd [56]

2.1. Function Quality

PHI use the functions of hearing aids to compensate for their hearing deficits [57]. The quality of these functions signifies the quality of sound information reception for them. Clear and consistent information is a significant influencing factor in interpersonal communication [58]. Therefore, the features of the hearing aids affect communication outcomes [59]. Many studies have also confirmed that the better the performance of hearing aids (such as noise suppression, clarity compensation, etc.), the better the communication outcomes for PHI in various scenarios [28,60–63]. Hence, this study proposes the following hypothesis:

Hypothesis 1 (H1). *The functional quality of AR smart glasses has a positive impact on the communication outcomes of PHI.*

2.2. Perceived Interaction Speed

Research indicates that in interpersonal communication, the speed of interaction between people (speaking rate, cohesion speed, pause intervals, etc.) is one of the three main dimensions for achieving smooth communication. There is a significant relationship between the speed of interaction and the quality of communication [64–66]. For PHI, due to their hearing loss, they cannot communicate directly with those without hearing impairments but must do so mediated by hearing aids. Therefore, hearing aid products are considered an additional pair of ears for PHI [67]; the interaction speed of the hearing aids signifies the sensitivity and reaction speed of their "ears". Gugenheimer, Plaumann [59] found that interruptions in conversation reduce communication quality. Conversely, if the device's real-time interaction speed is fast enough, synchronous dialogue can be achieved [68], reducing interruptions during communication and thereby enhancing communication quality. Therefore, the faster the interaction speed of the AR smart glasses, the better the communication outcome. Based on this, this study proposes the following hypothesis:

Hypothesis 2 (H2). *The perceived interaction speed of AR smart glasses by PHI has a positive impact on communication outcomes.*

2.3. Perceived Ease of Use

In this study, perceived ease of use refers to the degree of ease or difficulty that users with hearing impairments feel when using AR glasses. The literature has already confirmed that there is a significant relationship between perceived ease of use and communication [69,70]. Additionally, some studies have proven that the perceived ease of use of technology products designed for social communication has a positive impact on communication outcomes [71,72]. For example, Chan, Yong, and Harmizi [72] examined the relationship between the use of WhatsApp by students at private higher education institutions in Malaysia and interpersonal communication, confirming a positive correlation between perceived ease of use and interpersonal communication. Based on this, this study proposes the following hypothesis:

Hypothesis 3 (H3). *The perceived ease of use of AR smart glasses has a positive impact on the communication of PHI.*

2.4. Communication Effectiveness

Being able to communicate with people who have unimpaired hearing is crucial for those with hearing impairments [59]. Many studies have confirmed that good communication interactions positively influence confidence enhancement [73,74]. Blood, Blood [75] pointed out in their study that stuttering adolescents may lack confidence in their communication abilities due to communication difficulties. Conversely, smooth communication can boost self-confidence. In the field of assistive hearing device research, enhancing the communication capabilities of users with hearing impairments through relevant products, technologies, and services can alleviate the anxiety and stress caused by fear [76,77], which in turn can further boost the confidence of users with hearing impairments [78–80].

There is a close relationship between communication and social image [81–84]. Lin and Bhattacherjee [54] confirmed in their study that users' social communication with others in social networks positively impacts the creation of a favorable social image. Heffernan, Coulson [85] pointed out that the stigmatization and damage to the social image of PHI often result from communication difficulties. By achieving normal and free communication through technology without revealing their unique health status, PHI can avoid being seen as disabled, thus sidestepping stigmatized views and attitudes, and achieving equality and respect [86], which translates to a positive social image. Therefore, when AR hearing-assistive glasses help users with hearing impairments to communicate smoothly and avoid stigmatization, they can help these users establish a good social image. Hence, this study proposes the following hypotheses:

Hypothesis 4 (H4). *Communication effectiveness has a positive impact on the shaping of the social image of PHI.*

Hypothesis 5 (H5). *Communication effectiveness has a positive impact on the confidence of PHI.*

2.5. Social Image

Social image is defined as the extent to which users can obtain opinions and respect from their peers, family members, or others in their social relationships [87]. There is also a close relationship between social image and confidence. Confidence, in the context of personal motivation, explains why and to what extent people care about their self and social image, indicating that social image has a positive effect on confidence [88]. Lubis and Fazira [89] pointed out in their study that there is a significant positive correlation between social support (which includes the concept of social image) and confidence. In disability research, the role of social image in confidence is even more evident [90]. Simsek, Evli [91], in the context of chronic illness research, found a positive correlation between body image and confidence. Therefore, consistent with previous research, a good social image can enhance the confidence of the hearing-impaired group.

The study of social image in interactive products is of great significance. As the image of users comes from the opinions and views of others, users will thus decide on subsequent actions based on these views [92]. Some of the literature has confirmed that the social image produced by users using products or systems will significantly affect the subsequent intention to use [54,87,93]. Bispo and Branco [94] pointed out that the design of assistive technology for people with disabilities might change their social image. The same is true for hearing-assistive products—non-stigmatizing design may stimulate users' desire and behavior to use [33]. AR smart glasses are generally not associated with one's mental image of disability; this can reduce stigmatization, thus forming a good social image. To maintain this good social image, PHI may continue to choose to use AR glasses in the future. Based on the above discussion, this study proposes the following hypotheses:

Hypothesis 6 (H6). *The social image formed by PHI during the use of AR glasses has a positive impact on their confidence.*

Hypothesis 7 (H7). *The social image formed by PHI during the use of AR glasses has a positive impact on their behavioral intention.*

2.6. Confidence

Confidence can be defined as an individual's belief in their abilities, a state of certainty about the success of a specific behavior [95]. The relationship between confidence and behavioral intention has been confirmed in many studies [96–98]. For instance, Kim, Ahn, and No [97] pointed out in their study that confidence in one's physical health affects the choice and execution of behavior. Chai, Lin [98] found in their research that confidence in AI technology is positively correlated with the intention to continue using AI devices. In line with previous studies, this research believes that the confidence of PHI in the AR glasses technology assisting them in smooth communication has a positive impact on the intention to continue using AR glasses. Therefore, this article proposes the following hypothesis:

Hypothesis 8 (H8). *The confidence gained from social communication through AR glasses has a positive impact on PHI's intention to continue using AR glasses.*

Based on the discussions in the previous sections, this study formulates eight hypotheses. The path and hypothesis model are shown in Figure 1.

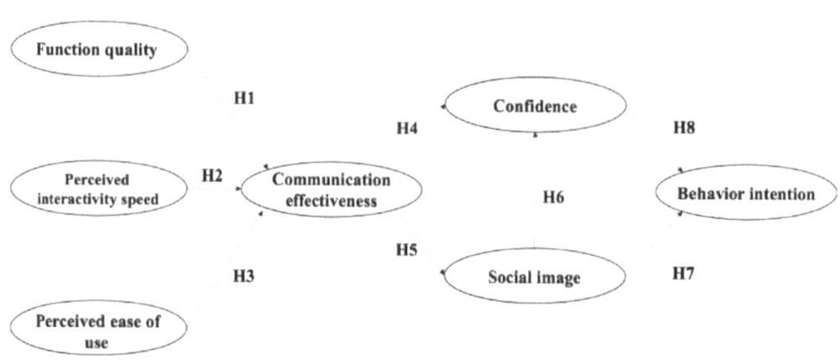

Figure 1. Research model.

3. Questionnaire Design and Data Collection

3.1. Questionnaire Design

This study combined the product features of AR hearing aid glasses with the characteristics of the research to design a literature-validated questionnaire (see Table 2). After completing the initial questionnaire design, we conducted a pretest with 30 participants and adjusted the questionnaire based on their feedback. The final version included basic information and an assessment of factors influencing the use of AR hearing aid glasses. (using a Likert's seven-point scale).

Table 2. Measurement scale of influencing factors of PHI using AR hearing assistant glasses.

Constructs	Items	Content	Source
Function quality	FQ1	I feel that the speech-to-text accuracy of AR glasses is very high.	Shanahan, Tran and Taylor [99], Wang, Wang [100]
	FQ2	I feel that the speech-to-text quality of AR glasses is high.	
	FQ3	I believe that the information output from the AR glasses is reliable.	
	FQ4	I believe the functionality quality of the AR glasses meets my requirements.	
Perceived interaction speed	PIS1	I feel that the speech-to-text speed of AR glasses is very fast.	Huang, Chiu [101]
	PIS2	I believe the process of speech-to-text with AR glasses is very smooth.	
	PIS3	I believe the speech-to-text speed of AR glasses is almost synchronous with the speed of the other person's speech.	
	PIS4	I feel that the response speed of the AR glasses is fast when communicating with others.	
Perceived ease of use	PEU1	Learning how to use AR glasses is easy for me.	Khlaisang, Songkram [102]
	PEU2	Interacting with AR glasses doesn't require much effort.	
	PEU3	I can use AR glasses proficiently in communication.	
Communication effectiveness	CE1	With the help of AR glasses, I communicate with others more easily and comfortably.	Sweeney, Morrison [53], Lam and Campbell [103]
	CE2	With the assistance of AR glasses, I can communicate better with others.	
	CE3	AR glasses help me understand others more effortlessly.	
	CE4	With the assistance of AR glasses, I can communicate with others smoothly and without barriers.	
Social image	SI1	By using AR glasses, I have shed the image of being hearing-impaired.	Yang, Yu [104]
	SI2	By using AR glasses, others see me as a normal person.	
	SI3	Using AR glasses gives others the impression that I am a regular individual.	
Confidence	CO1	With the help of AR glasses, I now have the confidence to handle the entire communication process.	Hong, Hwang [96]
	CO2	Compared to before, with the help of AR glasses, I believe my communication performance is better.	
	CO3	Compared to before, with the assistance of AR glasses, I will communicate with others more confidently.	
Behavioral intention	BI1	I am willing to use AR glasses as my hearing assistance device.	Rajeh, Abduljabbar [105], Hong, Lin and Hsieh [106]
	BI2	I would recommend AR glasses to my hearing-impaired friends.	
	BI3	I will continue to use AR glasses in the future.	

3.2. Data Collection

The research and experimentation for this study spanned eight months. During the preliminary preparation phase from January to April 2023, we conducted an initial screening of hearing-impaired subjects, visited multiple locations, tested and selected experimental tools, and designed and evaluated the questionnaire. From May to August 2023, we carried out formal questionnaire surveys at hearing centers and service institutions in Wuxi, Xiamen, Hangzhou, and other cities in China, using both offline experiences and online questionnaires. We employed a cluster sampling technique. Conducting surveys through established hearing centers and service institutions provided practical benefits, as it allowed for us to efficiently recruit a large number of participants within the given timeframe. Additionally, this approach enabled us to capture a broad range of experiences and perspectives from participants across various locations.

We used the LEION HEY AR smart glasses as the testing tool and invited participants to complete the questionnaire after experiencing the product for more than 15 min. After screening, a total of 189 valid questionnaires were collected. The demographic information of the respondents is shown in Table 3.

Table 3. Demographic information of the respondents.

Category	Group	Number	Percentage
Gender	Male	73	38.624%
	Female	116	61.376%
Age	<18	12	6.349%
	18–30	100	52.910%
	31–40	36	19.048%
	41–50	24	12.698%
	51–60	14	7.407
	>60	3	1.587
Education	High school or technical secondary school and below	55	29.101%
	junior college	63	33.333%
	Undergraduate	65	34.392%
	Graduate and above	6	3.175%
Degrees of hearing impairment	Mild	107	56.614%
	Moderate	77	40.741%
	Severe	5	2.646%

4. Data Analysis and Results

This study employs the partial least squares structural equation modeling (PLS-SEM) research method. As a flexible multivariate analysis approach, PLS-SEM is utilized for constructing and validating complex structural equation models [107]. Therefore, this study utilized the PLS-SEM algorithm in SmartPLS 4 V4.0.9.2, employing a weighted path scheme, with a maximum of 3000 iterations and default initial weights. Further, we used path analysis techniques to verify the eight proposed hypotheses. Finally, we integrated the empirical data and conducted an in-depth analysis within the existing theoretical framework, and then drew rigorous conclusions.

This study employed the SmartPLS software to calculate the reliability and validity of constructs, specifically considering three indicators: Cronbach's alpha, composite reliability, and average variance extracted (AVE). As shown in Table 4, the Cronbach's alpha value for each construct in this study exceeded 0.7, and the rho_c value also exceeded 0.7, indicating that all the constructs used have good reliability. Next, this study used AVE to measure convergent validity. The usual standard is for AVE to be greater than 0.5. All the indicators in this study meet this requirement [108]. Therefore, the constructs in this study exhibit good convergent validity.

If the square root of the AVE value of each construct is greater than the correlation coefficients between itself and other constructs, it suggests that the scale has good discriminant validity [109]. As shown in Table 5, the bold numbers on the diagonal represent the square root of the AVE values for each construct, which are all greater than the correlation coefficients, which indicates that there is good discriminant validity between the constructs used in this study.

Table 4. Loadings, AVE, composite reliability, and Cronbach's alpha.

Constructs	Items	Loadings	Cronbach's Alpha	Composite Reliability (rho_a)	Composite Reliability (rho_c)	AVE
Function quality	FQ1 FQ2 FQ3 FQ4	0.852 0.844 0.834 0.847	0.866	0.869	0.909	0.713
Perceived interaction speed	PIS1 PIS2 PIS3 PIS4	0.845 0.868 0.832 0.848	0.87	0.874	0.911	0.72
Perceived ease of use	PEU1 PEU2 PEU3	0.839 0.824 0.853	0.79	0.797	0.877	0.703
Communication effectiveness	CE1 CE2 CE3 CE4	0.851 0.86 0.843 0.832	0.868	0.868	0.91	0.717
Social image	SI1 SI2 SI3	0.825 0.903 0.869	0.833	0.838	0.9	0.75
Confidence	CO1 CO2 CO3	0.876 0.881 0.861	0.843	0.845	0.905	0.761
Behavioral intention	BI1 BI2 BI3	0.854 0.897 0.915	0.867	0.869	0.919	0.791

Table 5. Discriminant validity: Fornell–Larcker criterion.

	FQ	PIS	PEU	CE	SI	CO	BI
FQ	**0.844**						
PIS	0.771	**0.848**					
PEU	0.609	0.606	**0.839**				
CE	0.708	0.705	0.733	**0.847**			
SI	0.593	0.593	0.571	0.685	**0.866**		
CO	0.589	0.569	0.616	0.707	0.724	**0.873**	
BI	0.589	0.586	0.645	0.763	0.683	0.748	**0.889**

Note: Bold numbers is the square root of the AVE values for each construct.

This study also uses the HTMT (heterotrait/monotrait ratio) method to evaluate the discriminant validity of the constructs [110]. According to previous research, the HTMT value must be less than 0.9 [111]. As shown in Table 6, the HTMT values for all constructs are less than 0.9. Therefore, all constructs in this study have good discriminant validity.

Table 6. Discriminant validity: heterotrait/monotrait ratio (HTMT).

	FQ	PIS	PEU	CE	SI	CO	BI
FQ							
PIS	0.887						
PEU	0.731	0.721					
CE	0.812	0.808	0.878				
SI	0.696	0.695	0.698	0.805			
CO	0.684	0.660	0.755	0.825	0.861		
BI	0.675	0.672	0.772	0.879	0.801	0.875	

Also, during this stage, additional measures were evaluated, namely, the determination coefficient (R^2) and predictive relevance (Q^2) [108]. As shown in Table 7, the R^2 values between the constructs range from 46.9% to 66.9%. R^2 values greater than 26% are considered significant [112]. In this study, the Q^2 values of the constructs (calculated only for dependent variables) are all non-zero. Therefore, the hypothesized model in this study has acceptable predictive relevance [113]. Additionally, indicators such as the standardized root mean square residual (SRMR) and the normed fit index (NFI) were used to evaluate the fit of the structural equation model (see Table 8). The SRMR value is 0.082, which is below the threshold of 0.10, and the NFI value is 0.804, where an NFI value close to 1 indicates a good model fit. These fit indices suggest that the hypothesized model proposed in this study performs well in explaining the data structure.

Table 7. Results of R^2 and Q^2.

Construct	R^2	Q^2
Communication effectiveness	0.669	0.472
Social image	0.469	0.348
Confidence	0.608	0.454
Behavior intention	0.602	0.471

Table 8. Model fit indices.

Indices	Estimated Model
SRMR	0.082
d_ULS	2.007
d_G	0.598
Chi square	648.539
NFI	0.804

The bootstrapping procedure (with 5000 bootstrap resampling) was applied to further test the proposed hypotheses. The results of the model path analysis are shown in Figure 2, and the regression coefficient results of the structural equation model are shown in Table 9. The results indicate that all hypotheses of this study are supported. Furthermore, the full collinearity test results show that the variance inflation factor (VIF) ranges between 1.000 and 2.674. All the VIFs are below the recommended threshold of 5 [108], confirming that there is no multicollinearity issue in the estimated model of this study.

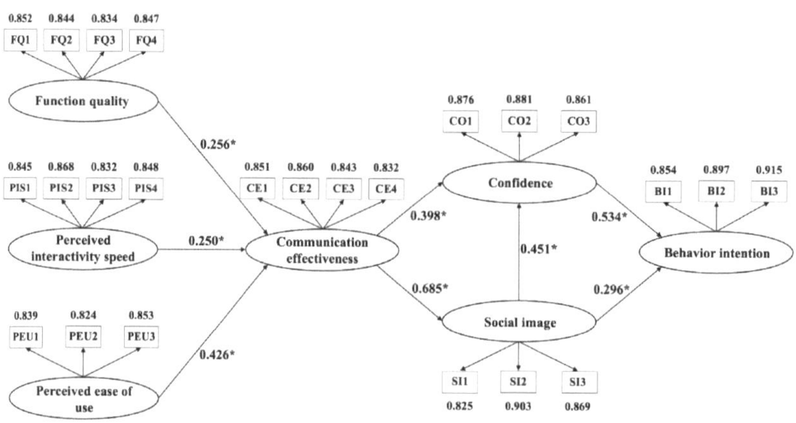

Figure 2. Results of path analysis. (* The level of significance is below 0.05).

Table 9. Path coefficients and the results of the significance tests.

Hypothesis	Path	Std Beta	*t* Statistics	*p* Values	VIF	Results
H1	FQ → CE	0.256	3.329	0.0001	2.674	Support
H2	PIS → CE	0.250	3.449	0.0001	2.655	Support
H3	PEU → CE	0.426	7.618	0.0000	1.715	Support
H4	CE → CO	0.398	6.298	0.0000	1.882	Support
H5	CE → SI	0.685	16.194	0.0000	1.000	Support
H6	SI → CO	0.451	7.337	0.0000	1.882	Support
H7	SI → BI	0.296	3.683	0.0000	2.101	Support
H8	CO → BI	0.534	7.314	0.0000	2.101	Support

5. Discussion

According to the research results, function quality and perceived interactivity speed have a significant positive impact on communication effectiveness (H1 and H2 are supported). The previous literature has pointed out that hearing aids can be considered an additional pair of ears for users with hearing impairments [67]. The quality and speed of their functions are equivalent to the clarity and sensitivity of these "ears". AR hearing aid glasses serve as an intermediary for PHI to interact with external sounds. The higher the functional quality of AR hearing aid glasses, the clearer the external sounds they read, and the more accurate the converted text information, leading to better communication effectiveness for the user. Similarly, if AR hearing aid glasses can quickly capture, process, and present visual information, enabling PHI to swiftly acquire conversation content, speech-to-text information, and respond accordingly, this instant feedback helps reduce delays and misunderstandings in communication. This allows for a synchronized rhythm with others, avoiding interruptions in conversations, making the entire communication process more natural, relaxed, and smooth [59], thereby enhancing the communication effectiveness for PHI.

Perceived ease of use has a significant positive impact on communication effectiveness (H3 is supported). Unlike traditional hearing aids, which users cannot control independently, AR hearing aid glasses offer more functions, meaning there may be many aspects requiring user operation. Although most functions are set up before communication interactions, the complexity of social situations and the unpredictability of human behavior can lead to changes in social communication conditions and needs [114]. This, in turn, necessitates adjustments to the AR hearing aid glasses, such as font size, color, and contrast, as well as turning on the device or adjusting the volume. If these adjustments can be easily made during conversations, PHI can focus more on the communication itself, thereby enhancing the effectiveness and experience of their interactions.

It is worth noting that even though function quality, perceived interaction speed, and perceived ease of use all have significant positive impacts on communication effectiveness, and perceived ease of use has a stronger influence on communication effectiveness (0.426 > 0.256 > 0.250). The reason for this might be related to the unique ways PHI receive information and their cognitive processing methods. PHI are not completely deaf; they still retain some degree of hearing ability. Before using hearing aids, PHI might intentionally or unintentionally employ various skills to complement this portion of sound information. For example, they imagine and reason to fill in the details not fully heard in conversations, especially for unclear words and phrases. They may also use non-verbal strategies to enhance communication, such as observing the speaker's lip movements, body language, facial expressions, and contextual environment to infer the meaning, emotions, and attitudes in the conversation [115–117]. By utilizing these techniques, PHI can combine their existing knowledge, memory, and experience to partially fill in the missing information and deduce the logical conclusions of the conversation [118]. Thus, for AR hearing-assistive glasses, even if the accuracy of voice-to-text isn't very high or the conversion speed is slow, individuals can still construct a complete dialogue scene using their imagination and reasoning skills. In contrast, the perceived ease of use of AR hearing-assistive glasses has a more significant effect on communication. On the one hand, the usage method of AR hearing aid glasses differs significantly from traditional hearing aids. Traditional hearing aids require little to no manual operation during daily use, whereas AR hearing aid glasses necessitate user interaction. This interaction can occur at any stage before, during, or after communication, emphasizing the importance of ease of use. On the other hand, the user's operation of the glasses is explicit and visible to both parties. If the glasses are challenging to use, users might need to adjust them repeatedly during conversations, not only wasting time and causing communication delays but also diverting their attention. Not focusing on the interlocutor during a conversation is considered impolite and might make the other party feel disrespected [119]. Therefore, the influence of perceived ease of use on communication effectiveness can create a chain reaction, much like the butterfly effect, resulting in a stronger impact.

Secondly, communication effectiveness has a significant positive impact on both social image and confidence (H4 and H5 are supported). With the assistance of AR glasses, effective two-way communication enables clear understanding and expression of information, preventing many awkward situations such as being unable to participate in group conversations, missing important information, or not responding promptly. This helps to avoid feelings of marginalization and inferiority, thereby enhancing conversational confidence. Furthermore, the stigmatization and negative social image of those with hearing impairments are often directly related to communication challenges [85]. With the support of AR hearing-assistive glasses, PHI can establish effective two-way communication, build a positive image, and gain more recognition, respect, and equality in social life, education, and career development [86].

Social image has a significant positive impact on confidence (H6 is supported), which is consistent with the findings of previous studies [89–91]. According to Tajfel and Turner [120], when individuals feel recognized and affirmed within their social group, their confidence is boosted. PHI often do not consider themselves having a disability [121]. Therefore, they desire to establish an image of capability equal to those with without impaired hearing. However, this desire often contradicts the use of hearing-assistive devices because the distinctive appearance of most of these devices inadvertently reveals their hearing deficiencies. Unlike other hearing aids that might expose one's hearing challenges, AR glasses possess high social acceptability and low stigmatization. They can enhance communication abilities without disclosing hearing impairments. Once this positive social image is recognized by others, it can boost positive emotions and confidence.

Lastly, both social image and confidence have a significant positive impact on the intention to use (H7 and H8 are supported). In social life, individuals not only perceive themselves as independent entities but also as members of social groups, and they seek recognition from these groups [120]. Therefore, the social image is crucial. When PHI gain a wholesome social image by using AR glasses, integrating them into the mainstream group, they are more likely to accept and adopt hearing-assistive technology. Conversely, devices that expose their hearing deficiencies are likely to be rejected [122]. Furthermore, compared to social image, confidence has a stronger impact on the intention to use (0.534 > 0.296). This might be due to confidence serving as an intrinsic factor, exerting a more direct inner drive on usage intention, while the social image, as an external factor, primarily plays a supporting role. The construction of social image is rooted in others' perceptions and attitudes, an external push. This external force typically undergoes self-awareness, filtration, absorption, and rational analysis before it internalizes and influences behavior. Throughout this process, users filter some external factors based on their self-perception, reducing the impact of these factors to some extent. In contrast, confidence, being an intrinsic driver, can directly influence behavior choices [123], and hence has a more potent influence.

6. Contributions and Limitations

This study, based on sociotechnical systems theory, explores the factors influencing the intention of PHI to use AR glasses as hearing aid devices from a comprehensive perspective of technological, social, and individual levels. It identifies the real needs and decision-making mechanisms of PHI, enriching the theoretical foundation of the hearing aid design field and providing practical guidance and insights.

6.1. Theoretical Contributions

(1). This study enriches the field of behavioral research in hearing impairment and design. By introducing sociotechnical systems theory into the study of hearing impairment behavior, it explores how the interaction between technological, social, and individual dimensions affects the experience of PHI using AR hearing aid glasses, thereby influencing their subsequent adoption intentions. This research provides a new explanatory pathway for the behavior of PHI using AR hearing glasses and offers a theoretical framework for further understanding and recognizing the deep needs of PHI. It also provides theoretical support for the development and design of hearing impairment treatments, services, and related products. Furthermore, this study helps overcome the limitations of technocentrism and partial perspectives in hearing impairment research.

(2). Through quantitative analysis, this study elucidates the intrinsic mechanisms and decision-making pathways for PHI choosing AR glasses as hearing aid devices. Specifically, it identifies that social image and confidence are the decisive factors influencing users' intention to use AR hearing aid glasses, while the technical aspects of functional quality, perceived interactivity speed, and perceived ease of use are merely necessary prerequisites and foundations and do not directly determine the intention to use AR hearing aid glasses. This finding aligns with the general direction of existing research on hearing impairment and hearing aid technology, providing further empirical evidence. Additionally, by examining specific aspects and more tangible product targets, this study clarifies the intrinsic relationships and influencing mechanisms between variables at the technical, social, and individual levels and the intention to use AR hearing glasses. This provides more targeted theoretical guidance for strategy formulation and practical implementation in the field of hearing aid technology and services.

6.2. Practical Contributions

In terms of practical implications, the results of this study make tangible contributions to expanding the market for AR hearing-assistive glasses and sustainable development. By clarifying various factors influencing the use of AR glasses as hearing-assistive devices by PHI, this study provides a research foundation and guiding direction for the development of AR hearing-assistive glasses and other hearing-assistive products. It offers recommendations and design strategies for optimizing their design, mainly including the following:

(1). In the development of AR hearing-assistive glasses, special attention should be given to the interactive ease-of-use design of the AR glasses. The basic operations of the AR glasses should be simplified to prevent users from abandoning their use due to difficulty. Consideration can even be given to employing the most advanced intelligent proactive interactive methods, allowing for the device to autonomously complete interactions based on circumstances. This avoids tedious operations during communication and allows for users to focus on communicating, thereby enhancing the communication experience.

(2). It is essential to integrate as many functions as possible, such as noise reduction, multi-directional microphone pickups, and adaptive light brightness adjustments and ensure the high quality of these features to assist PHI in communicating normally in various environments. It is also vital to improve the interaction speed of AR hearing-assistive glasses, such as the response speed for keyword activation and the speed of voice-to-text, so that PHI can maintain a consistent rhythm with their counterparts during communication.

(3). The design of AR glasses should closely resemble regular glasses used in daily life. The lens can adopt a single-sided design to ensure the virtual interface is not visible to others, thus avoiding excessive attention. This helps PHI rid themselves of the "special" label, thereby building social confidence. It is also essential to design the text information's display size, color, transparency, and position well, so users can clearly view the text while not obscuring the eyes and non-verbal actions of others. This facilitates more eye contact during communication, allowing for users to express their sincerity, earn the respect of others, establish a positive social image, and better integrate into various aspects of life, education, and work.

6.3. Research Limitations

While this study offers valuable contributions both theoretically and practically, there are still some limitations. On one hand, due to objective constraints such as culture, funding, geography, and time, we encountered many obstacles when trying to locate PHI, making it difficult to expand our sample size. On the other hand, since AR hearing-assistive glasses are an emerging product, most of our respondents were completely unfamiliar with them. This may lead to self-report biases and potential errors in data validity. Although we made efforts to minimize these biases by providing product descriptions, allowing participants to try the glasses and offering guidance as necessary before they filled out the questionnaire, we still recognize that this limitation could mislead our study's results. Therefore, when interpreting and promoting the findings of this study, potential uncertainties arising from data biases should be carefully considered. Moreover, there are numerous areas for further detailed research. For instance, PHI from different age groups may have varied attitudes towards AR glasses. Our study, with its limited sample, did not differentiate the intention to use based on age groups. Secondly, different genders might have different preferences for the design and aesthetics of hearing-assistive devices. Thirdly, acceptance of AR hearing-assistive glasses might be influenced to different degrees in various countries and cultural environments. Future research can build upon the foundation of this study and further segment personal attributes and societal scopes, allowing for more targeted and in-depth exploration of AR hearing-assistive glasses.

Author Contributions: Conceptualization, L.D.; Methodology, J.C.; Resources, D.L.; Data curation, L.D.; Writing—original draft, L.D.; Writing—review & editing, D.L.; Supervision, D.L. All authors have read and agreed to the published version of the manuscript.

Funding: This research received no external funding.

Institutional Review Board Statement: The study was conducted in accordance with the Declaration of Helsinki, and approved by the Institutional Review Board (or Ethics Committee) of Changshu Institute of Technology Ministry of Social Science (protocol code No. CIT MSS-E-2023-011 and date of 25 May 2023 approval).

Informed Consent Statement: Informed consent was obtained from all subjects involved in this study.

Data Availability Statement: The data that support the findings of this study are available from the corresponding author upon reasonable request.

Acknowledgments: We would like to thank Jiangnan University and Changshu Institute of Technology for providing the equipment and technical support for this research. Special thanks to Weiwei from Changshu Institute of Technology for offering detailed ethical guidance and supervision in the design of the questionnaire and the standardization of the experimental process.

Conflicts of Interest: The authors declare no conflicts of interest.

References

1. Roizen, N.J. Nongenetic causes of hearing loss. *Ment. Retard. Dev. Disabil. Res. Rev.* **2003**, *9*, 120–127. [CrossRef] [PubMed]
2. Daniel, E. Noise and Hearing Loss: A Review. *J. Sch. Health* **2007**, *77*, 225–231. [CrossRef] [PubMed]
3. Willems, P.J. Genetic Causes of Hearing Loss. *N. Engl. J. Med.* **2000**, *342*, 1101–1109. [CrossRef]
4. Tonelli, M.; Warick, R. Focusing on the Needs of People with Hearing Loss During the COVID-19 Pandemic and Beyond. *JAMA* **2022**, *327*, 1129–1130. [CrossRef]

5. Kim, S.Y.; Min, C.; Yoo, D.M.; Chang, J.; Lee, H.-J.; Park, B.; Choi, H.G. Hearing Impairment Increases Economic Inequality. *Clin. Exp. Otorhinolaryngol.* **2021**, *14*, 278–286. [CrossRef] [PubMed]
6. World Health Organization. *World Report on Hearing: Executive Summary*; World Health Organization: Geneva, Switzerland, 2021.
7. Swanepoel, W.; De Sousa, K.C.; Smits, C.; Moore, D.R. Mobile applications to detect hearing impairment: Opportunities and challenges. *Bull. World Health Organ.* **2019**, *97*, 717–718. [CrossRef] [PubMed]
8. Miao, L.; Wang, B.; Zhang, J.; Yin, L.; Pu, Y. A functional SNP in miR-625-5p binding site of AKT2 3′UTR is associated with noise-induced hearing loss susceptibility in the Chinese population. *Environ. Sci. Pollut. Res.* **2021**, *28*, 40782–40792. [CrossRef]
9. Olusanya, B.O.; Davis, A.C.; Hoffman, H.J. Hearing loss: Rising prevalence and impact. *Bull. World Health Organ.* **2019**, *97*, 646–646a. [CrossRef] [PubMed]
10. Shukla, A.; Harper, M.; Pedersen, E.; Goman, A.; Suen, J.J.; Price, C.; Applebaum, J.; Hoyer, M.; Lin, F.R.; Reed, N.S. Hearing Loss, Loneliness, and Social Isolation: A Systematic Review. *Otolaryngol. Head Neck Surg.* **2020**, *162*, 622–633. [CrossRef]
11. Ohlenforst, B.; Zekveld, A.A.; Jansma, E.P.; Wang, Y.; Naylor, G.; Lorens, A.; Lunner, T.; Kramer, S.E. Effects of hearing impairment and hearing aid amplification on listening effort: A systematic review. *Ear Hear.* **2017**, *38*, 267. [CrossRef] [PubMed]
12. World Health Organization. Deafness and Hearing Loss. 2023. Available online: https://www.who.int/news-room/fact-sheets/detail/deafness-and-hearing-loss (accessed on 2 February 2024).
13. Sawyer, C.S.; Armitage, C.J.; Munro, K.J.; Singh, G.; Dawes, P.D. Correlates of hearing aid use in UK adults: Self-reported hearing difficulties, social participation, living situation, health, and demographics. *Ear Hear.* **2019**, *40*, 1061–1068. [CrossRef] [PubMed]
14. Takaki, K.; Nozaki, E.; Kanai, T.; Hautasaari, A.; Kashio, A.; Sato, D.; Kamogashira, T.; Uranaka, T.; Urata, S.; Koyama, H. asEars: Designing and Evaluating the User Experience of Wearable Assistive Devices for Single-Sided Deafness. In Proceedings of the 2023 CHI Conference on Human Factors in Computing Systems, New York, NY, USA, 23–28 April 2023; pp. 1–17.
15. Kawata, N.; Nouchi, R.; Oba, K.; Matsuzaki, Y.; Kawashima, R. Auditory cognitive training improves brain plasticity in healthy older adults: Evidence from a randomized controlled trial. *Front. Aging Neurosci.* **2022**, *14*, 140. [CrossRef]
16. Putri, S.S.; Supena, A.; Yatimah, D. Utilization of Internet Media by Deaf Persons for Language Learning (Case study on 11-year-old child at SLB B Tunas Kasih 2, Bogor City, West Java). In Proceedings of the International Conference on Education, Science and Technology, West Sumatera, Indonesia, 13–16 March 2019; pp. 151–157.
17. Chung, S.-H.; Jeong, S.W.; Kim, L.-S. A case of auditory neuropathy caused by pontine hemorrhage in an adult. *J. Audiol. Otol.* **2017**, *21*, 107. [CrossRef]
18. Wu, H.C.; Thallmayer, T.; Deal, J.A.; Betz, J.F.; Reed, N.S.; Lin, F.R. Prevalence Trends in Hearing Aid Use among US Adults Aged 50 to 69 Years with Hearing Loss—2011 to 2016 vs. 1999 to 2004. *JAMA Otolaryngol. Head Neck Surg.* **2021**, *147*, 831–832. [CrossRef]
19. Gagné, J.-P.; Southall, K.; Jennings, M.B. Stigma and self-stigma associated with acquired hearing loss in adults. *Hear. Rev.* **2011**, *18*, 16–22.
20. KochKiN, S. MarkeTrak VIII: The key influencing factors in hearing aid purchase intent. *Hear. Rev.* **2012**, *19*, 12–25.
21. Kochkin, S. MarkeTrak VII: Obstacles to adult non-user adoption of hearing aids. *Hear. J.* **2007**, *60*, 24–51. [CrossRef]
22. Jenstad, L.; Moon, J. Systematic review of barriers and facilitators to hearing aid uptake in older adults. *Audiol. Res.* **2011**, *1*, e25. [CrossRef] [PubMed]
23. Meister, H.; Walger, M.; Brehmer, D.; von Wedel, U.-C.; von Wedel, H. The relationship between pre-fitting expectations and willingness to use hearing aids. *Int. J. Audiol.* **2008**, *47*, 153–159. [CrossRef] [PubMed]
24. David, D.; Werner, P. Stigma regarding hearing loss and hearing aids: A scoping review. *Stigma Health* **2016**, *1*, 59. [CrossRef]
25. Southall, K.; Gagné, J.-P.; Jennings, M.B. Stigma: A negative and a positive influence on help-seeking for adults with acquired hearing loss. *Int. J. Audiol.* **2010**, *49*, 804–814. [CrossRef] [PubMed]
26. Ruusuvuori, J.E.; Aaltonen, T.; Koskela, I.; Ranta, J.; Lonka, E.; Salmenlinna, I.; Laakso, M. Studies on stigma regarding hearing impairment and hearing aid use among adults of working age: A scoping review. *Disabil. Rehabil.* **2021**, *43*, 436–446. [CrossRef]
27. Xu, M.; Li, J. Design of an AR Realistic Interactive Hearing Aid System Based on Digital Construction. *Packag. Eng.* **2023**, *44*, 404–410. (In Chinese) [CrossRef]
28. Mehra, R.; Brimijoin, O.; Robinson, P.; Lunner, T. Potential of Augmented Reality Platforms to Improve Individual Hearing Aids and to Support More Ecologically Valid Research. *Ear Hear.* **2020**, *41*, 140s–146s. [CrossRef] [PubMed]
29. Ridha, A.M.; Shehieb, W. Assistive technology for hearing-impaired and deaf students utilizing augmented reality. In Proceedings of the 2021 IEEE Canadian Conference on Electrical and Computer Engineering (CCECE), Virtual, 12–17 September 2021; pp. 1–5.
30. Amlani, A.M.; Taylor, B.; Levy, C.; Robbins, R. Utility of smartphone-based hearing aid applications as a substitute to traditional hearing aids. *Hear. Rev.* **2013**, *20*, 16–18.
31. Slaney, M.; Lyon, R.F.; Garcia, R.; Kemler, B.; Gnegy, C.; Wilson, K.; Kanevsky, D.; Savla, S.; Cerf, V.G. Auditory measures for the next billion users. *Ear Hear.* **2020**, *41*, 131S–139S. [CrossRef]
32. Ochsner, B.; Spöhrer, M.; Stock, R. Rethinking assistive technologies: Users, environments, digital media, and app-practices of hearing. *NanoEthics* **2022**, *16*, 65–79. [CrossRef]
33. dos Santos, A.D.P.; Ferrari, A.L.M.; Medola, F.O.; Sandnes, F.E. Aesthetics and the perceived stigma of assistive technology for visual impairment. *Disabil. Rehabil. Assist. Technol.* **2022**, *17*, 152–158. [CrossRef]
34. Dufraux, A.; Vincent, E.; Hannun, A.; Brun, A.; Douze, M. Lead2Gold: Towards exploiting the full potential of noisy transcriptions for speech recognition. In Proceedings of the 2019 IEEE Automatic Speech Recognition and Understanding Workshop (ASRU), Singapore, 14–18 December 2019; pp. 78–85.

35. Chang, P.F.; Tucker, R.V. Assistive Communication Technologies and Stigma: How Perceived Visibility of Cochlear Implants Affects Self-Stigma and Social Interaction Anxiety. *Proc. ACM Hum. Comput. Interact.* **2022**, *6*, 77. [CrossRef]
36. Chang, V.; Wang, Y.; Wills, G. Research investigations on the use or non-use of hearing aids in the smart cities. *Technol. Forecast. Soc. Change* **2020**, *153*, 119231. [CrossRef]
37. Desjardins, J.L.; Sotelo, L.R. Self-Reported Reasons for the Non-Use of Hearing Aids among Hispanic Adults with Hearing Loss. *Am. J. Audiol.* **2021**, *30*, 709–716. [CrossRef] [PubMed]
38. Sawyer, C.S.; Munro, K.J.; Dawes, P.; O'Driscoll, M.P.; Armitage, C.J. Beyond motivation: Identifying targets for intervention to increase hearing aid use in adults. *Int. J. Audiol.* **2019**, *58*, 53–58. [CrossRef] [PubMed]
39. Brown, K.; Pullin, G. Uncovering Nuance: Exploring Hearing Aids and Super Normal Design. *Des. J.* **2019**, *22*, 589–599. [CrossRef]
40. Ioannou, A.; Constantinou, V. Augmented reality supporting deaf students in mainstream schools: Two case studies of practical utility of the technology. In *Interactive Mobile Communication Technologies and Learning: Proceedings of the 11th IMCL Conference*; Springer International Publishing: Cham, Switzerland, 2018; pp. 387–396.
41. Federici, S.; Meloni, F.; Borsci, S. The abandonment of assistive technology in Italy: A survey of users of the national health service. *Eur. J. Phys. Rehabil. Med.* **2016**, *52*, 516–526. [PubMed]
42. Petrie, H.; Carmien, S.; Lewis, A. Assistive technology abandonment: Research realities and potentials. In *Computers Helping People with Special Needs: 16th International Conference, ICCHP 2018, Linz, Austria, 11–13 July 2018, Proceedings, Part II 16*; Springer International Publishing: Cham, Switzerland, 2018; pp. 532–540.
43. Choi, J.E.; Ma, S.M.; Park, H.; Cho, Y.-S.; Hong, S.H.; Moon, I.J. A comparison between wireless CROS/BiCROS and soft-band BAHA for patients with unilateral hearing loss. *PLoS ONE* **2019**, *14*, e0212503. [CrossRef]
44. de Jonge, D.; Aplin, T.; Larkin, S.; Ainsworth, E. The aesthetic appeal of assistive technology and the economic value baby boomers place on it: A pilot study. *Aust. Occup. Ther. J.* **2016**, *63*, 415–423. [CrossRef] [PubMed]
45. Trist, E.L. *The Evolution of Socio-Technical Systems*; Ontario Quality of Working Life Centre: Toronto, ON, Canada, 1981; Volume 2.
46. van Eijnatten, F.M. Developments in socio-technical systems design (STSD). In *A Handbook of Work and Organizational Psychology*; Psychology Press: London, UK, 2013; pp. 61–88.
47. Maguire, M. Socio-technical systems and interaction design—21st century relevance. *Appl. Ergon.* **2014**, *45*, 162–170. [CrossRef]
48. Sony, M.; Naik, S. Industry 4.0 integration with socio-technical systems theory: A systematic review and proposed theoretical model. *Technol. Soc.* **2020**, *61*, 101248. [CrossRef]
49. Punch, J.L.; Hitt, R.; Smith, S.W. Hearing loss and quality of life. *J. Commun. Disord.* **2019**, *78*, 33–45. [CrossRef]
50. Wang, S.M.; Chuan-Chuan Lin, J. The effect of social influence on bloggers' usage intention. *Online Inf. Rev.* **2011**, *35*, 50–65. [CrossRef]
51. Steuer, J.; Biocca, F.; Levy, M.R. Defining virtual reality: Dimensions determining telepresence. *Commun. Age Virtual Real.* **1995**, *33*, 37–39. [CrossRef]
52. Davis, F.D. New Measures for Three User Acceptance Constructs: Attitude Toward Using, Perceived Usefulness, and Perceived Ease of Use. Student Thesis, University of Michigan, Ann Arbor, MI, USA, 1987.
53. Sweeney, A.D.; Morrison, M.D.; Jarratt, D.; Heffernan, T. Modeling the constructs contributing to the effectiveness of marketing lecturers. *J. Mark. Educ.* **2009**, *31*, 190–202. [CrossRef]
54. Lin, C.P.; Bhattacherjee, A. Extending technology usage models to interactive hedonic technologies: A theoretical model and empirical test. *Inf. Syst. J.* **2010**, *20*, 163–181. [CrossRef]
55. Wilkes, R.E. A structural modeling approach to the measurement and meaning of cognitive age. *J. Consum. Res.* **1992**, *19*, 292–301. [CrossRef]
56. Taylor, S.; Todd, P.A. Understanding information technology usage: A test of competing models. *Inf. Syst. Res.* **1995**, *6*, 144–176. [CrossRef]
57. Batool, K.; Iqbal, M.N.; Mushtaq, R.; Shakeel, M. Effectiveness of Assistive Technology in Teaching Mathematics to the Students with Hearing Impairment at Primary Level. *VFAST Trans. Educ. Soc. Sci.* **2022**, *10*, 93–99.
58. Bambacas, M.; Patrickson, M. Interpersonal communication skills that enhance organisational commitment. *J. Commun. Manag.* **2008**, *12*, 51–72. [CrossRef]
59. Gugenheimer, J.; Plaumann, K.; Schaub, F.; Vito, P.D.C.S.; Duck, S.; Rabus, M.; Rukzio, E. The Impact of Assistive Technology on Communication Quality Between Deaf and Hearing Individuals. In Proceedings of the 2017 ACM Conference on Computer Supported Cooperative Work and Social Computing, Portland, OR, USA, 25 February–1 March 2017; pp. 669–682.
60. Sockalingam, R.; Holmberg, M.; Eneroth, K.; Shulte, M. Binaural hearing aid communication shown to improve sound quality and localization. *Hear. J.* **2009**, *62*, 46–47. [CrossRef]
61. Reddy, C.K.A.; Shankar, N.; Bhat, G.S.; Charan, R.; Panahi, I. An Individualized Super-Gaussian Single Microphone Speech Enhancement for Hearing Aid Users with Smartphone as an Assistive Device. *IEEE Signal Process. Lett.* **2017**, *24*, 1601–1605. [CrossRef] [PubMed]
62. López-Espejo, I.; Tan, Z.-H.; Jensen, J. Improved external speaker-robust keyword spotting for hearing assistive devices. *IEEE/ACM Trans. Audio Speech Lang. Process.* **2020**, *28*, 1233–1247. [CrossRef]
63. Ganguly, A.; Küçük, A.; Panahi, I. Real-time smartphone application for improving spatial awareness of hearing assistive devices. In Proceedings of the 2018 40th Annual International Conference of the IEEE Engineering in Medicine and Biology Society (EMBC), Honolulu, HI, USA, 18–21 July 2018; pp. 433–436.

64. Skehan, P. Processing perspectives on task performance. In *Processing Perspectives on Task Performance*; John Benjamins Publishing Company: Amsterdam, The Netherlands, 2014; pp. 1–278.
65. Tavakoli, P.; Skehan, P. 9. Strategic planning, task structure and performance testing. In *Planning and Task Performance in a Second Language*; John Benjamins: Amsterdam, The Netherlands, 2005; pp. 239–273.
66. Hilton, H. Oral fluency and spoken proficiency: Considerations for research and testing. *Meas. L2 Profic. Perspect. SLA* **2014**, *27*, 53.
67. Niparko, J.K.; Marlowe, A. Hearing aids and cochlear implants. In *Oxford Handbook of Auditory Science: The Ear*; Oxford University Press: Oxford, UK, 2010; pp. 409–436. [CrossRef]
68. Gao, Q.; Rau, P.-L.P.; Salvendy, G. Measuring perceived interactivity of mobile advertisements. *Behav. Inf. Technol.* **2010**, *29*, 35–44. [CrossRef]
69. Arshad, M.; Akram, M.S. Social media adoption by the academic community: Theoretical insights and empirical evidence from developing countries. *Int. Rev. Res. Open Distrib. Learn.* **2018**, *19*, 244–262. [CrossRef]
70. Abdullah, D.; Jayaraman, K.; Shariff, D.; Bahari, K.A.; Nor, N.M. The effects of perceived interactivity, perceived ease of use and perceived usefulness on online hotel booking intention: A conceptual framework. *Int. Acad. Res. J. Soc. Sci.* **2017**, *3*, 16–23.
71. Jiarui, W.; Xiaoli, Z.; Jiafu, S. Interpersonal Relationship, Knowledge Characteristic, and Knowledge Sharing Behavior of Online Community Members: A TAM Perspective. *Comput. Intell. Neurosci.* **2022**, *2022*, 4188480. [CrossRef] [PubMed]
72. Chan, T.J.; Yong, W.K.; Harmizi, A. Usage of WhatsApp and interpersonal communication skills among private university students. *J. Arts Soc. Sci.* **2020**, *3*, 15–25.
73. Mittal, S.; Gera, R.; Batra, D.K. An evaluation of an integrated perspective of perceived service quality for retail banking services in India. *Int. J. Bank Mark.* **2015**, *33*, 330–350. [CrossRef]
74. Jin, H.K.; Park, S.H.; Kang, J.E.; Choi, K.S.; Kim, H.A.; Jeon, M.S.; Rhie, S.J. The influence of a patient counseling training session on pharmacy students' self-perceived communication skills, confidence levels, and attitudes about communication skills training. *BMC Med. Educ.* **2019**, *19*, 172. [CrossRef]
75. Blood, G.W.; Blood, I.M.; Tellis, G.; Gabel, R. Communication apprehension and self-perceived communication competence in adolescents who stutter. *J. Fluen. Disord.* **2001**, *26*, 161–178. [CrossRef]
76. Power, M.R.; Power, D.; Horstmanshof, L. Deaf people communicating via SMS, TTY, relay service, fax, and computers in Australia. *J. Deaf Stud. Deaf Educ.* **2007**, *12*, 80–92. [CrossRef]
77. Pilling, D.; Barrett, P. Text communication preferences of deaf people in the United Kingdom. *J. Deaf Stud. Deaf Educ.* **2008**, *13*, 92–103. [CrossRef] [PubMed]
78. Sexton, J. Empowering adolescents who are deaf and hard of hearing. *N. Carol. Med. J.* **2017**, *78*, 129–130. [CrossRef]
79. Dawes, P.; Maslin, M.; Munro, K.J. 'Getting used to'hearing aids from the perspective of adult hearing-aid users. *Int. J. Audiol.* **2014**, *53*, 861–870. [CrossRef] [PubMed]
80. Backenroth, G.A.; Ahlner, B.H. Quality of life of hearing-impaired persons who have participated in audiological rehabilitation counselling. *Int. J. Adv. Couns.* **2000**, *22*, 225–240. [CrossRef]
81. Khairani, A.; Ahmad, R.; Marjohan, M. Contribution of self image to interpersonal communication between students in the schools. *J. Couns. Educ. Technol.* **2019**, *2*, 65–70. [CrossRef]
82. Rodriguez Mosquera, P.M.; Uskul, A.K.; Cross, S.E. The centrality of social image in social psychology. *Eur. J. Soc. Psychol.* **2011**, *41*, 403–410. [CrossRef]
83. Lee, S.; Park, H.; Ahn, Y. The influence of tourists' experience of quality of street foods on destination's image, life satisfaction, and word of mouth: The moderating impact of food neophobia. *Int. J. Environ. Res. Public Health* **2020**, *17*, 163. [CrossRef]
84. Li, H.; Lien, C.-H.; Wang, S.W.; Wang, T.; Dong, W. Event and city image: The effect on revisit intention. *Tour. Rev.* **2021**, *76*, 212–228. [CrossRef]
85. Heffernan, E.; Coulson, N.S.; Henshaw, H.; Barry, J.G.; Ferguson, M.A. Understanding the psychosocial experiences of adults with mild-moderate hearing loss: An application of Leventhal's self-regulatory model. *Int. J. Audiol.* **2016**, *55*, S3–S12. [CrossRef] [PubMed]
86. Barak, A.; Sadovsky, Y. Internet use and personal empowerment of hearing-impaired adolescents. *Comput. Hum. Behav.* **2008**, *24*, 1802–1815. [CrossRef]
87. Lin, C.-P.; Huang, H.-N.; Joe, S.-W.; Ma, H.-C. Learning the Determinants of Satisfaction and Usage Intention of Instant Messaging. *CyberPsychol. Behav.* **2008**, *11*, 262–267. [CrossRef]
88. Bénabou, R.; Tirole, J. Self-confidence and personal motivation. *Q. J. Econ.* **2002**, *117*, 871–915. [CrossRef]
89. Lubis, L.; Fazira, E. Connection Management Self-Concept and Social Support with Student Confidence. *Nidhomul Haq: J. Manaj. Pendidik. Islam* **2022**, *7*, 31–38. [CrossRef]
90. Foustanos, A.; Pantazi, L.; Zavrides, H. Representations in Plastic Surgery: The Impact of Self-Image and Self-Confidence in the Work Environment. *Aesthetic Plast. Surg.* **2007**, *31*, 435–442. [CrossRef]
91. Simsek, N.; Evli, M.; Uzdil, N.; Albayrak, E.; Kartal, D. Body Image and Sexual Self-confidence in Patients with Chronic Urticaria. *Sex. Disabil.* **2020**, *38*, 147–159. [CrossRef]
92. Venkatesh, V.; Morris, M.G. Why don't men ever stop to ask for directions? Gender, social influence, and their role in technology acceptance and usage behavior. *MIS Q.* **2000**, *24*, 115–139. [CrossRef]

93. Kim, H.-W.; Gupta, S.; Koh, J. Investigating the intention to purchase digital items in social networking communities: A customer value perspective. *Inf. Manag.* **2011**, *48*, 228–234. [CrossRef]
94. Bispo, R.; Branco, V. *Designing out Stigma: A New Approach to Designing for Human Diversity*; European Academy of Design: Porto, Portugal, 2011.
95. Stankov, L.; Lee, J.; Luo, W.; Hogan, D.J. Confidence: A better predictor of academic achievement than self-efficacy, self-concept and anxiety? *Learn. Individ. Differ.* **2012**, *22*, 747–758. [CrossRef]
96. Hong, J.-C.; Hwang, M.-Y.; Tai, K.-H.; Tsai, C.-R. An Exploration of Students' Science Learning Interest Related to Their Cognitive Anxiety, Cognitive Load, Self-Confidence and Learning Progress Using Inquiry-Based Learning with an iPad. *Res. Sci. Educ.* **2017**, *47*, 1193–1212. [CrossRef]
97. Kim, H.-S.; Ahn, J.; No, J.-K. Applying the Health Belief Model to college students' health behavior. *Nutr. Res. Pract.* **2012**, *6*, 551–558. [CrossRef] [PubMed]
98. Chai, C.S.; Lin, P.Y.; Jong, M.S.y.; Dai, Y.; Chiu, T.K.F.; Huang, B. Factors Influencing Students' Behavioral Intention to Continue Artificial Intelligence Learning. In Proceedings of the 2020 International Symposium on Educational Technology (ISET), Bangkok, Thailand, 24–27 August 2020; pp. 147–150.
99. Shanahan, T.; Tran, T.P.; Taylor, E.C. Getting to know you: Social media personalization as a means of enhancing brand loyalty and perceived quality. *J. Retail. Consum. Serv.* **2019**, *47*, 57–65. [CrossRef]
100. Wang, Y.-Y.; Wang, Y.-S.; Lin, H.-H.; Tsai, T.-H. Developing and validating a model for assessing paid mobile learning app success. *Interact. Learn. Environ.* **2019**, *27*, 458–477. [CrossRef]
101. Huang, L.-T.; Chiu, C.-A.; Sung, K.; Farn, C.-K. A comparative study on the flow experience in web-based and text-based interaction environments. *Cyberpsychol. Behav. Soc. Netw.* **2011**, *14*, 3–11. [CrossRef]
102. Khlaisang, J.; Songkram, N.; Huang, F.; Teo, T. Teachers' perception of the use of mobile technologies with smart applications to enhance students' thinking skills: A study among primary school teachers in Thailand. *Interact. Learn. Environ.* **2023**, *31*, 5037–5058. [CrossRef]
103. Lam, C.; Campbell, K.S. Follow the Leader? The Impact of Leader Rapport Management on Social Loafing. *Bus. Prof. Commun. Q.* **2021**, *84*, 181–204. [CrossRef]
104. Yang, H.; Yu, J.; Zo, H.; Choi, M. User acceptance of wearable devices: An extended perspective of perceived value. *Telemat. Inform.* **2016**, *33*, 256–269. [CrossRef]
105. Rajeh, M.T.; Abduljabbar, F.H.; Alqahtani, S.M.; Waly, F.J.; Alnaami, I.; Aljurayyan, A.; Alzaman, N. Students' satisfaction and continued intention toward e-learning: A theory-based study. *Med. Educ. Online* **2021**, *26*, 1961348. [CrossRef]
106. Hong, J.-C.; Lin, P.-H.; Hsieh, P.-C. The effect of consumer innovativeness on perceived value and continuance intention to use smartwatch. *Comput. Hum. Behav.* **2017**, *67*, 264–272. [CrossRef]
107. Deng, L.; Wei, W.; Chen, J. A Study on the Impact Mechanisms of Users' Behavioral Intentions Towards Augmented Reality Picture Books for Adult Readers. *Int. J. Hum. Comput. Interact.* **2024**, 1–18. [CrossRef]
108. Hair, J.F.; Risher, J.J.; Sarstedt, M.; Ringle, C.M. When to use and how to report the results of PLS-SEM. *Eur. Bus. Rev.* **2019**, *31*, 2–24. [CrossRef]
109. Fornell, C.; Larcker, D.F. Evaluating structural equation models with unobservable variables and measurement error. *J. Mark. Res.* **1981**, *18*, 39–50. [CrossRef]
110. Henseler, J.; Ringle, C.M.; Sarstedt, M. A new criterion for assessing discriminant validity in variance-based structural equation modeling. *J. Acad. Mark. Sci.* **2015**, *43*, 115–135. [CrossRef]
111. Gold, A.H.; Malhotra, A.; Segars, A.H. Knowledge management: An organizational capabilities perspective. *J. Manag. Inf. Syst.* **2001**, *18*, 185–214. [CrossRef]
112. Henseler, J.; Ringle, C.M.; Sinkovics, R.R. The use of partial least squares path modeling in international marketing. In *New Challenges to International Marketing*; Emerald Group Publishing Limited: Bingley, UK, 2009; Volume 20, pp. 277–319.
113. Cohen, J. *Statistical Power Analysis for the Behavioral Sciences*; Lawrence Erlbaum: Hillsdale, NJ, USA, 1988; pp. 75–108.
114. Eksvärd, S.; Falk, J. Evaluating Speech-to-Text Systems and AR-glasses: A study to develop a potential assistive device for people with hearing impairments. Student Thesis, Uppsala University, Uppsala, Sweden, 2021.
115. Helvik, A.-S.; Jacobsen, G.; Svebak, S.; Hallberg, L.R.M. Hearing Impairment, Sense of Humour and Communication Strategies. *Scand. J. Disabil. Res.* **2007**, *9*, 1–13. [CrossRef]
116. Barrenas, M.-L.; Holgers, K.-M. A clinical evaluation of the hearing disability and handicap scale in men with noise induced hearing loss. *Noise Health* **2000**, *2*, 67. [PubMed]
117. de Miranda, R.S.; Shubert, C.O.; Machado, W.C.A. Communication with people with hearing disabilities: An integrative review. *Rev. Pesqui. Cuid. Fundam. Online* **2014**, *6*, 1695–1706. [CrossRef]
118. Hines, J. Communication problems of hearing-impaired patients. *Nurs. Stand. (Through 2013)* **2000**, *14*, 33. [CrossRef]
119. Bion, W.R. *Attention and Interpretation*; Jason Aronson: Lanham, MD, USA, 1995.
120. Tajfel, H.; Turner, J.C. The social identity theory of intergroup behavior. In *Political Psychology*; Psychology Press: London, UK, 2004; pp. 276–293.
121. Vicars, W.G. Is Being Deaf a Disability? Available online: https://www.lifeprint.com/asl101/topics/disability-deafness.htm (accessed on 2 February 2024).

122. Faucett, H.A.; Ringland, K.E.; Cullen, A.L.; Hayes, G.R. (In) visibility in disability and assistive technology. *ACM Trans. Access. Comput. (TACCESS)* **2017**, *10*, 1–17. [CrossRef]
123. Bandura, A. Self-efficacy: Toward a unifying theory of behavioral change. *Psychol. Rev.* **1977**, *84*, 191. [CrossRef]

behavioral sciences

MDPI

Article

Links between Vaccination Fear-, Anxiety-, Alexithymia-, and Type D Personality-Related Vaccination Decisions: A Network Analysis in a Multicultural Sample

Olga Malas [1,*], Nada Mallah Boustani [2], Mirko Duradoni [3], Dayo Omotoso [4], Asiye Şengül Avşar [5], Anastasiia Shyroka [6], Giulia Colombini [3] and Maria Dolores Tolsá [7]

1 Department of Psychology, Sociology and Social Work, University of Lleida, Avinguda de l'Estudi General, 4, 25001 Lleida, Spain
2 Faculty of Business and Management, Saint Joseph University, Mar Mikhael, Beirut 1104 2020, Lebanon
3 Department of Education, Languages, Interculture, Literatures and Psychology, University of Florence, Via di San Salvi, 12, Building 26, 50135 Florence, Italy
4 Department of Human Anatomy, Redeemer's University, Ede 232103, Osun State, Nigeria
5 Department of Measurement and Evaluation in Education, Recep Tayyip Erdoğan University, Campus Zihni Derin, Fener Mahallesi, 53100 Rize, Turkey
6 Department of Psychology and Psychotherapy, Ukrainian Catholic University, Sventsitskogo 17, 79011 Lviv, Ukraine
7 eHealth, Research Centre, C/Cristofol de Boleda, 1-2, 25006 Lleida, Spain
* Correspondence: author: olga.malas@udl.cat

Abstract: This study examines the links between vaccination status, fear of vaccination (cognitive and somatic symptoms), anxiety, alexithymia, and type D personality (negative affect and social inhibition), to propose policies to increase vaccination rates. A sample of university students (n = 2535; mean age = 20.59, SD = 2.04; male: 26.75%, female: 73.25%) from Spain, Italy, Lebanon, Nigeria, Turkey, and Ukraine completed the Vaccination Fear Scale (VFS-6), the Generalised Anxiety Disorder scale (GAD-7), the Perth Alexithymia Questionnaire—Short Form (PAQ-S), the Type D Scale (DS14), and also a question on vaccination status. Correlation, regression, and network analyses were applied. Cognitive symptoms of fear of vaccination and negative affect were the most significant in the correlation and regression analyses. In the network analysis, negative affect showed the highest values in all centrality indices and positive relationships with other nodes. Vaccination status showed negative relationships with fear of vaccination, alexithymia, and social inhibition. The network structure is similar between the sexes but varies between cultures and sexes within cultures. The relationship between vaccination status and cognitive symptoms of fear of vaccination was the most consistent, allowing for interventions at this level to be advised across cultures. For more specific interventions, cultural context must be considered for optimal results.

Keywords: vaccination; fear; anxiety; personality type D; alexithymia; network analysis

1. Introduction

There is consensus that vaccination constitutes a crucial intervention that prevents between two and three million deaths per year, standing out as one of the most economically efficient strategies for the prevention of infectious diseases [1,2]. Despite these clear benefits, vaccination rates have seen a decline in recent years, emerging as one of the top ten threats to global health [2]. Consequently, the imperative to improve vaccination rates has been captured in the strategic framework supporting the Sustainable Development Goals (SDGs) outlined in the 2030 Agenda, a commitment made by all member states of the United Nations [1].

The existing literature on vaccine hesitancy and resistance primarily focuses on describing sociodemographic factors. In this context, risk factors for vaccine resistance have been identified as being young, female [3,4], single, childless, from rural areas [5], with a low educational level [5], low income [5,6], without health insurance [3], and belonging to a minority ethnic group [5,6]. Additionally, mistrust of authorities and health experts and certain political views [7–9], religious or personal beliefs against vaccination [3,10], and other conspiracy beliefs [11–13] have also been described.

Studies on psychopathological factors or mood states are less common. Among specific phobias, trypanophobia, or fear of needles, has been described as a factor of reluctance [11,12,14]. An underlying factor in vaccine refusal is fear of vaccination [15–17], which has been shown to be a more significant predictor than vaccine hesitancy [18] or fear of becoming infected with the disease [16]. Therefore, as symptoms of fear are easily identifiable and interventions exist to manage them, researchers in this field suggest developing strategies to reduce fear of vaccination [19].

Fear and anxiety often show a good correlation, but there are no data to establish a positive relationship between anxiety and vaccination status [20]. Theoretically, people with anxiety disorders tend to overestimate threats [21], have a greater intolerance of uncertainty [22], and may be more hesitant than those without anxiety problems [23], which could affect their decision to get vaccinated. In any case, studies conducted during the COVID-19 pandemic, when health authorities were urging vaccination, show that anxious and non-anxious individuals did not differ in terms of COVID-19 vaccine hesitancy and acceptance [24]. There are also data indicating that COVID-19-related anxiety was positively associated with vaccination [20]. This contrasts with other studies suggesting that the fear of vaccination correlates positively with generalised anxiety [25].

It is known that personality traits exert a considerable influence on health behaviour [26]. In this context, traits which are regarded as risk factors for vaccine rejection include paranoid tendencies and low levels of conscientiousness, agreeableness, emotional stability, and empathy [8,27]. Similarly, studies indicate that individuals with lower levels of emotional stability, conscientiousness, and agreeableness, but higher levels of openness to experience, expressed less confidence in the safety of vaccines [3,5]. Openness to experience, conscientiousness, extraversion, agreeableness, and negative emotionality were associated with COVID-19 vaccine rejection; however, the facets of agreeableness, conscientiousness, and openness tended to lose importance in favour of negative emotionality and extraversion as the circumstances of the pandemic changed [28]. These results suggest a possible connection between type D personality and alexithymia with vaccine hesitancy.

There is little evidence on the impact of alexithymia or type D personality on vaccine hesitancy. Both are known to be risk factors for anxiety, depression [29,30], and various physical pathologies [29]. Alexithymia is a multidimensional personality trait characterised by difficulties in identifying and describing emotions, an impoverished fantasy life, and an outward-oriented thinking style, which could be relevant to vaccine hesitancy [31,32]. The rationale for suggesting a predictive role of alexithymia in vaccine hesitancy is based on the concept that the lack of access to personal emotions and emotional empathy compromises the ability to understand the emotional significance of protecting oneself and others from infection through vaccination [33]. Type D personality was defined by Denollet et al. [34] as a distressed personality construct characterised by the simultaneous and synergistic interplay of its two components: negative affectivity (NA), or a tendency towards negative thoughts and emotions, and social inhibition (SI), or difficulty in expressing such thoughts and emotions. SI has been associated with high negative emotionality and personal distress [35] and has a high, significant, and negative correlation with extraversion [36]. When individuals experience a life-threatening situation, negative affect (expressed as fear and anxiety) can motivate them to act in the interest of their health [37] and promote vaccination [38]. However, a recent study revealed that negative affect correlated negatively with intentions to vaccinate against COVID-19 [39], which aligns with the hypothesis that in uncertain and uncontrollable situations, individuals focus on reducing negative affect rather than reducing potential threats through behavioural changes [40]. Therefore, fostering vaccination intentions through an individual's negative affect may stimulate more fear and the inability to adopt preventive measures such as vaccination [39,41].

In this way, the objective of this study was to investigate the relationships of potentially relevant factors such as fear of vaccination, generalised anxiety, alexithymia, type D personality (negative affect and social inhibition), related to vaccination status, taking into account the sex and culture of the study population The ultimate goal is to identify common factors, regardless of context, that influence the decision to get vaccinated, enabling the design of pro-vaccination campaigns that are applicable across different settings, making them more cost-effective and feasible in public health.

The network analysis was applied in the present study. This methodology has already been used in previous studies to investigate the association between different psychological alterations, e.g., [42,43]. This type of analysis is characterised by providing a comprehensive visual representation of the complex relationships between the variables under study, which facilitates a deeper understanding of the direct and indirect interactions between variables from a data-driven perspective. This is challenging when using more traditional multivariate techniques [42,43]. Additionally, it offers the advantage of identifying central and influential variables within the structure, bridge nodes that specifically connect the variables under study, and the strength of the interconnections [42,44]. This can help to underpin specific interventions and strategies for addressing these issues [43].

2. Methods

2.1. Participants

The sample comprised college students from Spain (n = 388), Italy (n = 376), Lebanon (n = 487), Nigeria (n = 561), Turkey (n = 410), and Ukraine (n = 313). Of the pooled data set (n = 2535) which included less than 25-year-old students only (M_{age} = 20.59, SD = 2.04), 73.25% were females while 26.75% were males. Table 1 shows additional background information.

Table 1. Descriptive and frequency analysis (TS: total sample, n = 2535; 1. Spain, n = 388; 2. Italy, n = 376; 3. Lebanon, n = 487; 4. Nigeria, n = 561; 5. Turkey, n = 410; and 6. Ukraine, n = 313).

Variable		TS	Sample Nationality 1	2	3	4	5	6	X^2/df p
Vaccination (%)	Yes	76.41	96.40	96.01	87.47	37.61	92.93	58.79	707.27
	No	23.59	3.60	3.99	12.53	62.39	7.07	41.21	<0.001
VFS-6	Median	11.0	8.0	8.0	11.0	14.0	13.0	9.0	66.78
	IR	8.0–15.0	7.0–12.0	7.0–11.0	8.0–16.0	10.0–18.0	9.0–17.0	7.0–13.0	<0.001
VFS1	Median	7.0	5.0	5.0	7.0	9.0	9.0	6.0	62.54
	IR	4.0–10.0	4.0–8.0	4.0–7.0	5.0–9.0	6.0–12.0	5.0–11.0	4.0–9.0	<0.001
VFS2	Median	3.0	3.0	3.0	4.0	4.0	3.0	3.0	54.76
	IR	3.0–5.0	3.0–3.0	3.0–3.0	3.0–7.0	3.0–8.0	3.0–6.0	3.0–4.0	<0.001
GAD-7	Median	9.0	10.0	8.0	9.0	9.0	9.0	7.0	10.29
	IR	5.0–13.0	6.0–13.0	6.0–12.0	6.0–14.0	5.0–14.0	6.0–14.0	4.0–11.0	<0.001
PAQ-S	Median	18.0	16.5	16.0	21.0	22.0	15.0	17.0	47.71
	IR	13.0–24.0	11.0–22.0	12.0–21.0	16.0–27.0	16.0–28.0	10.0–21.2	12.0–22.0	<0.001
DS14	Median	37,0	35.0	38.0	35.0	40.0	38.0	34.0	17.26
	IR	30.0–44.0	28.0–41.0	30.0–47.0	30.0–43.0	33.0–46.5	30.7–45.0	27.0–42.0	<0.001
NA	Median	18.0	17.0	20.0	18.0	18.0	20.0	16.0	14.37
	IR	14.0–23.0	13.0–21.0	16.0–24.0	15.0–23.0	13.5–22.5	15.0–25.0	13.0–21.0	<0.001
SI	Median	18.0	18.0	18.5	17.0	22.0	18.0	18.0	39.17
	IR	15.0–23.0	14.0–20.7	14.0–24.0	15.0–21.0	18.0–25.0	13.7–22.0	13.0–22.0	<0.001

VFS-6: Vaccination Fear Scale. VFS1: cognitive fear measured with VFS-6. VFS2: somatic fear measured with VFS-6. GAD-7: generalised anxiety disorder. PAQ-S: alexithymia. DS14: type D personality. NA: negative affect measured with DS14. SI: social inhibition measured with DS14. IR = interquartile range; X^2/df = Kruskal–Wallis test expressed as Chi-square/df.

The inclusion/exclusion criteria were being a university student under 25 years of age and being fluent in the language used in the forms. University students were selected to ensure homogeneous samples with respect to academic level and other social characteristics. A sample size of 250 or more per country was required because simulation studies have shown that sample sizes of 250 are generally sufficient for networks of up to 10 to 25 nodes [45,46]. In this case, the network consists of 7 nodes (1 binary and 6 continuous), so the sample size is considered appropriate for the current study.

2.2. Procedure

The countries included in this study (Spain, Italy, Lebanon, Nigeria, Turkey, and Ukraine) were selected through an open call for researchers interested in collaborating on the study. Those who participated voluntarily accepted the invitation, demonstrating their commitment to contributing to the research.

The data were collected in 2023, during the final phase of the COVID-19 pandemic, prior to the WHO declaration of the end of the health crisis, when a booster vaccination was recommended but not mandatory. The articles found on this topic were written before the pandemic or during its critical phases, when the perception of disease risk was high, and the importance of immunisation was significant. However, there are few studies focused on the final phase of the pandemic, when the risk perception still existed but was lower, and there was more information about the safety and effectiveness of the vaccines that would be received. Hence, this research could be timely in offering evidence-based updates on predictive vaccination variables in the absence of a pandemic emergency, which could be relevant for any vaccination programme.

The questionnaire was administered in the official language of each participating country (Spanish, Italian, Arabic, English, Turkish, and Ukrainian). The scales are already validated in these languages, so cross-cultural adaptation was not required. The questionnaire was administered online. The link to the questionnaire was sent to university professors, requesting their voluntary collaboration in the study. Those who agreed forwarded the link to their students. Students who voluntarily clicked on the link first accessed the informed consent document. This document informed potential participants about the study's objectives, the intended use of the data, and the measures taken to ensure the confidentiality of the data collected. Explicitly providing informed consent was a necessary requirement for continuing and participating in the study. The Ethical Review Committee of the University of Lleida was responsible for granting ethical approval for this study (study authorisation number: CERT23).

2.3. Instruments

Vaccination Status: A binary question (yes/no) was included to determine whether the participant had received the vaccine.

Vaccination Fear Scale (VFS-6; [16,25]): This scale consists of 6 items, divided into two correlated factors with 3 items each. The first factor assesses cognitive symptoms of the fear of vaccination (F1: items 1, 2, and 4), while the second factor evaluates somatic symptoms (F2: items 3, 5, and 6). The items are rated on a 5-point Likert scale, ranging from 1 (strongly disagree) to 5 (strongly agree), with total scores ranging from 6 to 30. Higher scores indicate higher levels of fear of vaccination. The items are applicable to any vaccine; in this case, they were adapted to assess fear of the COVID-19 vaccine. In this study, the scale from Spain, Italy, Lebanon, Nigeria, Turkey, and Ukraine revealed a Cronbach's α from 0.83 to 0.88; a cognitive factor from 0.80 to 0.89; and a somatic factor from 0.81 to 0.91.

Generalised Anxiety Disorder (GAD-7; [47]): This scale comprises 7 items that assess symptoms such as feeling nervous or anxious; excessive worry about various things; easy irritability; or a sense of fear that something terrible might happen. The items are scored on a 4-point Likert scale, ranging from 0 (not at all) to 3 (every day), with total scores ranging from 0 to 21. Scores above 10 are considered to be in the clinical range. In this study, Cronbach's α values of 0.86 to 0.91 were obtained for the scales used in Spain, Italy, Lebanon, Nigeria, Turkey, and Ukraine.

Type D Personality Scale (DS14; [48]): The DS14 is a 14-item scale with two subscales. One subscale measure negative affectivity (NA: items 2, 4, 5, 7, 9, 12, and 13), and the other measure social inhibition (SI: items 1, 3, 6, 8, 10, 11, and 14). Items are rated on a 5-point Likert scale ranging from 0 = false to 4 = true (items 1 and 3 are reverse-scored). In this study, the Cronbach's alpha obtained for the total sample was 0.86 and 0.80 for NA and SI, respectively. In this study, the scale from Spain, Italy, Lebanon, Nigeria, Turkey, and Ukraine revealed a Cronbach's α from 0.83 to 0.90; an NA factor from 0.80 to 0.89; and an SI factor from 0.66 to 0.88.

Perth Alexithymia Questionnaire—Short Form (PAQ-S; [49]): This is a unidimensional scale consisting of 6 items, scored on a 7-point Likert scale ranging from 1 (completely disagree) to 7 (completely agree). Higher scores indicate higher levels of alexithymia. In the total sample of this study, the Cronbach's alpha obtained was 0.83, indicating good internal consistency. In this study, the scale from Spain, Italy, Lebanon, Nigeria, Turkey, and Ukraine revealed a Cronbach's α from 0.79 to 0.87.

2.4. Statistical Analysis

Descriptive, frequency, and inferential analyses were conducted using the SPSS v.28 software. The quantitative variables on a ratio scale were subjected to the Kolmogorov–Smirnov normality tests ($n > 50$). None of the variables fulfilled the assumption of normality ($p < 0.05$), so they were analysed through non-parametric inferential tests. Consequently, for the analysis of differences, medians and interquartile ranges were calculated for continuous variables, such as scores on the applied scales, while frequencies were computed for categorical variables, such as vaccination status. Subsequently, the Kruskal–Wallis test was applied to compare the medians of continuous variables and the Chi-square test to compare the frequencies of categorical variables. Spearman's *Rho* coefficient was used to evaluate the correlations between the main variables. The strength of the association and its directionality were assessed by Gamma (Γ) and Somers' *d* statistics, respectively. Finally, the predictive capacity of the variables on vaccination status was determined by hierarchical regression analyses. Due to the absence of prior studies providing a specific order of importance for the variables in our particular context, we opted to use the SPSS automatic stepwise approach. This method allows us to evaluate the incremental contribution of each variable, providing valuable information about their relative influence in the model.

Following this, using the JASP v.0.18.3.0 package, network analysis was applied to elucidate and confirm the factorial structure of the different scales used in the study and their independence (based on the items from the different applied scales). Subsequently, network analysis was conducted for the data on vaccination status, fear of vaccination measured with the VFS-6 as cognitive fear and somatic fear, generalised anxiety disorder measured with the GAD-7, alexithymia measured with the PAQ-S, and type D personality measured with the DS14 as negative affect and social inhibition.

The analysis was conducted following the recommendations of Epskamp et al. [50]. The first step involved the use of a pairwise Markov random field (PMRF; [51]). Specifically, a Mixed Graphical Model (MGM) with regularised estimation using the extended Bayesian information criterion (EBIC) was used [50]. MGM is applied as it is the most appropriate technique for processing data that contain continuous and categorical variables [52]. An EBIC is used to estimate model parameters and select the most appropriate network structure while avoiding overfitting by allowing for simpler and more parsimonious models to be chosen [50].

When used to conduct network psychometrics, in the MGM, using PMRF, the variables are represented as nodes in a graph, and connections or relationships between variables are represented as edges. These edges are grouped into ordered and related subnetworks, forming clusters similar to latent variables [53], indicating the degree to which they represent a dimension, thereby demonstrating whether the components significantly measure a construct [54]. In the second case, the analysis is applied to elucidate the network structure of the continuous and categorical variables in the study. The network plot was used to establish the conditional dependence of each node considering all other nodes in the network [55]. To obtain information about the relevance of each node, four centrality indices were estimated: betweenness, closeness, strength, and expected influence [50]. In this study, particular attention was paid to the edges between nodes, both positive and negative, and edge weights that represent the strength of the conditional association between nodes. Finally, following Hevey's [55] recommendations, the stability of the nodes was also examined using the subset bootstrap procedure based on 1000 iterations [50].

3. Results

3.1. Descriptive, Frequency, and Inferential Analysis

The descriptive and frequency analysis are shown in Table 1. The results reveal statistically significant differences between the countries for all analysed variables ($p < 0.001$). Vaccination rates vary widely, from 37.61% in Nigeria to 96.40% in Spain. Analysis of vaccination fear (VFS-6) shows medians ranging from 8.0 in Spain and Italy to 14.0 in Nigeria. The cognitive fear component (VFS1) has medians of 5.0 in Spain and Italy, and 9.0 in Nigeria and Turkey, while the somatic fear (VFS2) shows less variability, with medians of 3.0 in most countries and 4.0 in Lebanon and Nigeria. The medians for generalised anxiety disorder (GAD-7) are relatively homogeneous, varying between 7.0 in Turkey and 10.0 in Spain. For alexithymia (PAQ-S) and type D personality, medians range from 15.0 and 34.0 in Turkey to 22.0 and 40.0 in Nigeria, respectively, reflecting differences in emotional regulation and levels of negative affect and social inhibition between the countries.

In summary, countries with high vaccination rates, such as Spain and Italy, show the lowest medians for vaccination fear. In contrast, Nigeria, with the lowest vaccination rate, has the highest medians for vaccination fear, as well as for alexithymia, negative affect, and social inhibition.

3.2. Correlation and Regression Analysis

As detailed in Table 2, and as expected, all analysed variables show significant Spearman Rho correlation with each other and with vaccination status, with significance levels at 0.01 (two-tailed). Among these variables, cognitive fear (VFS1) exhibits the most notable correlation with vaccination status ($Rho = -0.311$), indicating a moderate negative relationship. The importance of this relationship is further supported by the directionality and strength of the association ($\Gamma = -0.454$; $d = -0.239$). Following this, alexithymia (PAQ-S), cognitive fear (VFS2), and social inhibition (SI) present weaker negative correlations, with directionality and strength of association values consistent with these results. Although significant, negative affect (NA) and anxiety (GAD) show much weaker positive correlations.

Table 2. Correlations, strength, and directionality between the analysed variables and vaccination state.

	Spearman Rho Correlations									Strength & Directionality		
	VS	VFS	VFS1	VFS2	GAD	PAQ	DS	NA	SI	*p*	Γ	*d*
VS	--									--	--	--
VFS	−0.280	--								--	--	--
VFS1	−0.311	0.953	--							<0.001	−0.454	−0.239
VFS2	−0.124	0.748	0.547	--						<0.001	−0.223	−0.109
GAD	0.021	0.165	0.133	0.181	--					0.285	0.031	0.016
PAQ	−0.142	0.263	0.212	0.283	0.315	--				<0.001	−0.199	−0.105

Table 2. *Cont.*

	Spearman Rho Correlations									Strength & Directionality		
	VS	VFS	VFS1	VFS2	GAD	PAQ	DS	NA	SI	*p*	Γ	*d*
DS	−0.031	0.244	0.216	0.211	0.447	0.471	--			--	--	--
NA	0.069	0.217	0.189	0.187	0.533	0.419	0.872	--		<0.001	0.098	0.051
SI	−0.122	0.209	0.183	0.192	0.230	0.406	0.848	0.497	--	<0.001	−0.174	−0.091

Note: All correlations were significant at the 0.01 level (two-tailed) VS: vaccination state. VFS: fear measured with VFS-6. VFS1: cognitive fear measured with VFS-6. VFS2: somatic fear measured with VFS-6. DS: type D personality measured with DS14. NA: negative affect measured with DS14. SI: social inhibition measured with DS14.

The results for hierarchical regression analysis (see Table 3) indicated that vaccination status was more strongly associated with the cognitive factor of fear of vaccination (VFS1), thereby explaining the 10.3% vaccination status in the total sample, during the final phase of the pandemic. The introduction of the other variables step by step allowed for an increase in explained variance to 15.8%. Generalised anxiety did not increase the explained variance in the total sample, confirming the results obtained in the correlation analysis.

Table 3. Hierarchical regression analysis for vaccination state versus analysed variables.

Model		*B*	*B* IC95%		*t*	*p*	r^2	Δr^2
1	VFS1	−0.321	−0.043	−0.034	−17.036	<0.001	0.103	0.103
2	VFS1	−0.344	−0.046	−0.037	−18.170	<0.001	0.120	0.017
	NA	0.133	0.006	0.012	6.996	<0.001		
3	VFS1	−0.330	−0.044	−0.035	−17.541	<0.001	0.139	0.020
	NA	0.212	0.012	0.017	9.879	<0.001		
	SI	−0.163	−0.015	−0.009	−7.577	<0.001		
4	VFS1	−0.316	−0.042	−0.033	−16.763	<0.001	0.151	0.011
	NA	0.247	0.014	0.020	11.135	<0.001		
	SI	−0.131	−0.013	−0.006	−5.930	<0.001		
	PAQ	−0.124	−0.009	−0.004	−5.839	<0.001		
5	VFS1	−0.367	−0.049	−0.039	−16.893	<0.001	0.158	0.007
	NA	0.239	0.013	0.019	10.810	<0.001		
	SI	−0.136	−0.013	−0.007	−6.173	<0.001		
	PAQ	−0.140	−0.010	−0.005	−6.557	<0.001		
	VFS2	0.104	0.009	0.023	4.643	<0.001		

VFS1: cognitive fear measured with VFS-6. VFS2: somatic fear measured with VFS-6. PAQ: alexithymia measured with PAQ-S. NA: negative affect measured with DS14. SI: social inhibition measured with DS14.

3.3. Psychometric Network Analysis

The results of the network analysis, after introducing all the items from the questionnaires (VFS-6, GAD-7, PAQ-S, and DS16), can be seen in Figure 1. The items were clearly grouped as expected, in ordered and related subnetworks, forming clusters that corresponded to the latent variables of this study. This demonstrated that the components significantly measured their corresponding constructs, indicating good independence among them.

The network analysis, depending on sex, showed the same clusters, but with a sparsity (related nodes/total nodes) of 0.648 in males and 0.593 in females (being 0.589 in the total sample). This suggested a greater interrelation among items from different scales and subscales in females than in males. The network analysis, depending on the country, revealed the same node grouping and clusters, but with a sparsity ranging from 0.746 to 0.636. This suggested a more complex interrelation among items in the Lebanese sample, followed by the Nigerian, Ukrainian, Turkish, Spanish, and Italian samples, respectively.

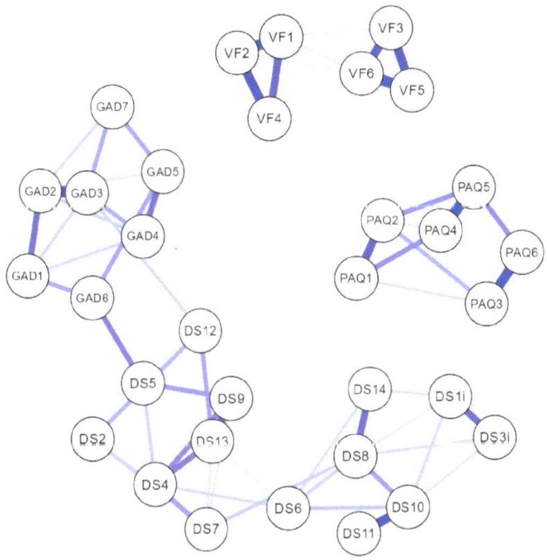

Figure 1. The network obtained for the total sample. VF: VFS-6 items. GAD: GAD-7 items. PAQ: PAQ-S items. DS: DS14 items.

Strong relationships were observed between certain items of the GAD-7 (items 3 and 6) and NA (items 5 and 12), particularly in the Ukrainian sample and to a lesser extent in the Lebanese sample. In contrast, in the Lebanese sample, the items of the DS14 formed a well-defined cluster, but not the NA and SI subnetworks, which, although ordered in proximity as expected, exhibited complex relationships among their items and also with the PAQ-S and VFS-6. The results of this analysis can be found in the Supplementary Material.

3.4. Network Analysis

The NwA plot, incorporating the total scores of the VFS-6, GAD-7, PAQ-S, and DS14 scales and subscales (continuous variables), as well as responses to the dichotomous vaccination status question (categorical variable), is shown in Figure 2. The network displayed seven nodes, with a sparsity of 0.048, indicating a clear interrelation among all the nodes.

The network weight matrix and centrality measures for the total sample can be seen in Table 4. Centrality plots are available in Figure 3. The node showing the highest centrality in the network was negative affect, followed by vaccination status. Negative affect was positively connected with vaccination status ($r = 0.251$; $p < 0.05$), anxiety ($r = 0.438$; $p < 0.05$), and all other nodes in the network.

Table 4. Network weight matrix and centrality measures for total sample ($n = 2535$).

	Weight Matrix							Centrality Measures			
Variable	**VS**	**VFS1**	**VFS2**	**GAD**	**PAQ**	**NA**	**SI**	**Betweenness**	**Closeness**	**Strength**	**Expected Influence**
VS	0.000							1.303	1.305	0.410	−1.555
VFS1	−0.398	0.000						0.391	−0.205	0.357	−0.619
VFS2	0.105	0.493	0.000					−0.521	−1.106	−0.454	0.683
GAD	0.000	0.020	0.019	0.000				−0.977	−0.805	−1.422	0.038
PAQ	−0.172	−0.038	0.172	0.108	0.000			−0.521	−0.218	−0.379	−0.029
NA	0.251	0.101	0.032	0.438	0.205	0.000		1.303	1.464	1.799	1.644
SI	−0.163	−0.027	0.060	−0.065	0.206	0.396	0.000	−0.977	−0.435	−0.310	−0.163

VS: vaccination State. VFS1: cognitive fear measured with VFS-6. VFS2: somatic fear measured with VFS-6. GAD: generalised anxiety disorder measured with GAD-7. PAQ: alexithymia measured with GAD-7. NA: negative affect measured with DS14. SI: social inhibition measured with DS14.

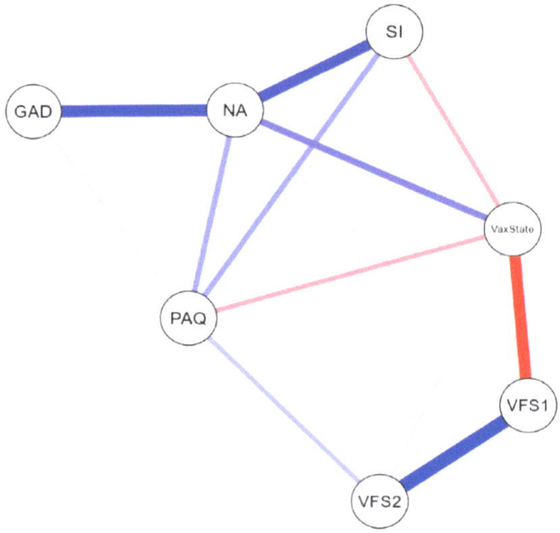

Figure 2. Total sample network plot (n = 2.535). VFS1: cognitive fear measured with VFS-6. VFS2: somatic fear measured with VFS-6. GAD: generalised anxiety disorder measured with GAD-7. PAQ: alexithymia measured with PAQ-S. NA: negative affect measured with DS14. SI: social inhibition measured with DS14.

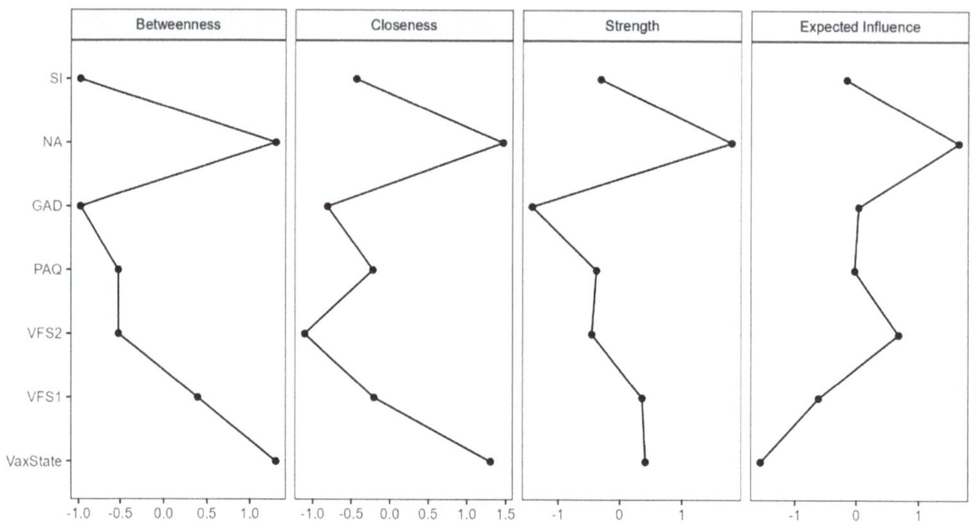

Figure 3. Centrality plots for total sample network analysis (n = 2535). VFS1: cognitive fear measured with VFS-6. VFS2: somatic fear measured with VFS-6. GAD: generalised anxiety disorder measured with GAD-7. PAQ: alexithymia measured with GAD-7. NA: negative affect measured with DS14. SI: social inhibition measured with DS14.

On the other hand, vaccination status, besides exhibiting a strong positive relationship with negative affect, showed negative edges with the cognitive factor of vaccination fear ($r = -0.398$; $p < 0.05$), social inhibition ($r = -0.163$; $p < 0.05$), and alexithymia ($r = -0.172$; $p < 0.05$).

Anxiety lacked centrality, but it exhibited positive values of expected influence in the network. Similarly, the somatic factor of vaccination fear did not show adequate centrality values, but it could exert its effect through the cognitive factor, which displayed positive values of strength and betweenness centrality, explaining the weight matrix between factors (VFS2/VFS1: $r = 0.493$; $p < 0.05$; VFS2/VS: $r = 0.105$; $p < 0.05$).

The stability data of the nodes, after applying a subset bootstrap procedure based on 1000 iterations, were very adequate (see Figure 4), confirming the adequacy of the sample size.

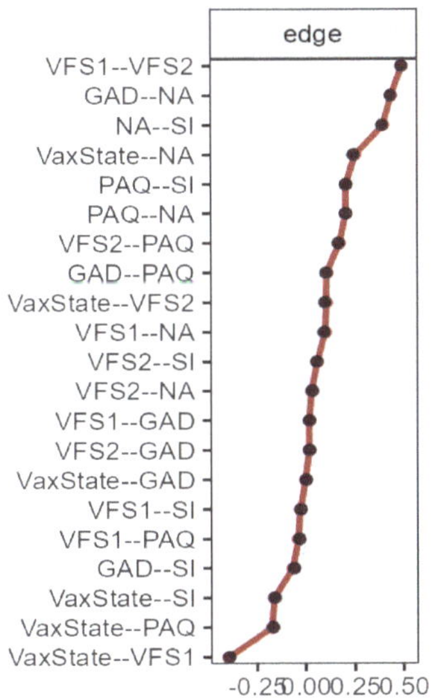

Figure 4. Edge stability for total sample network analysis ($n = 2535$). The edge weights, with each horizontal line representing an edge, are represented by the red line, and the 95% confidence intervals by the grey area. VS: vaccination state. VFS1: cognitive fear measured with VFS-6. VFS2: somatic fear measured with VFS-6. GAD: generalised anxiety disorder measured with GAD-7. PAQ: alexithymia measured with GAD-7. NA: negative affect measured with DS14. SI: social inhibition measured with DS14.

3.5. Network Analysis for Sex and Cultures

The network analysis depending on sex resulted in an equivalent network structure between the male and female samples and with the total sample. However, there was a lower sparsity value in females compared to males (0.143/0.238), indicating a greater number of relationships between items among females. On the contrary, the network analysis depending on culture resulted in network structures with significant differences between them and with the total sample. The results of this analysis can be found in the Supplementary Material.

The sparsity values ranged from 0.238 in Spain, Italy, and Lebanon to 0.381 in the Turkish sample, 0.429 in the Nigerian sample, and 0.476 in the Ukrainian sample (from more to fewer relationships between items). Similarly, to the total sample, negative affect exhibits the highest centrality in all samples, except for the Spanish sample, where it only appeared in the female sample. On the other hand, vaccination status retained some of its indices only in certain samples. Anxiety showed good, expected influence in all samples, regardless of sex, with notable centrality observed for all its indices in the Spanish sample of both sexes, and for some of its indices in the Nigerian, Turkish, and Ukrainian samples. Additionally, notable centrality was observed for alexithymia in the Lebanese sample and social inhibition in the Turkish sample. In general, the factors of vaccination fear became important, as they exhibit positive values in some of their centrality indices across all samples. The edge analysis revealed the presence of positive edges of negative affect with all or some of the other nodes in the network, but with a less significant weight matrix in its relationship with vaccination status. On the other hand, vaccination status showed negative edges with cognitive fear in the Nigerian, Turkish, and Ukrainian samples of both sexes and in the Italian and Lebanese samples of females. It also exhibited negative edges with somatic fear of vaccination in the Spanish male sample. Negative edges were also observed with anxiety in the Spanish female sample and with alexithymia in the Lebanese female sample and the Ukrainian male sample.

4. Discussion

The study involved researchers from Spain, Italy, Lebanon, Nigeria, Turkey, and Ukraine. Although the sample was not intentionally selected, it provides valuable geographical and cultural diversity, enriching the analysis of how factors such as vaccine fear, generalised anxiety, alexithymia, and type D personality influence vaccination decisions. The most significant differences pertain to the individualistic or collectivist characteristics of their societies, trust in health authorities, vaccine accessibility, and the type of vaccine administered. Spain and Italy, with an individualistic orientation, focus on personal decision-making [56]. In contrast, Lebanon and Nigeria exhibit more collectivist traits, where health decisions are often based on social norms and community expectations, as well as the opinions of community, family, or religious leaders [57–63]. Turkey and Ukraine, on the other hand, have mixed characteristics [56], leading to a combination of individual and collective influences on vaccination. Trust in health authorities also varies significantly among these countries, particularly in the context of the COVID-19 pandemic. In Spain, Italy, and Turkey, trust in health authorities was relatively high; in contrast, trust was lower in Lebanon and Nigeria, with misinformation significantly impacting vaccine acceptance [58,59]. In Ukraine, before the conflict, there was generally a positive disposition towards vaccines, though trust in authorities could be variable depending on the local context [59]. Vaccine accessibility also varied. In Ukraine, access to vaccines was relatively universal before the conflict [58,59], but this changed afterwards. In Nigeria, vaccine accessibility was more uneven due to challenges in health infrastructure and distribution [60]. In Lebanon, universities played a crucial role in providing vaccines to students, thereby improving accessibility for this demographic group [61]. Regarding specific vaccines administered, Pfizer-BioNTech was used in Spain, Italy, Turkey, Lebanon, and Ukraine; Moderna in Spain and Italy; AstraZeneca in Spain, Italy, Turkey, Lebanon, and Nigeria; Janssen in Spain, Italy, and Nigeria; Sinovac (CoronaVac) in Turkey and Ukraine; Sinopharm in Nigeria; and Sputnik V in Turkey and Ukraine [59–61]. Generally, Pfizer-BioNTech, Moderna, and AstraZeneca encountered less rejection compared to vaccines such as Sinovac, Sinopharm, and Sputnik V [62].

The results of the correlation analysis showed a significant and negative relationship between cognitive fear of vaccination and vaccination status. Directionality and strength results support this finding, indicating it as a factor to consider. Correlations were also negative, although of low magnitude, with alexithymia and social inhibition. These findings suggest that, although there is a relationship, it is relatively weak, indicating that these factors have limited influence on the decision to vaccinate. Contrary to expectations, negative affect showed a positive correlation, albeit of low magnitude. Therefore, its effect would have a very limited impact on vaccination status. Moreover, although the initial hypothesis suggested that generalised anxiety might be related to vaccination status, the results did not show a significant correlation between these variables. This finding could suggest that generalised anxiety is not a relevant predictor of vaccination behaviour in this specific sample. The regression analysis confirmed the results of the correlation analysis for cognitive symptoms of vaccination fear, indicating an explanatory capacity of 10.3%. However, the regression also showed that negative affect, despite its positive correlation, increases the explained variance of the model from 10.3% to 12%, suggesting an additional significant predictive effect. Similarly, social inhibition and alexithymia increase the explained variance up to 15.8%, reflecting their predictive importance.

The network analysis can provide an explanation for these results. This analysis allowed for the identification of central variables and the most influential interactions within the network structure generated by the study variables. This approach provided a deeper understanding of how the studied factors interrelate, highlighting negative affect as a central node that connects all variables to each other. Thus, while it presented a positive edge with vaccination status, it also exhibited edges with anxiety, alexithymia, social inhibition, and the vaccination fear factors. Therefore, although it has a direct positive effect, indirectly it could have a negative effect, explaining its capacity to increase the explained variance in vaccination status.

The results of this study suggested that vaccination fear, especially the cognitive fear factor, was significantly related to vaccination status. This finding is consistent with previous research that identifies fear as a crucial factor in vaccine hesitancy [15–17], with fear of vaccination being a stronger predictor compared to hesitancy [18] or fear of the targeted disease [16]. The negative association between cognitive fear and vaccination status indicated that those with higher levels of cognitive fear are less likely to get vaccinated, underscoring the need for specific interventions to reduce this type of fear, in particular, because fear symptoms were relatively identifiable and manageable [19].

Contrary to the hypothesis proposed, generalised anxiety did not show a significant correlation with vaccination status. This finding aligns with studies conducted during the COVID-19 pandemic, where no significant differences in vaccine hesitancy were found between anxious and non-anxious individuals [24]. Thus, while some studies have found positive correlations between anxiety and vaccination fear [16,25], others suggested that anxiety about COVID-19 may be positively associated with vaccination [20]. The lack of a significant correlation could indicate that generalised anxiety is not a reliable predictor of the intention to vaccinate in the context of the final phase of the pandemic. This may also be because its variability overlapped with that of other variables, not providing additional relevant information to explain the variability of the dependent variable. In any case, the network analysis indicated that, although anxiety lacks centrality, it exhibited positive values of expected influence in the network, suggesting that it may exert its effect through other variables.

The results also suggested that difficulty in identifying and expressing emotions (a characteristic of alexithymia) and a tendency to avoid social interaction (typical of type D personality) may contribute to vaccine hesitancy. These findings are consistent with studies that reported that a lack of access to personal emotions and emotional empathy can compromise the ability to understand the importance of vaccination [33]. Additionally, although negative affect showed positive relationships with vaccination status, it also exhibited them with alexithymia and social inhibition. Denollet [48] described how in type D personality, the combination of negative affect and social inhibition can result in avoidance behaviours. However, in the context of vaccination, the NA component alone can drive preventive behaviour, which would be consistent with the hypothesis of Ferrer and Klein [56], who suggested that individuals with a high perception of risk are more likely to adopt preventive behaviours. In the current study, it is observed that negative affect without the presence of high social inhibition could motivate vaccination, which is consistent with the finding of a positive correlation between negative affect and vaccination.

The descriptive analysis revealed significant differences among samples from different countries in terms of sex, vaccination fear, anxiety, alexithymia, and type D personality. On the other hand, network analysis provided a detailed insight into how variables interrelate depending on sex and cultural context. Thus, no significant differences were observed between sexes, but differences were found between cultures. In all analysed countries, vaccination status showed a significant negative edge with the cognitive fear factor of vaccination. This indicated consistency in how vaccination fear negatively influences vaccination status across diverse cultures. Negative affect also emerged as a central node (in all samples except among Spanish males) thereby underscoring its importance in the network of analysed variables. Additionally, specific nodes and edges highlighted the importance of anxiety in the Spanish, Turkish, and Ukrainian samples; alexithymia in the Italian, Lebanese, Nigerian, and Ukrainian samples; and social inhibition in the Turkish and Ukrainian samples. These differences underscored the importance of cultural and sociodemographic factors when designing strategies to increase vaccination rates.

In any case, the most significant finding of our study is that, regardless of national characteristics such as collectivism versus individualism, trust in the healthcare system, or vaccine availability, fear of vaccination emerges as the most central factor in the decision to get vaccinated. This result could be extrapolated to other countries, suggesting that, regardless of context, fear of vaccination has a significant influence on vaccine acceptance. Therefore, countries facing similar challenges with vaccine acceptance could use these data to focus their communication and education strategies on addressing vaccine-related fears.

Limitations and Conclusions

There were several limitations that need to be addressed. Firstly, the research findings can only be generalised to university students under the age of 25. It is unclear whether the results would also be applicable to the general population. Second, the non-directed selection of participating countries also presents limitations. The sample is not representative of all regions of the world, which may restrict the generalisability of the results to other geographic areas not included in the study. Therefore, it is recommended that future research consider a more strategic selection of countries to validate and expand these findings. Third, while fear of vaccination has been identified as a central factor in vaccine acceptance, the results were obtained specifically within the context of COVID-19 vaccination. Therefore, to determine whether these findings are applicable to other vaccines, additional research in those specific contexts is needed.

Another limitation of the study is that the questions about vaccination were designed with binary response options (yes/no), which did not capture variations in the reception of one or multiple doses of the vaccine or differences in vaccination schedules between countries. This simplified approach allowed for efficient and uniform data collection among participants, facilitating general comparisons of vaccine acceptance. However, it may have overlooked important factors influencing vaccination perception and acceptance, such as the number of doses received or variations in vaccination schedules. Additionally, the study was conducted during the final phase of the pandemic, when attitudes towards vaccination might have changed compared to the more critical phases of the health crisis. Therefore, it is possible that these aspects influenced the results, and a more detailed exploration of these variables in future research could provide a more comprehensive understanding of vaccine acceptance.

In any case, this study underscores the importance of fear, especially cognitive fear, in vaccine hesitancy. While generalised anxiety does not appear to be a significant predictor of vaccination intention, alexithymia and type D personality do, albeit to a lesser extent. Additionally, cultural and sociodemographic differences highlight the need for personalised approaches to increase vaccination rates. Network analysis emerges as a valuable tool for understanding the complex interactions among factors influencing vaccination, providing a solid foundation for future public health interventions and strategies.

Supplementary Materials: Network analysis supporting information can be downloaded at https://www.mdpi.com/article/10.3390/bs14090761/s1.

Author Contributions: Conceptualisation, O.M. and M.D.T.; methodology, O.M. and M.D.T.; formal analysis, O.M. and M.D.T.; investigation, O.M., N.M.B., M.D., D.O., A.Ş.A., A.S. and G.C.; data curation, O.M.; writing—original draft preparation, O.M.; writing—review and editing, N.M.B., M.D., D.O., A.Ş.A. and A.S.; project administration, M.D.T. All authors have read and agreed to the published version of the manuscript.

Funding: This research received no external funding.

Institutional Review Board Statement: The study was conducted in accordance with the Declaration of Helsinki and approved by the Ethical Review Committee of the University of Lleida (study authorisation number: CERT23, dated 12 July 2023).

Informed Consent Statement: Informed consent was obtained from all subjects involved in the study.

Data Availability Statement: Data will be made available upon request.

Conflicts of Interest: The authors declare no conflicts of interest.

References

1. World Health Organization. Health in the 2030 Agenda for Sustainable Development. Sixty-Ninth World Health Assembly. Document A69/15. April 2016. Available online: https://apps.who.int/gb/e/e_wha69.html (accessed on 9 May 2024).
2. World Health Organization. Immunization Coverage. July 2022. Available online: https://www.who.int/news-room/fact-sheets/detail/immunization-coverage (accessed on 9 May 2024).
3. Lin, F.Y.; Wang, C.H. Personality and individual attitudes toward vaccination: A nationally representative survey in the United States. *BMC Public Health* **2020**, *20*, 1759. [CrossRef] [PubMed]
4. Salali, G.D.; Uysal, M.S. COVID-19 vaccine hesitancy is associated with beliefs on the origin of the novel coronavirus in the UK and Turkey. *Psychol. Med.* **2022**, *52*, 3750–3752. [CrossRef]
5. Lee, C.H.; Duck, I.M.; Sibley, C.G. Personality and demographic correlates of New Zealanders' confidence in the safety of childhood vaccinations. *Vaccine* **2017**, *35*, 6089–6095. [CrossRef] [PubMed]
6. Jeudin, P.; Liveright, E.; Del Carmen, M.G.; Perkins, R.B. Race, ethnicity, and income factors impacting human papillomavirus vaccination rates. *Clin. Therap.* **2014**, *36*, 24–37. [CrossRef]
7. Cadeddu, C.; Daugbjerg, S.; Ricciardi, W.; Rosano, A. Beliefs towards vaccination and trust in the scientific community in Italy. *Vaccine* **2020**, *38*, 6609–6617. [CrossRef]
8. Candio, P.; Violato, M.; Clarke, P.M.; Duch, R.; Roope, L.S. Prevalence, predictors and reasons for COVID-19 vaccine hesitancy: Results of a global online survey. *Health Policy* **2023**, *137*, 104895. [CrossRef]
9. Fridman, A.; Gershon, R.; Gneezy, A. COVID-19 and vaccine hesitancy: A longitudinal study. *PLoS ONE* **2021**, *16*, e0250123. [CrossRef] [PubMed]
10. Amin, A.B.; Bednarczyk, R.A.; Ray, C.E.; Melchiori, K.J.; Graham, J.; Huntsinger, J.R.; Omer, S.B. Association of moral values with vaccine hesitancy. *Nat. Hum. Behav.* **2017**, *1*, 873–880. [CrossRef]
11. Freeman, D.; Lambe, S.; Yu, L.M.; Freeman, J.; Chadwick, A.; Vaccari, C.; Waite, F.; Rosebrock, L.; Petit, A.; Vanderslott, S.; et al. Injection fears and COVID-19 vaccine hesitancy. *Psychol. Med.* **2023**, *53*, 1185–1195. [CrossRef]
12. Hornsey, M.J.; Harris, E.A.; Fielding, K.S. The psychological roots of anti-vaccination attitudes: A 24-nation investigation. *Health Psychol.* **2018**, *37*, 307. [CrossRef]
13. Malas, O. Influence of fear on anti-vaccine conspiracy theories and behaviour against vaccination. *Rev. Psicol. Salud* **2023**, *11*, 179–192. [CrossRef]
14. Malas, O.; Tolsá, M.D. Needle-related fear versus vaccination fear, vaccination intention, and declared reasons for avoiding vaccination. *Clínica Salud* **2022**, *33*, 101–107. [CrossRef]
15. Kahan, D.M.; Braman, D.; Cohen, G.L.; Gastil, J.; Slovic, P. Who fears the HPV vaccine, who doesn't, and why? An experimental study of the mechanisms of cultural cognition. *Law Hum. Behav.* **2010**, *34*, 501–516. [CrossRef]
16. Malas, O.; Tolsá, M.D. Vaccination Fear Scale (VFS-6): Development and Initial Validation. *Medit. J. Clin. Psychol.* **2021**, *9*. [CrossRef]
17. Peretti-Watel, P.; Raude, J.; Sagaon-Teyssier, L.; Constant, A.; Verger, P.; Beck, F. Attitudes toward vaccination and the H1N1 vaccine: Poor people's unfounded fears or legitimate concerns of the elite? *Soc. Sci. Med.* **2014**, *109*, 10–18. [CrossRef] [PubMed]
18. Duradoni, M.; Veloso, M.V.; La Gamma, M.; Monciatti, A.M.; Guazzini, A. Italian version of the Vaccination Fear Scale (VFS-6): Internal and external validation. *Medit. J. Clin. Psychol.* **2022**, *10*, 1–19. [CrossRef]
19. Ochnik, D.; Rogowska, A.M.; Benatov, J.; Arzenšek, A. Adaptation and Preliminary Validation of the Fear of Coronavirus Vaccination Scale in the Prospective Study among a Representative Sample of Polish, Israeli, Slovenian, and German Adults during the COVID-19 Pandemic. *Int. J. Environ. Res. Public Health* **2022**, *19*, 11587. [CrossRef] [PubMed]
20. Bendau, A.; Plag, J.; Petzold, M.B.; Ströhle, A. COVID-19 vaccine hesitancy and related fears and anxiety. *Int. Immunopharmacol.* **2021**, *97*, 107724. [CrossRef]
21. Ferreri, F.; Lapp, L.K.; Peretti, C.S. Current research on cognitive aspects of anxiety disorders. *Curr. Opi. Psychiatry* **2011**, *24*, 49–54. [CrossRef]
22. Oglesby, M.E.; Schmidt, N.B. The role of threat level and intolerance of uncertainty (IU) in anxiety: An experimental test of IU theory. *Behav. Ther.* **2017**, *48*, 427–434. [CrossRef]
23. Birrell, J.; Meares, K.; Wilkinson, A.; Freeston, M. Toward a definition of intolerance of uncertainty: A review of factor analytical studies of the Intolerance of Uncertainty Scale. *Clin. Psychol. Rev.* **2011**, *31*, 1198–1208. [CrossRef] [PubMed]
24. McNeil, A.; Purdon, C. Anxiety disorders, COVID-19 fear, and vaccine hesitancy. *J. Anxiety Disord.* **2022**, *90*, 102598. [CrossRef]

25. Malas, O.; Boustani, N.M.; Duradoni, M.; Omotoso, D.; Avşar, A.Ş.; Shyroka, A.; Colombini, G.; Blanch, A. The Vaccination Fear Scale (VFS-6): Adaptation, Cross-Cultural Validation, and Invariance among Genders and Six Different Cultures, Applying Classical Test Theory (CTT) and Item Response Theory (IRT). *Eur. J. Investig. Health Psychol. Educ.* **2024**, *14*, 808–822. [CrossRef]
26. Turiano, N.A.; Hill, P.; Graham, E.K.; Mroczek, D.K. 22 associations between personality and health behaviors across the life span. In *The Oxford Handbook of Integrative Health Science*, 2nd ed.; Ryff, C.D., Krueger, R.F., Eds.; Oxford University Press: New York, NY, USA, 2018; p. 305. [CrossRef]
27. Pfattheicher, S.; Petersen, M.B.; Böhm, R. Information about herd immunity through vaccination and empathy promote COVID-19 vaccination intentions. *Health Psychol.* **2022**, *41*, 85. [CrossRef] [PubMed]
28. Baker, M.N.; Merkley, E. Dynamic role of personality in explaining COVID-19 vaccine hesitancy and refusal. *Front. Psychol.* **2023**, *14*, 1163570. [CrossRef]
29. Pedersen, S.S.; Denollet, J. Type D personality, cardiac events, and impaired quality of life: A review. *Eur. J. Prev. Cardiol.* **2003**, *10*, 241–248. [CrossRef] [PubMed]
30. Tselebis, A.; Kosmas, E.; Bratis, D.; Moussas, G.; Karkanias, A.; Ilias, I.; Tzanakis, N. Prevalence of alexithymia and its association with anxiety and depression in a sample of Greek chronic obstructive pulmonary disease (COPD) outpatients. *Ann. Gen. Psychiatry.* **2010**, *9*, 1–7. [CrossRef]
31. Barchetta, S.; Martino, G.; Craparo, G.; Salehinejad, M.A.; Nitsche, M.A.; Vicario, C.M. Alexithymia is linked with a negative bias for past and current events in healthy humans. *Int. J. Environ. Res. Public Health* **2021**, *18*, 6696. [CrossRef]
32. Vicario, C.M.; Martino, G.; Marcuzzo, A.; Craparo, G. No evidence of perceptual pseudoneglect in Alexithymia. *Brain Sci.* **2021**, *11*, 376. [CrossRef]
33. Vicario, C.M.; Mucciardi, M.; Faraone, G.; Lucifora, C.; Schade, H.M.; Falzone, A.; Nitsche, M.A. Individual predictors of vaccine hesitancy in the Italian post COVID-19 pandemic era. Hum. *Vaccines Immunother.* **2024**, *20*, 2306677. [CrossRef]
34. Denollet, J.; Rombouts, H.; Gillebert, T.C.; Brutsaert, D.L.; Sys, S.U.; Stroobant, N. Personality as independent predictor of long-term mortality in patients with coronary heart disease. *Lancet* **1996**, *347*, 417–421. [CrossRef] [PubMed]
35. Eisenberg, N.; Fabes, R.A.; Murphy, B.C. Relations of shyness and low sociability to regulation and emotionality. *J. Pers. Soc. Psychol.* **1995**, *68*, 505. [CrossRef]
36. De Fruyt, F.; Denollet, J. Type D personality: A five-factor model perspective. *Psychol. Health* **2002**, *17*, 671–683. [CrossRef]
37. Tugade, M.M.; Fredrickson, B.L. Resilient individuals use positive emotions to bounce back from negative emotional experiences. *J. Pers. Soc. Psychol.* **2004**, *86*, 320. [CrossRef] [PubMed]
38. Lin, T.T.; Bautista, J.R. Predicting intention to take protective measures during haze: The roles of efficacy, threat, media trust, and affective attitude. *J. Health Commun.* **2016**, *21*, 790–799. [CrossRef] [PubMed]
39. Zou, X.; Chen, Q.; Zhang, Y.; Evans, R. Predicting COVID-19 vaccination intentions: The roles of threat appraisal, coping appraisal, subjective norms, and negative affect. *BMC Public Health* **2023**, *23*, 230. [CrossRef] [PubMed]
40. Lerner, J.S.; Keltner, D. Fear, anger, and risk. *J. Pers. Soc. Psychol.* **2001**, *81*, 146. [CrossRef]
41. Chou, W.Y.S.; Budenz, A. Considering emotion in COVID-19 vaccine communication: Addressing vaccine hesitancy and fostering vaccine confidence. *Health Commun.* **2020**, *35*, 1718–1722. [CrossRef]
42. Cheung, T.; Jin, Y.; Lam, S.; Su, Z.; Hall, B.J.; Xiang, Y.T. Network analysis of depressive symptoms in Hong Kong residents during the COVID-19 pandemic. *Transl. Psychiatry* **2021**, *11*, 460. [CrossRef]
43. Sardella, A.; Varallo, G.; Agus, M.; Lenzo, V.; Zagaria, A.; Terrone, G.; Franceschini, C. Anxiety, depression, emotion regulation, and daytime sleepiness: Are there links between these factors? Network analysis on an Italian sample during the COVID-19 pandemic. *Clin. Neuropsychiatry* **2023**, *20*, 395. [CrossRef]
44. Jones, P.J.; Ma, R.; McNally, R.J. Bridge centrality: A network approach to understanding comorbidity. *Multivar. Behav. Res.* **2021**, *56*, 353–367. [CrossRef]
45. Epskamp, S. Brief report on estimating regularized gaussian networks from continuous and ordinal data. *arXiv* **2016**, arXiv:1606.05771. [CrossRef]
46. Van Borkulo, C.D.; Borsboom, D.; Epskamp, S.; Blanken, T.F.; Boschloo, L.; Schoevers, R.A.; Waldorp, L.J. A new method for constructing networks from binary data. *Sci. Rep.* **2014**, *4*, 5918. [CrossRef] [PubMed]
47. Spitzer, R.L.; Kroenke, K.; Williams, J.B.W.; Löwe, B. A brief measure for assessing generalized anxiety disorder the GAD-7. *Arch. Intern. Med.* **2006**, *166*, 1092–1097. [CrossRef] [PubMed]
48. Denollet, J. DS14: Standard assessment of negative affectivity, social inhibition, and Type D personality. *Psychosom. Med.* **2005**, *67*, 89–97. [CrossRef] [PubMed]
49. Preece, D.A.; Mehta, A.; Petrova, K.; Sikka, P.; Bjureberg, J.; Chen, W.; Becerra, R.; Allan, A.; Robinson, K.; Gross, J.J. The Perth Alexithymia Questionnaire-Short form (PAQ-S): A 6-item measure of alexithymia. *J. Affect. Disord.* **2023**, *325*, 493–501. [CrossRef] [PubMed]
50. Epskamp, S.; Borsboom, D.; Fried, E.I. Estimating psychological networks and their accuracy: A tutorial paper. *Behav. Res. Methods* **2018**, *50*, 195–212. [CrossRef]
51. Robinaugh, D.J.; Millner, A.J.; McNally, R.J. Identifying highly influential nodes in the complicated grief network. *J. Abnorm. Psychol.* **2016**, *125*, 747. [CrossRef]
52. Haslbeck, J.M.B.; Waldorp, L.J. MGM: Estimating time-varying mixed graphical models in high-dimensional data. *J. Stat. Softw.* **2020**, *93*, 1–46. [CrossRef]

53. Epskamp, S.; Rhemtulla, M.; Borsboom, D. Generalized network psychometrics: Combining network and latent variable models. *Psychometrika* **2017**, *82*, 904–927. [CrossRef]
54. Christensen, A.P.; Golino, H.; Silvia, P.J. A psychometric network perspective on the validity and validation of personality trait questionnaires. *Eur. J. Personal.* **2020**, *34*, 1095–1108. [CrossRef]
55. Hevey, D. Network analysis: A brief overview and tutorial. *Health Psychol. Behav. Med.* **2018**, *6*, 301–328. [CrossRef] [PubMed]
56. Triandis, H.C. *Individualism and Collectivism*; Routledge: London, UK, 2018.
57. Schwartz, S.H. A Theory of Cultural Value Orientations: Explication and Applications. *Compar. Sociol.* **2006**, *5*, 137–182. [CrossRef]
58. Leigh, J.P.; Moss, S.J.; White, T.M.; Picchio, C.A.; Rabin, K.H.; Ratzan, S.C.; Wyka, K.; El-Mohandes, A.; Lazarus, J.V. Factors affecting COVID-19 vaccine hesitancy among healthcare providers in 23 countries. *Vaccine* **2022**, *40*, 4081–4089. [CrossRef]
59. Lazarus, J.V.; Wyka, K.; White, T.M.; Picchio, C.A.; Gostin, L.O.; Larson, H.J.; Rabin, K.; Ratzan, S.C.; Kamarulzaman, A.; El-Mohandes, A. A survey of COVID-19 vaccine acceptance across 23 countries in 2022. *Nat. Med.* **2023**, *29*, 366–375. [CrossRef]
60. Olu-Abiodun, O.; Abiodun, O.; Okafor, N. COVID-19 vaccination in Nigeria: A rapid review of vaccine acceptance rate and the associated factors. *PLoS ONE* **2022**, *17*, e0267691. [CrossRef]
61. Hamdan, M.B.; Singh, S.; Polavarapu, M.; Jordan, T.R.; Melhem, N.M. COVID-19 vaccine hesitancy among university students in Lebanon. *Epidemiol. Infect.* **2021**, *149*, e242. [CrossRef]
62. Rahman, M.M.; Masum, M.H.U.; Wajed, S.; Talukder, A. A comprehensive review on COVID-19 vaccines: Development, effectiveness, adverse effects, distribution and challenges. *Virusdisease* **2022**, *33*, 1–22. [CrossRef] [PubMed]
63. Ferrer, R.A.; Klein, W.M. Risk perceptions and health behavior. *Curr. Opin. Psychol.* **2015**, *5*, 85–89. [CrossRef] [PubMed]

behavioral sciences

MDPI

Article

The Impact of Home Medication Management Practices on Medication Adherence

Lisa Gualtieri [1,*], Meredith Steinfeldt [2], Eden Shaveet [3], Brandon Estime [4] and Meera Singhal [5]

1 Tufts University School of Medicine, Boston, MA 02111, USA
2 Nicklaus Children's Health System, Miami, FL 33155, USA; meredith.steinfeldt@nicklaushealth.org
3 Cornell University, New York, NY 10044, USA; ems486@cornell.edu
4 Children's National Hospital, Washington, DC 20010, USA; bestime@childrensnational.org
5 Lewis Katz School of Medicine, Temple University, Philadelphia, PA 19140, USA; meera.singhal@temple.edu
* Correspondence: lisa.gualtieri@tufts.edu; Tel.: +1-781-330-9456

Abstract: Medication adherence is a vexing challenge, with over 50% of US adults not adhering to their prescribed medication regimen. Most medications are self-administered by patients at home, requiring them to independently develop and manage their own medication routines. By understanding these home-based practices, such as where patients store their medications and how different storage locations impact adherence, we can develop targeted interventions to improve adherence rates. Our goal was to identify and categorize self-reported home medication management practices and determine which practices are associated with self-reported medication adherence. From the 1673 total survey respondents we learned that the most common places people store their medications at home are nightstand drawers (28%), on top of nightstands (27%), kitchen cabinets (22%), and bathroom medicine cabinets (20%). Kitchen cabinets and bathroom vanities were significantly associated with increased odds of having ever forgotten to take a medication. On the other hand, desks, dining room tables, and the inside of nightstand drawers were associated with the greatest statistically significant decrease in odds of having ever forgotten to take a medication. Almost all (96%) respondents were receptive to receiving guidance from healthcare providers on how to store medications. Patients are largely responsible for creating their own home medication management practices, including deciding where to store their medication at home. Understanding which home storage locations are associated with medication adherence can lead to innovative approaches to improve adherence, including personalized guidance to patients from their healthcare providers for patients.

Keywords: medication adherence; home medication management; survey; digital health; user-centered design

1. Introduction

1.1. Definition and Importance

Medication adherence, defined as the extent to which patients take medication as prescribed, was highlighted as "a problem of striking magnitude" by the World Health Organization (WHO) [1]. Studies indicate that 50% or fewer US adults are adherent to their medication, which has contributed to deaths and hospital admissions [2–4]. The problem of medication nonadherence is growing across all ages, racial/ethnic groups, and sexes [5]. With the prevalence of nonadherence and the severity of the health consequences, the WHO states that enhancing the efficacy of medication adherence interventions could have a more significant impact on population health than advancements in specific medical treatments [6].

1.2. Medication Adherence

More medications are self-administered at home than in hospitals and clinics combined [7]. Consequently, understanding home medication management is critical for improving medication adherence. Numerous barriers to medication adherence have been identified, including medication cost, limited access to pharmacies, and poor health literacy skills [8–12]. Adherence is also influenced by factors that evolve as a patient progresses through different phases of their medication regimen [13]. The Ascertaining Barriers to Compliance (ABC) taxonomy identifies the stages of adherence as initiation, which is the consumption of the first dose of a prescribed medication; implementation, which refers to adherence to the prescribed dosing regimen from initiation until the final dose of the medication; and discontinuation, which occurs when a patient stops taking the medication for any reason [14]. The taxonomy further distinguishes between intentional and unintentional nonadherence to illustrate the complex nature of adherence [15]. One of the most common unintentional reasons for nonadherence is forgetfulness [16].

Throughout the stages of the medication lifecycle, healthcare providers have multiple opportunities to guide patients in establishing or improving medication management practices. Given the in-depth knowledge providers have of their patient's health and medication histories, coupled with the trust patients place in them, they are arguably the best sources for this guidance [17,18]. Interventions to improve adherence also include pharmacist counseling and home visits to provide tailored guidance on medication regimens [19–21]. However, most patients have limited opportunities to receive guidance due to constraints on provider time and the costs associated with these interventions. Guidance can also come from family and friends, and studies have shown the value of leveraging social contacts to engage patients in effective medication management [22]. For family and friends to be helpful, they need prior experience with adherence, comfort with discussing medication-related issues, and availability for ongoing communication.

Most patients must independently devise and implement their own home medication management practices, including decisions on where to store medications, how to establish medication-taking routines, and which containers, devices, or apps to use for adherence support. At the initiation phase, they may have little knowledge to build on.

Categorizing medication storage locations and determining which are associated with adherence are an understudied area [23]. Existing research and patient guidelines on storage primarily focus on safety, including how to store medications securely in homes with children or pets [13], avoiding environmental factors like heat, humidity, and light that can compromise medication stability [24]; preventing medication errors [14]; and reducing the risk of medication misuse due to poor medication management [15].

We describe our efforts to identify and categorize home medication management practices as a foundational step toward developing interventions aimed at improving medication adherence in patients' homes [25]. Other than prior studies on medication safety, this study is unique in identifying home storage locations and reporting which of these locations are associated with better medication adherence.

2. Methods

2.1. Study Sample

We designed a survey to learn about home medication management. Data were collected via participant self-reports through an online survey that was administered in English using Google Forms, an online survey platform that uses data encryption and advanced malware protection to protect user responses [26]. After the survey was designed and piloted, all protocols were submitted to and approved by the Tufts University Health Sciences Institutional Review Board (IRB) under STUDY00002224.

The survey was open between 18 November and 14 December 2021, and participants were recruited using social media platforms (Twitter, LinkedIn, Facebook, and Instagram) and through Tufts University's Osher Lifelong Learning Institute mailing list. Eligible participants were 18 years of age or older. Informed consent was obtained from all subjects.

Anyone who completed the survey was eligible to win one of ten USD $25 Amazon gift cards by random draw.

2.2. Procedures

A total of 1966 survey responses were collected. Of those, 1673 (85%) responses were deemed valid after screening for exclusion criteria (n = 293, 15%). Responses were dropped if they had any of the following qualities: consecutive sets of identical responses reported at the same time (n = 132); suspicious responses including identical open-text responses from the same day (n = 83); non-English responses (n = 59); or responses reported using an abnormal email address containing long strings of numbers, which were suspected to be fraudulently generated (n = 19).

2.3. Measures

The items included in our survey were designed to elicit respondents' experiences with managing their medication at home. The questions were either multiple choice, on a 5-point Likert scale, or free-text open-ended to collect participant experiences related to medication storage locations, self-reported medication adherence, and perceived importance of adherence. Data pertaining to age, race, ethnicity, sex, and highest level of education were also collected.

2.4. Medication Storage Location

One of the survey questions, "Where in your home do you store your prescriptions that you take on a regular basis?", was designed to elicit where respondents stored the medications taken regularly. Because an individual might use multiple locations, respondents could select one or more locations; the options were as follows: "Kitchen table", "Kitchen cabinet", "Kitchen counter", "Kitchen drawer", "In the refrigerator", "On the bathroom vanity", "In the vanity drawer or cabinet", "Bathroom medicine cabinet", "On top of the bedroom nightstand", "In the nightstand drawer", "Desk", "Dining room table", "Backpack, purse, or bag", and "Closet". An open text field was included for locations not in the list. Open-text responses were categorized by existing values via consensus coding to promote inter-rater reliability.

A separate question asked where respondents stored medications that they did not regularly take: "Where in your home do you store medications other than the ones that you take on a regular basis (such as over-the-counter medications, an extra supply of your medications, vitamins, etc.)?" Respondents could select from the same options provided above.

2.5. Analysis

The analysis of survey results assessed relative frequencies for all sample characteristics and variables listed in Measures. Bivariate analyses were performed for the home medication storage locations used by survey respondents, the perceived importance of medication adherence, and the variables indicating adherence to medications taken regularly. Bivariate analyses included chi^2 tests of homogeneity of proportions and bivariate logistic regression models.

3. Results

3.1. Sample Demographic Characteristics

Of the 1673 total respondents, the ages ranged from 18 to over 90 years old with most (65%) being between the ages of 20 and 39 years. For race/ethnicity, a majority identified as White (62%). For sex, over half (55%) identified as female. For the highest degree obtained, a majority (87%) had at least some college coursework experience with 45% having obtained a bachelor's, master's, or professional degree. The distribution of the sample is depicted in Table 1.

Table 1. Characteristics of sample by self-reported adherence (n = 1673).

Characteristic	Overall N (%)	Ever Forgot to Take a Medication (Row %)				Recently Forgot to Take a Medication [a] (Row %)			
		Yes	No	Chi^2 *	*p*	Yes	No	Chi^2 *	*p*
Overall	1673 (100)	60	40			38	62		
Age by decade									
<19	9 (<1)	67	33	81.44	<0.001	67	33	17.39	0.026
20–29	443 (26)	55	45			42	58		
30–39	641 (38)	54	46			38	62		
40–49	244 (15)	59	41			39	61		
50–59	127 (8)	75	25			35	65		
60–69	82 (5)	85	15			37	63		
70–79	84 (5)	86	14			23	77		
80–89 [b]	38 (2)	82	18			29	71		
90 [b]	5 (<1)	80	20			20	80		
Race/ethnicity [c]									
White	1040 (62)	61	39	0.38	0.536	35	65	12.86	<0.001
American Indian or Alaskan Native	254 (15)	47	53	20.95	<0.001	67	33	2.43	0.119
Black or African American	168 (10)	68	32	5.32	0.021	51	49	14.16	<0.001
Asian	138 (8)	68	32	3.94	0.047	54	46	15.94	<0.001
Hispanic or Latino	136 (8)	60	40	<0.01	0.980	46	54	4.53	0.033
Native Hawaiian or Other Pacific Islander	68 (4)	81	19	12.66	<0.001	66	34	24.20	<0.001
Sex [d]									
Female	910 (55)	64	36	19.92	<0.001	38	62	4.91	0.086
Male	765 (45)	55	45			37	63		
Highest education completed									
<High school diploma or equivalency	47 (3)	75	26	43.77	<0.001	62	38	21.63	0.001
High school diploma or equivalency	174 (10)	55	45			43	57		
Some college	444 (27)	50	50			36	64		
Associate's degree	182 (11)	56	44			45	55		
Bachelor's degree	390 (23)	65	35			34	65		
Master's or professional degree [b]	365 (22)	68	32			36	64		
Doctoral degree	71 (4)	73	27			34	66		
Receptivity to storage guidance [c]									
Receptive to guidance from at least one [e]	1606 (96)	60	40	0.87	0.350	38	62	2.67	0.103
From physician	909 (54)	57	43	6.35	0.012	35	65	4.93	0.026
From pharmacist	996 (60)	62	38	4.78	0.029	37	63	1.24	0.265
From mobile application or website	304 (18)	75	25	32.51	<0.001	46	54	9.83	0.002
From printed material (brochures)	221 (13)	76	24	28.16	<0.001	39	61	0.13	0.723
Not receptive to guidance from any listed source [f]	67 (4)	66	34	0.87	0.350	28	72	2.67	0.103

Table 1. *Cont.*

Characteristic	Overall N (%)	Ever Forgot to Take a Medication (Row %)				Recently Forgot to Take a Medication [a] (Row %)			
		Yes	No	Chi^2 *	*p*	Yes	No	Chi^2 *	*p*
Reason for choosing storage location									
Safety	714 (43)	47	53	84.01	<0.001	32	68	20.25	<0.001
Ease of access	620 (37)	73	27	69.85	<0.001	40	60	1.42	0.233
Visibility	612 (37)	53	47	21.17	<0.001	33	67	8.93	0.003
Proximity to items used every day	560 (33)	66	34	11.42	0.001	43	57	10.35	0.001
Proximity to food or drink	391 (23)	60	40	2.23	0.135	43	57	5.71	0.017
Household conditions	282 (17)	55	45	3.87	0.049	32	68	5.68	0.017
Other	3 (<1)	100	0	1.99	0.159	0	100	1.83	0.176

[a]: "Recently" was defined as forgetting to take a medication in the last two weeks. [b]: These values were combined due to the small sample size or similarity. [c]: These were not mutually exclusive; a single respondent may fall into several categories, except for composite values. [d]: <1% identified with a sex that was unlisted. [e]: Composite variable or value. [f]: Derived from absence of value selection. * Pearson chi^2: The *p*-values denote likelihood of observed chi^2, assuming homogeneity of the proportions. For the non-mutually exclusive items, chi^2 is calculated for each selection as a binary value by the binary adherence proxy.

3.2. Receptivity to Storage Guidance

Over 1600 respondents (N = 1606, 96%) reported being receptive to guidance on medication storage, with more than half (54%) saying they would be open to receiving guidance if it was from a physician. More respondents (60%) said they would be receptive to guidance from a pharmacist. Fewer said they would be open to receiving guidance from a mobile application or website (18%) or would be receptive to printed material, such as brochures (13%). Nearly two-thirds (65%) of those who reported being receptive to guidance from a physician said that they had not recently forgotten to take a medication ($p = 0.026$), while 54% of those who were open to guidance from a mobile application or website self-reported that they had not recently forgotten to take a medication ($p = 0.002$).

3.3. Storage Location

The most common home storage location for primary medications was in nightstand drawers (N = 475, 28%), followed closely by atop bedroom nightstands (N = 456, 27%). Other common storage locations for primary medications were kitchen cabinets (N = 372, 22%) and bathroom medicine cabinets (N = 330, 20%). Among these commonly reported storage locations, atop bedroom nightstands ($p = 0.005$), nightstand drawers ($p < 0.001$), and kitchen cabinets (p= 0.001), significantly fewer respondents reported recently forgetting to take their medication. Other storage locations for primary medications that had significantly fewer respondents recently forgetting to take their medication included the kitchen counter ($p = 0.013$), desk ($p = 0.040$), dining room table ($p = 0.042$), and closet ($p = 0.004$). Table 2 shows the primary medication storage locations for our sample.

The most common reasons respondents chose their medication storage locations were related to medication safety, visibility, and proximity. The majority of those who chose a storage location due to safety ($p < 0.001$), visibility ($p = 0.003$), proximity to items used daily ($p = 0.001$), proximity to food or drink ($p = 0.017$), and household conditions ($p = 0.017$) reported that they had not recently forgotten to take their medication. Those who chose safety were also less likely to report ever forgetting to take their medication ($p < 0.001$).

Table 2. Home medication storage by ever or recently forgetting to take medication (n = 1673).

Home Medication Storage Locations	Overall N (%)	Ever Forgot to Take a Medication (Row %)				Recently Forgot to Take a Medication ** (Row %)			
		Yes	No	Chi² *	*p*	Yes	No	Chi² *	*p*
Overall	1673 (100)	60	40			38	62		
Kitchen table	223 (13)	52	48	7.98	0.005	42	58	1.63	0.201
Kitchen cabinet	372 (22)	66	34	7.04	0.008	45	55	10.91	0.001
Kitchen counter	294 (18)	62	38	0.28	0.596	44	56	6.18	0.013
Kitchen drawer	298 (18)	54	46	6.39	0.011	42	58	3.05	0.081
In refrigerator	284 (17)	53	47	7.04	0.008	39	61	0.37	0.542
On bathroom vanity	196 (12)	75	25	20.32	<0.001	41	59	1.15	0.284
In vanity drawer or cabinet	245 (15)	61	39	0.05	0.829	38	62	<0.01	0.966
Bathroom medicine cabinet	330 (20)	62	38	0.86	0.355	36	64	0.76	0.385
Atop bedroom nightstand	456 (27)	50	50	24.88	<0.001	32	68	7.71	0.005
In the nightstand drawer	475 (28)	49	51	35.66	<0.001	29	71	19.72	<0.001
Desk	264 (16)	45	55	29.89	<0.001	32	68	4.24	0.040
Dining room table	161 (10)	45	55	16.39	<0.001	30	70	4.15	0.042
Backpack, purse, or bag	239 (14)	53	47	6.50	0.011	35	65	0.86	0.354
Closet	80 (5)	51	49	2.80	0.094	22	78	8.40	0.004
Unlisted location (Alone) ***	17 (1)	94	6	8.25	0.004	35	65	0.05	0.828

* *p*-values denote the likelihood of observed chi², assuming homogeneity of the proportions. For all values, chi² is calculated for each selection as a binary value (only affirmative displayed) by the binary adherence proxy. ** "Recently" is defined as forgetting to take a medication in the last two weeks. *** Inclusive of uncategorizable responses for which a categorizable response was not also provided.

3.4. Bivariate Analyses

Medication Storage Location and Ever or Recently Forgetting to Take a Medication

The home medication storage locations that were significantly associated with decreased odds of having ever forgotten to take a medication included kitchen tables (OR: 0.67, 95% CI: 0.50–0.88), kitchen drawers (OR: 0.72, 95% CI: 0.56–0.93), in the refrigerator (OR: 0.71, 95% CI: 0.55–0.91), atop the bedroom nightstand (OR: 0.58, 95%CI: 0.46–0.72), in the nightstand drawer (OR: 0.52, 95% CI: 0.42–0.65), desks (OR: 0.48, 95% CI: 0.37–0.63), dining room tables (OR: 0.51, 95% CI: 0.37–0.71), and a backpack, purse, or bag (OR: 0.70, 95% CI: 0.53–0.92). The two medication storage locations that were significantly associated with increased odds of having ever forgotten to take a medication were kitchen cabinets (OR: 1.39, 95% CI: 1.09–1.76) and bathroom vanities (OR: 2.15, 95% CI: 1.53–3.02).

Five home medication storage locations were significantly associated with having decreased odds of forgetting to take a medication within the two weeks prior to the survey: atop bedroom nightstand (OR: 0.73, 95% CI: 0.58–0.91), in the nightstand drawer (OR: 0.60, 95% CI: 0.48–0.75), desk (OR: 0.75, 95% CI: 0.56–0.99), on the dining room table (OR: 0.70, 95% CI: 0.49–0.99), and in the closet (OR: 0.46, 95% CI: 0.27–0.79). Two locations were significantly associated with increased odds of forgetting to take a medication in the two weeks prior to the survey: kitchen cabinets (OR: 1.48, 95% CI: 1.17–1.87) and kitchen counters (OR: 1.38, 95% CI: 1.17–1.78) This analysis is shown in Table 3.

Table 3. Bivariate associations between home medication storage location and self-reported medication adherence.

Home Medication Storage Location	Ever Forgot to Take a Medication (Row %)	Recently Forgot to Take a Medication ** (Row %)
	OR (95% CI)	OR (95% CI)
Kitchen table	0.67 (0.50–0.88) *	1.21 (0.91–1.61)
Kitchen cabinet	1.39 (1.09–1.76) *	1.48 (1.17–1.87) *
Kitchen counter	1.07 (0.83–1.39)	1.38 (1.07–1.78) *
Kitchen drawer	0.72 (0.56–0.93) *	1.25 (0.97–1.62)
In refrigerator	0.71 (0.55–0.91) *	1.08 (0.84–1.41)
On bathroom vanity	2.15 (1.53–3.02) *	1.18 (0.87–1.60)
In vanity drawer or cabinet	1.03 (0.78–1.36)	1.01 (0.76–1.33)
Bathroom medicine cabinet	1.12 (0.88–1.44)	0.89 (0.70–1.15)
Atop bedroom nightstand	0.58 (0.46–0.72) *	0.73 (0.58–0.91) *
In nightstand drawer	0.52 (0.42–0.65) *	0.60 (0.48–0.75) *
Desk	0.48 (0.37–0.63) *	0.75 (0.56–0.99) *
Dining room table	0.51 (0.37–0.71) *	0.70 (0.49–0.99) *
Backpack, purse, or bag	0.70 (0.53–0.92) *	0.87 (0.66–1.16)
Closet	0.68 (0.44–1.07)	0.46 (0.27–0.79) *

* $p < 0.05$. ** "Recently" is defined as forgetting to take a medication in the last two weeks.

3.5. Additional Findings

Some additional analysis of survey results found that nearly two-thirds (63%) of those who lived alone reported that they had ever forgotten to take their medication, compared to 64% of people living with 1–2 people, 55% of those living with 3–4 people, and 51% of those living with 5 or more people; $p = 0.002$. Over a third of the sample (N = 599, 36%) reported that they were responsible for helping one or more people they lived with manage their medication, while 15% of the sample said they helped one or more people they did not live with. Fewer respondents (N = 137, 8%) reported helping individuals that they did and did not live with, though this group had a significantly low rate of ever forgetting to take their medication (43%, $p < 0.001$).

Nearly half (48%) of the sample reported being reminded to take their medication by a spouse or a partner, the highest frequency among the sample. Over two-thirds of these respondents (68%) said they had not recently forgotten to take a medication. Respondents who reported that no one reminded them to take their medication had the lowest rate of historical medication adherence (only 87% said that they had forgotten to take a medication at least once in their life). These findings suggest that if one lives with others, living with a spouse or partner might be the most significant relationship for supporting adherent behavior.

4. Discussion

4.1. Receptivity to Storage Guidance

Nearly all (96%) of the respondents were receptive to receiving guidance on medication storage, and more than half (54%) of the sample reported that they would be open to receiving guidance from a physician. Two-thirds (65%) of these respondents reported that they had not recently forgotten to take a medication, indicating that their receptivity was not to reduce nonadherence but rather to improve their medication management practices. Although respondents desired guidance, changes in the healthcare system, such as shorter doctor's visits, may limit the opportunities for patients to receive counseling on medication adherence.

4.2. Storage Location

Our primary goals in planning this study were to learn which locations in the home patients use for medication storage and if any of those locations were associated with adherence. Nightstands were the most common location for respondents to store their medications, with respondents using nightstand drawers (28%) and atop nightstands (27%) more than other locations. Among those commonly used locations, both atop bedroom nightstands and within nightstand drawers were significantly associated with recent medication adherence.

Those who chose a storage location due to safety (43% of the sample) reported the highest rate of medication adherence (for both ever forgetting and recently forgetting). Visibility was also associated with adherence, with 67% of those who said they chose their medication storage location for visibility purposes reporting that they had not recently forgotten to take a medication.

These findings can inform the guidance provided to patients on where to store their medication and can also inform the design of devices tailored for specific storage locations. Additional characteristics of a location, such as whether a storage location is in a personal or shared space and its visibility, should be factored into counseling on home medication management.

5. Future Directions

5.1. Guidance from Physicians and Pharmacists

With most respondents (96%) expressing interest in receiving guidance, one future direction is to develop interventions to provide patients with personalized guidance on medication storage. Since half of respondents (54%) indicated they would be receptive to guidance from their physician, home medication storage discussions could occur during office visits. This would require physicians to allocate time for a discussion and ask key questions to personalize guidance to both a living situation and any past adherence history. Interventions could address patients' needs under three sets of circumstances: how to manage their first prescription, how to manage adding a prescription that increases the complexity of a medication regimen, and a review of current adherence practices.

An even larger number (60%) of respondents were interested in receiving guidance from a pharmacist. The combination of a prescription history, including frequency of prescription refills, in combination with key questions about home medication management, can identify patients who are nonadherent. Interventions could use these indicators to prompt pharmacists to provide guidance about home medication storage. However, guidance may require a different format for the almost 25% of the US population who have their medications shipped directly to their home, thereby removing opportunities for face-to-face interaction between patients and pharmacists [27]. Other changes that interventions need to accommodate include fewer prescriptions dropped off because of electronic prescribing and longer waits to talk to pharmacists who are administering vaccines.

5.2. Better Home and Device Design for Supporting Adherence

With nightstands being the most common place for respondents to store their medications and being the most significantly associated with recent medication adherence, innovative designs could support medication adherence. There are currently nightstands on the market with a spectrum of features designed to support charging devices and other technology-related activities. Novel nightstand designs could accommodate prescription bottles and pill containers to increase fit and visibility. Other settings in patients' homes could be designed to support medication adherence. One example is to relocate built-in medicine cabinets to a cooler and drier environment; another is to design a kitchen cabinet specifically for medication much like spice cabinets, which are designed to ease locating and removing containers of spice.

Our findings on where patients store their medications could lead to the design of location-specific containers or devices in the same way that lighting differs depending on location. A desktop lamp, a living room lamp, and a kitchen light all work for a specific setting. Another important consideration is that many digital devices use auditory or visual cues to provide time-based reminders to patients to take their medication. However, these reminders are only effective if a patient is in a position to see or hear them. To improve adherence, these alerts could be redesigned to align with home usage patterns, ensuring that reminders are noticed. Time-based notifications may not even be an effective approach for adherence reminders, especially when most medications do not need to be taken at a specific time and most patients have fluctuations in their schedules. A promising future direction is to apply principles similar to car seatbelts alerts, which emit an auditory notification if the seatbelt is unlatched when the ignition is turned on. This concept could be adapted for medication adherence by pairing sensors on prescription bottles or pill containers with sensors tied to everyday routines, such as making coffee or brushing teeth, to provide reminders precisely when they are needed [28].

6. Limitations

Using social media as our primary survey dissemination method restricted our respondent pool to those active on the platforms we utilized. Additionally, while the survey methodology was useful for gathering self-reported data, it did not allow for a deeper exploration of the underlying choices and behaviors. Despite these limitations, we successfully identified significant bivariate relationships between several rationales respondents cited for their choice of medication storage locations and their self-reported adherence.

7. Conclusions

This survey uncovered where people store their medications and identified which storage locations are associated with medication adherence. Other results center on the factors influencing patients' choice of medication storage locations and their receptivity to receiving guidance. These findings have inspired the development of interventions for healthcare professionals to provide adherence guidance, as well as innovative approaches to the design of homes, furnishings, and devices tailored to home medication management. The survey has further led to a follow-up study using in-depth interviews to explore the complex decisions patients make in managing their medications at home [29].

Author Contributions: L.G. initiated this research project, was responsible for developing and deploying the survey, and contributed to writing this paper. E.S. and M.S. (Meredith Steinfeldt) performed the primary analysis for the survey results and contributed to writing this paper. B.E. and M.S. (Meera Singhal) contributed to writing this paper. All authors approved the submitted version. All authors have read and agreed to the published version of the manuscript.

Funding: This research was funded by Tufts University through the Springboard Program and by the National Center for Advancing Translational Sciences, National Institutes of Health, Award Number UL1TR002544. The content is solely the responsibility of the authors and does not necessarily represent the official views of the NIH.

Institutional Review Board Statement: The study was conducted in accordance with the Declaration of Helsinki, and approved by the Tufts University Health Sciences Institutional Review Board (protocol code STUDY00002224, 18 November 2021).

Informed Consent Statement: The studies involving human participants were reviewed and approved by Tufts University Health Sciences Institutional Review Board in Boston, MA. Written informed consent for participation was not required for this study in accordance with the national legislation and the institutional requirements.

Data Availability Statement: The data that support the findings of this study are available from the corresponding author, L.G., upon reasonable request.

Acknowledgments: The authors offer their appreciation to the graduate and medical students at Tufts University School of Medicine who were instrumental in the discussions and literature reviews that led to this survey, most especially Avi Patel. The authors thank the students who contributed to the design of the survey and provided feedback on this paper, including Deelia Wang, Issac Baek, Justin Barton, Cheryl Croll, and Ricardo Boschetti. The authors thank Jeff Glenning for his editing of this paper.

Conflicts of Interest: The authors declare no conflict of interest.

References

1. WHO. *Adherence to Long-Term Therapies: Evidence for Action*; World Health Organization: Geneva, Switzerland, 2003; ISBN 978-92-4-154599-0.
2. Bouwman, L.; Eeltink, C.M.; Visser, O.; Janssen, J.J.W.M.; Maaskant, J.M. Prevalence and Associated Factors of Medication Non-Adherence in Hematological-Oncological Patients in Their Home Situation. *BMC Cancer* **2017**, *17*, 739. [CrossRef] [PubMed]
3. Stawarz, K.; Gardner, B.; Cox, A.; Blandford, A. What Influences the Selection of Contextual Cues When Starting a New Routine Behaviour? An Exploratory Study. *BMC Psychol.* **2020**, *8*, 29. [CrossRef] [PubMed]
4. Desai, R.; Thakkar, S.; Fong, H.K.; Varma, Y.; Ali Khan, M.Z.; Itare, V.B.; Raina, J.S.; Savani, S.; Damarlapally, N.; Doshi, R.P.; et al. Rising Trends in Medication Non-Compliance and Associated Worsening Cardiovascular and Cerebrovascular Outcomes Among Hospitalized Adults Across the United States. *Cureus* **2019**, *11*, e5389. [CrossRef] [PubMed]
5. OECD. *Investing in Medication Adherence Improves Health Outcomes and Health System Efficiency: Adherence to Medicines for Diabetes, Hypertension, and Hyperlipidaemia*; OECD Health Working Papers; OECD: Paris, France, 2018; Volume 105.
6. Brown, M.T.; Bussell, J.K. Medication Adherence: WHO Cares? *Mayo Clin. Proc.* **2011**, *86*, 304–314. [CrossRef] [PubMed]
7. Aspden, P.; Institute of Medicine (U.S.) (Eds.) *Preventing Medication Errors*; Quality Chasm Series; National Academies Press: Washington, DC, USA, 2007; ISBN 978-0-309-10147-9.
8. Kaul, S.; Avila, J.C.; Mehta, H.B.; Rodriguez, A.M.; Kuo, Y.; Kirchhoff, A.C. Cost-related Medication Nonadherence among Adolescent and Young Adult Cancer Survivors. *Cancer* **2017**, *123*, 2726–2734. [CrossRef]
9. McQuaid, E.L.; Landier, W. Cultural Issues in Medication Adherence: Disparities and Directions. *J. Gen. Intern. Med.* **2018**, *33*, 200–206. [CrossRef]
10. Park, Y.; Raza, S.; George, A.; Agrawal, R.; Ko, J. The Effect of Formulary Restrictions on Patient and Payer Outcomes: A Systematic Literature Review. *J. Manag. Care Spec. Pharm.* **2017**, *23*, 893–901. [CrossRef]
11. Wroe, A.L. Intentional and Unintentional Nonadherence: A Study of Decision Making. *J. Behav. Med.* **2002**, *25*, 355–372. [CrossRef]
12. Lindquist, L.A.; Go, L.; Fleisher, J.; Jain, N.; Friesema, E.; Baker, D.W. Relationship of Health Literacy to Intentional and Unintentional Non-Adherence of Hospital Discharge Medications. *J. Gen. Intern. Med.* **2012**, *27*, 173–178. [CrossRef]
13. Aslani, P.; Schneider, M.P. Adherence: The Journey of Medication Taking, Are We There Yet? *Int. J. Clin. Pharm.* **2014**, *36*, 1–3. [CrossRef]
14. Vrijens, B.; De Geest, S.; Hughes, D.A.; Przemyslaw, K.; Demonceau, J.; Ruppar, T.; Dobbels, F.; Fargher, E.; Morrison, V.; Lewek, P.; et al. A New Taxonomy for Describing and Defining Adherence to Medications. *Br. J. Clin. Pharmacol.* **2012**, *73*, 691–705. [CrossRef] [PubMed]
15. Khan, M.U.; Aslani, P. Exploring Factors Influencing Initiation, Implementation and Discontinuation of Medications in Adults with ADHD. *Health Expect.* **2021**, *24*, 82–94. [CrossRef] [PubMed]
16. Gadkari, A.S.; McHorney, C.A. Unintentional Non-Adherence to Chronic Prescription Medications: How Unintentional Is It Really? *BMC Health Serv. Res.* **2012**, *12*, 98. [CrossRef] [PubMed]
17. Edelman 2023 Edelman Trust Barometer. Available online: https://www.edelman.com/trust/2023/trust-barometer (accessed on 18 October 2023).
18. McHugh, J.; Elul, B.; Narayan, S. *The Prescription of Trust: Pharmacists Transforming Patient Care*; Columbia University Mailman School of Public Health: New York, NY, USA, 2022.
19. Centers for Disease Control and Prevention. *Pharmacist-Provided Medication Therapy Management in Medicaid*; U.S. Department of Health and Human Services: Washington, DC, USA, 2021.
20. Papastergiou, J.; Luen, M.; Tencaliuc, S.; Li, W.; Van Den Bemt, B.; Houle, S. Medication Management Issues Identified during Home Medication Reviews for Ambulatory Community Pharmacy Patients. *Can. Pharm. J.* **2019**, *152*, 334–342. [CrossRef] [PubMed]
21. Flanagan, P.S.; Barns, A. Current Perspectives on Pharmacist Home Visits: Do We Keep Reinventing the Wheel? *Integr. Pharm. Res. Pract.* **2018**, *7*, 141–159. [CrossRef]
22. Scheurer, D.; Choudhry, N.; Swanton, K.A.; Matlin, O.; Shrank, W. Association between Different Types of Social Support and Medication Adherence. *Am. J. Manag. Care* **2012**, *18*, e461–e467.
23. Conference Abstracts. Abstracts of the 26th Annual Meeting of ESPACOMP, The International Society for Medication Adherence, Berlin, Germany, 17–19 November 2022. *Int. J. Clin. Pharm.* **2023**, *45*, 250–280. [CrossRef]
24. Funk, O.G.; Yung, R.; Arrighi, S.; Lee, S. Medication Storage Appropriateness in US Households. *Innov. Pharm.* **2021**, *12*, 16. [CrossRef]

25. Gualtieri, L.; Wang, D. Hosting a Co-Design Workshop: Older Adults Ideate. In Proceedings of the 27th Annual Meeting of ESPACOMP International Society for Medication Adherence, Budapest, Hungary, 30 November–1 December 2023.
26. Google Forms: Online Form Creator. Available online: https://www.google.com/forms/about/ (accessed on 18 November 2021).
27. Rupp, M.T. Attitudes of Medicare-Eligible Americans Toward Mail Service Pharmacy. *J. Manag. Care Spec. Pharm.* **2013**, *19*, 564–572. [CrossRef]
28. Gualtieri, L.; Rosenbluth, S. Can Technology Solve the Problem of Medication Nonadherence? *Mayo Clin. Proc. Digit. Health* **2024**, *2*, 34–37. [CrossRef]
29. Gualtieri, L.; Rigby, M.; Wang, D.; Mann, E. Medication Management Strategies to Support Medication Adherence: Interview Study with Older Adults. *Interact. J. Med. Res.* **2024**, *13*, e53513. [CrossRef] [PubMed]

behavioral sciences

MDPI

Article

Considering the Role of Behavioural Fatigue in the COVID-19 Lockdown Debates in Great Britain: A Retrospective Analysis of a National Survey Assessing the Relationships between Capability, Opportunity, Motivation, and Behaviour

Saval Khanal [1], Kelly Ann Schmidtke [2,*], Kaloyan Haralampiev [3] and Ivo Vlaev [4,*]

[1] Health Economics Consulting, University of East Anglia, East Anglia, Norwich NR4 7TJ, UK; s.khanal@uea.ac.uk
[2] Liberal Arts, College of Arts and Sciences, University of Health Sciences and Pharmacy, St. Louis, MO 63110, USA
[3] Department of Sociology, Faculty of Philosophy, Sofia University "St. Kliment Ohridski", 1504 Sofia, Bulgaria; k_haralampiev@phls.uni-sofia.bg
[4] Warwick Business School, University of Warwick, Coventry CV4 7AL, UK
* Correspondence: kelly.schmidtke@uhsp.edu (K.A.S.); ivo.vlaev@wbs.ac.uk (I.V.)

Abstract: During the COVID-19 pandemic, the term "behavioural fatigue" became the centre of policy debates in Great Britain. These debates involved deciding when to go into lockdown and whether behavioural interventions could be effective. Behavioural interventions can only succeed where people's Capabilities, Opportunities, and Motivations to perform target behaviours are supported. Our retrospective data analyses examine the relationships between people's Capabilities, Opportunities, Motivations, and Behaviours, i.e., adherence to lockdown guidelines. Our cross-sectional analyses include 17,962 unique participants in Great Britain who completed a survey over the initial 30 days of the first lockdown (April 2020). We examine trends in responses to each scale and then the relationships between the scales using Granger's causality test with tests for stationarity and cointegration. A mixture of increasing and decreasing trends was identified for Capabilities and Opportunities. Decreasing trends were identified for Motivation and Behaviour. Granger's causality tests found that Capability forecasts Opportunity and Behaviour and that Motivation forecasts Opportunity. The discussion reiterates that to realise and maintain Behaviour changes, policies surrounding people's Capabilities, Opportunities, and Motivations must continue to support target behaviours.

Keywords: behaviour; COVID-19; nudge systems thinking; retrospective; United Kingdom

1. Background

In the absence of medical interventions, government guidance around the world aimed to decrease COVID-19 infections by changing people's behaviours [1,2]. How policymakers conceptualise behaviour change inevitably influences the policies they develop. Broadly speaking, two policy strategies could inform government interventions, which, in line with Rose's seminal work, we refer to as "high-risk prevention strategies" and "population prevention strategies" [3]. According to Rose, high-risk prevention strategies seek to reduce the health impact of the diseases in target areas while allowing population immunity to increase eventually resulting in lower case numbers. Given a high-risk prevention strategy, governments could ask people at higher risk to stay home while those at lower risk could continue traveling to work. In contrast, population strategies seek to reduce the number of infections until transmissions cease naturally or acceptable medical interventions become available. Given a population strategy, governments could encourage everyone to stay home in a national lockdown until an effective vaccine is available.

The present text does not assume that governments explicitly considered Rose's distinction between high-risk and population strategies before developing policies; rather, we propose that policies could be described accordingly. For instance, governments in Brazil initially applied more high-risk strategies with local lockdowns, and in South Korea initially applied more population strategies with national lockdowns [4,5]. Initially, the government in Great Britain appeared to consider a high-risk strategy, suggesting a more local lockdown approach may be taken when and where breakout infections occurred to quickly contain local outbreaks. On the 9 March 2020, Chief Medical Officer Chris Whitty explained that "Anything we do, we have got to be able to sustain. Once we have started these things, we have to continue them through the peak, and there is a risk that, if we go too early, people will understandably get fatigued, and it will be difficult to sustain this over time" [6]. His choice of the word "fatigue" possibly describes the way governments conceptualised behaviour change, which if true could render rapid local lockdowns a rational policy choice. Specifically, if any behaviour change is likely to stop over time, then policy actions to change behaviour must be carefully timed to coincide with the periods of highest risk.

The word choice of "fatigue" was quickly criticised. On the 16th of March, 681 behavioural scientists penned an open letter arguing against the idea that "behavioural fatigue" had scientific underpinnings and urged the government to adopt actions better aligned with a population strategy [7]. Additionally, Ferguson's (2020) [8] mathematical models were published comparing the potential health impacts of each strategy. These models suggest that a population strategy could dramatically reduce hospitalisations and deaths. On the 23rd of March, Prime Minister Boris Johnson announced the first national lockdown in Great Britain, wherein people were ordered to stay at home except for the following four purposes [9]: (1) "shopping for basic necessities, as infrequently as possible," (2) "one form of exercise a day—for example a run, walk, or cycle—alone or with members of your household," (3) "any medical need, to provide care or to help a vulnerable person," and (4) "travelling to and from work, but only where this is absolutely necessary and cannot be done from home."

The open letter penned by behavioural scientists did not say that behavioural fatigue did not exist; rather, they were "not convinced that enough is known about behavioural fatigue or to what extent these insights apply to the current exceptional circumstances." A more critical review states that behavioural fatigue "is not a real phenomenon: it must be either a naïve construct or a policy contrivance" [10]. A related critique outlines three senses of fatigue (tiredness, impairment, and distress), none of which were supported across the COVID-19 lockdowns [11]. The concept of behavioural fatigue remains contentious, partly due to its vague definition during the early pandemic. Instead of viewing it as an immutable psychological determinant, this paper suggests that behavioural fatigue could be understood as a dynamic outcome shaped by the Capability, Opportunity, and Motivation of individuals—a framework captured by the COM-B model. The COM-B model, developed by Michie et al. [12], posits that Capability (skills and knowledge), Opportunity (external factors), and Motivation (internal processes) interact to influence Behaviour. By applying this model, we can better assess the factors that drive or hinder adherence to public health guidance.

The COM-B model describes these three interrelated factors that must be present at a sufficient level for a target behaviour to occur [13]. Compared to other models of behaviour (e.g., the common-sense models, the health beliefs model [14], or the theory of planned behaviour) [15], the COM-B model offers a more comprehensive assessment [16]. Capability has to do with an individual's physical (e.g., skills) or psychological (e.g., awareness) capacity to perform the behaviour. Opportunity has to do with the physical environment (e.g., objects) and social (e.g., social norms) factors that lie outside the individuals that may enable or prompt them to perform the behaviour. Motivation has to do with an individual's reflective mental processes (e.g., planning) and automatic mental processes (e.g., emotions) that energise the behaviour.

The 2011 COM-B model is redrawn from Michie's paper in Figure 1. The model anticipates that all three components influence behaviour. It further specifies that Capability and Opportunity influence Motivation (but not the reverse). And lastly, feedback loops are anticipated, where the performance (or non-performance) of a target Behaviour may influence ongoing Capabilities, Opportunities, and Motivations. The model is largely used to understand individual behaviour. The present paper extends the model to population trends.

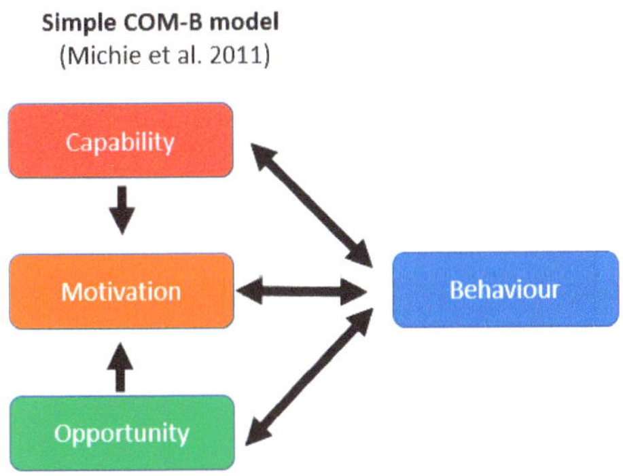

Figure 1. Redrawn COM-B model figures from [12].

The present paper assesses data collected about people's Capabilities, Opportunities, and Motivations to adhere to government guidance (Behaviour) during the first lockdown in Great Britain. First, we aim to assess trends in people's Capabilities, Opportunities, Motivations, and Behaviours. A decreasing trend in Behaviour could support a descriptive interpretation of behavioural fatigue. Second, we aim to assess the associations between people's Capabilities, Opportunities, Motivations, and Behaviours.

2. Methods

2.1. Study Design

The present study is a retrospective analysis of cross-sectional surveys conducted by YouGov. YouGov is an internet-based market research and data analytics company. A search of YouGov's publications between April 2020 and July 2020 finds eight publications that could have been informed by the present data and could have influenced government policy. None include a comprehensive analysis of behaviour change according to people's Capabilities, Opportunities, and Motivations. A publication in April 2020 looks at daily moods but not behaviour change [17]. A publication in May 2020 looks at exercise Behaviours but not Capabilities or Opportunities [18]. A publication in June 2020 looks at changes in Behaviour after news leaked of a public official not following the rules, which could change Motivation but not Capability or Opportunity [19]. Additional publications were about charitable donations [20] and stores openings [21–23]. The final publication was about whether government policy makes us do what they want us to do, which contained no data analysis [24].

Participation in the present study was voluntary. Participants provided consent for their anonymised data to be used in future analyses and received points they could redeem for prizes on YouGov's website. The University of Warwick approved this study as a secondary analysis (ID: 110.20-21).

2.2. Participants and Setting

The online surveys took place over the first 30 days of the first national lockdown in Great Britain, which started on the 1 April 2020 [25]. YouGov's recruitment strategy aimed for a representative sample each day in terms of age, gender, social class, and education in terms of the most recent census [26], but these demographics were not connected to individual responses analysed by the present research team. Participants could only take part in one survey. Eligible participants were at least 18 years old and lived in Great Britain. The sample size for the present study was a convenience sample from this retrospective data.

2.3. Variables

The selected survey items and their response options appear in Table 1. These survey items were not designed by the present research team but were selected by co-author IV in agreement with the research team to capture each COM-B component. IV has over 25 years of experience conducting behavioural science and policy research. Two items capture the Capability component regarding how knowledgeable participants felt about social distancing and limiting their risks. Two items capture the Opportunity component regarding how easy participants thought it was to follow the social distancing guidelines. Two items capture the Motivation component regarding how worried participants felt about the virus generally and personally. Lastly, four items capture the behaviour change component regarding how often participants were seeing friends, seeing family, going to work, and using public transit. The Opportunity items were only featured in the first 21 days. The remaining items were featured in all 30 days.

Table 1. Survey Items.

COM-B Component	Item	Response Options as Coded in Present Analyses
Capability	How well informed, if at all, do you feel you are about what social distancing is and how it applies to you?	Very well informed (4), Fairly well informed (3); Not very informed (2); Not informed at all (1)
Capability	I know what I need to do to limit my risk of contracting coronavirus.	Strongly agree (5); Agree (4); Neither agree nor disagree (3); Disagree (2); Strongly disagree (1)
Opportunity	How easy or difficult are you finding it to stick to social distancing rules?	Very easy (4); Fairly easy (3); Fairly difficult (2); Very difficult (1); Do not know (participants removed from analyses)
Opportunity	How easy or difficult do you think other people around you are finding it to stick to social distancing rules?	Very easy (4); Fairly easy (3); Fairly difficult (2); Very difficult (1); Do not know (participants removed from analyses)
Motivation	Overall, how worried are you about coronavirus?	Extremely worried (5); Very worried (4); Somewhat worried (3); Not very worried (2); Not at all worried (1); Don't know (participants removed from analyses)
Motivation	To what extent do you think coronavirus poses a risk to you personally?	Major risk (5); Significant risk (4); Moderate risk (3); Minor risk (2); No risk at all (1); Don't know (participants removed from analyses)
Behaviour	Please look at the list of activities below and, for each one, say whether you have reduced how much you are doing it: Seeing Friends	I am still doing this as much as usual (1); I am still doing this, but have cut it down a little (2); I am still doing this, but have cut down a lot (3); I have stopped doing this entirely (4); Not applicable, I did not do this anyway (participants removed from analyses)
Behaviour	Seeing members of my	I am still doing this as much as usual (1); I am still doing this, but have cut it down a little (2); I am still doing this; but have cut down a lot (3); I have stopped doing this entirely (4); Not applicable, I did not do this anyway (participants removed from analyses)
Behaviour	Going to your place of work	I am still doing this as much as usual (1); I am still doing this, but have cut it down a little (2); I am still doing this; but have cut down a lot (3); I have stopped doing this entirely (4); Not applicable, I did not do this anyway (participants removed from analyses)
Behaviour	Using public transit	I am still doing this as much as usual (1); I am still doing this, but have cut it down a little (2); I am still doing this; but have cut down a lot (3); I have stopped doing this entirely (4); Not applicable, I did not do this anyway (participants removed from analyses)

2.4. Statistical Methods

The items composing each COM-B component were aggregated using means. Participants responding "don't know" (for the Opportunity or Motivation items) or "not applicable, I did not do this anyway" (for the Behaviour items) were omitted from all analyses. Response scales for Opportunity and Behaviour ranged from 1 to 4, for Motivation ranged from 1 to 5, and for Capability from 1 to 4.5. Higher scores for Capability and Opportunity indicate that participants felt more informed about or had more Opportunities to comply with social distancing guidelines. Higher scores for Motivation indicate that participants felt more concerned about the coronavirus. Higher scores for Behaviour change indicate greater changes in Behaviour compared to before the lockdown commenced.

2.4.1. Tests for Overall Trends

For each COM-B component, graphs displaying the daily mean component scores were visually examined and fitted for best-fit model trend lines. Seven models were compared, including exponential, linear, or polynomial (2nd–6th-degree fits). The model with the largest adjusted R Square and/or the smallest Akaike Information Criterion (AIC)/Bayesian Information Criterion (BIC) scores was selected. When there was a discrepancy between criteria, the BIC was used because it better protects against overfitting [27]. These tests were conducted using Microsoft (R) Excel (R) LTSC MSO (16.0.14332.20771) 64-bit.

2.4.2. Tests for Relationships

The relationships between the COM-B components were analysed using the Granger's causality test with tests for stationarity and cointegration using eViews (R) 10+ [28]. Note that assessments for Granger "causality" are not equivalent to randomised controlled trial assessments of causality. Granger's causality establishes whether the necessary temporal order for causation is present. The test is used for retrospective data analyses. Specifically, it tests whether the preceding levels of two factors, say X and Y, better predict later levels of Y than preceding levels of Y alone. If so, then X is said to "granger-cause" Y [29]. For example, if preceding levels of Capability and Behaviour change are better predictors of Behaviour change than Behaviour change alone, then Capability could be said to "granger-cause" Behaviour change. Granger's causality test is a particularly powerful associative analysis because the temporal order of granger causes need not be the same in the reverse. That is, while X could granger-cause Y, Y might not granger-cause X.

A flow chart is provided in Figure 2 showing how the data were processed. Each pair of COM-B components were assessed separately. The first series of tests assess whether the data in each pair are stationary, i.e., an assumption for the most straightforward Granger's causality test. Stationarity is tested for with the Augmented Dickey–Fuller (ADF) with an alpha value of 0.05 (top diamond in Figure 2); the null hypothesis is that the data have a single root, i.e., are not stationary. In many retrospective data sets, particularly in finance and macroeconomics, this assumption is often not met as the data are integrated (Granger, 2003, p. 361) [30]. Here, data were not stationary and, as is common practice, we transformed non-stationary time-series data by first differencing to make the series stationary (Baker, al., 2015, p. 145) [31].

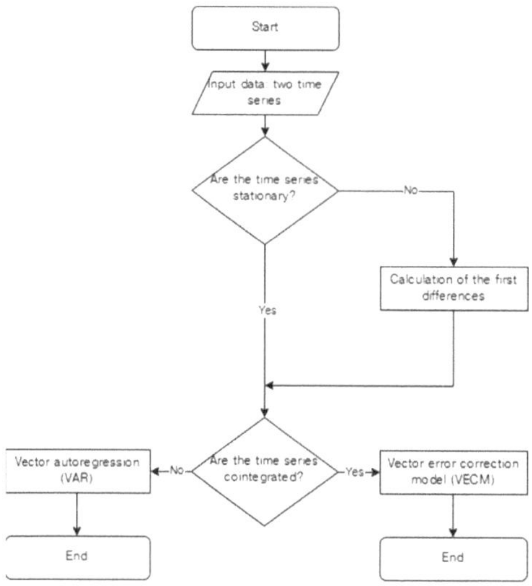

Figure 2. General algorithm of the relationship analyses.

The next series of tests assessed whether the transformed data in each pair were cointegrated using the Johansen Cointegration Test with an alpha value of 0.05 (bottom diamond in Figure 2); the null hypothesis is that there was no cointegration. Where data were not cointegrated, a vector autoregression model was used to assess relationships. Where data were cointegrated, we generated a vector error-correction model. In the vector error correction model, the change in one of the series is explained in terms of the lag difference between the series. If a pair of series is cointegrated at least one lag, one variable is said to be a [granger-]cause of the other (Granger, 2003, p. 366) [30]. In the present analyses, a lag of one day is applied.

3. Results

3.1. Participants

Of the 49,321 responders who took part in YouGov's original surveys, 31,359 (63.6%) were omitted from the analyses. Nearly half were omitted (49.0%) for responding "not applicable" to at least one Behaviour item; this response was most common for the Behaviour item about using public transportation (41.1% of all responders), followed by items about going to work (36.2% of all responders), seeing friends (6.7% of all responders) and seeing members of my family they did not live with (6.0% of all responders). Fewer responders were removed for saying "I don't know" to an Opportunity (5.6% of all responders) or a Motivation (2.2% of all responders) item.

For the remaining 17,962 participants (36.4%), the average number of participants each day was 598.73, with a standard deviation of 28.92.

3.2. Outcome of Trend Tests

A summary of the trend analyses for each component of the COM-B model is provided. Tables of the results for the six models compared are in Supplementary Files S1.

3.2.1. Capability—Trends Significantly Increasing and Decreasing

The mean daily Capability scores are in Figure 3a. Visual examinations of the graph show participants' Capabilities scores starting and ending at about 4 out of 4.5. Descriptively, the mean participant had a high sense of knowledge over the first 30 days of lockdown. Statistical tests locate significant increasing and decreasing trends. A third-degree polynomial was the best-fit model (Adjusted R square = 0.39; AIC = −130.64;

BIC = −126.43). In the first 7 days, Capability increases. Then, it decreases from days 8 to 24. Lastly, from days 25 to 30, Capability increases again.

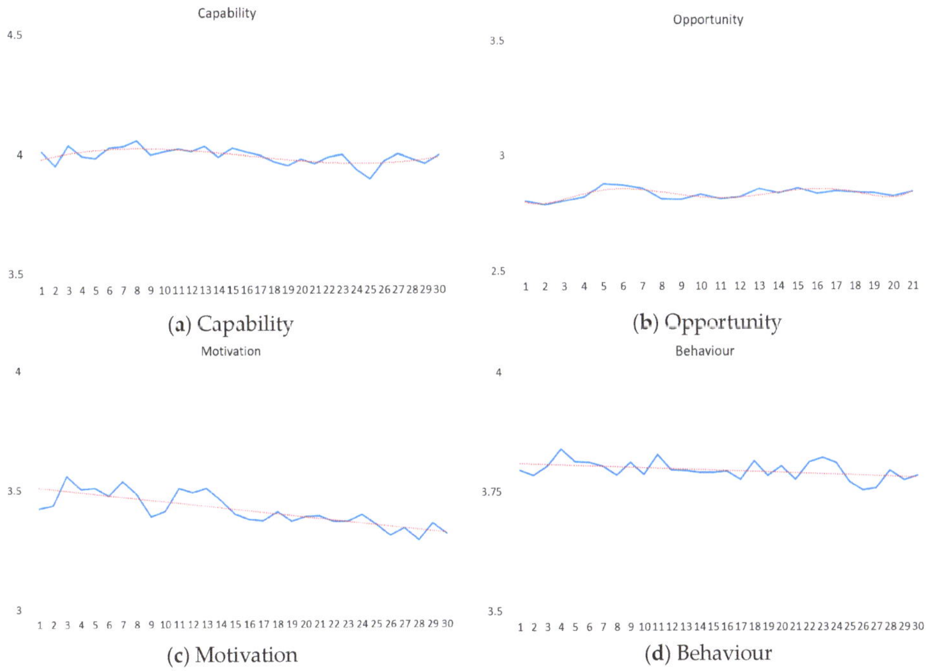

(**a**) Capability (**b**) Opportunity (**c**) Motivation (**d**) Behaviour

Figure 3. The mean daily scores with a best-fit model line for each COM-B component.

3.2.2. Opportunity—Significantly Increasing and Decreasing Trends

The mean daily Opportunity scores are in Figure 3b. Visual examinations of the graph show participants' Opportunity scores starting and ending at slightly under 3 out of 4. Descriptively, the mean participant thought it was fairly easy to follow the guidelines over the first 30 days of lockdown. Statistical tests locate several significant increasing and decreasing trends. The sixth-degree polynomial was the best-fit model (Adjusted R square = 0.47; AIC = −108.17; BIC = −101.90). Participants reported Opportunity decreases from days 1 to 2. Then, it increases from days 3 to 6 before decreasing from days 7 to 11. Then, Opportunity increases again from days 12 to 16 before again decreasing from days 17 to 20. Lastly, on the 21st day, Opportunity again increases.

3.2.3. Motivation—A Significantly Decreasing Trend

The mean daily Motivation scores are in Figure 3c. Visual examinations of the graph show participants' Motivation scores starting at around 3.5 out of 5 and slightly decreasing thereafter. The mean participant's Motivations were between being very and somewhat worried, and slightly decreasing towards being less worried over the first 30 days of lockdown. A linear model was the best-fit model (Adjusted R square = 0.64; AIC = −104.60; BIC = −103.20). The average daily decrease is 0.007.

3.2.4. Behaviour—Trend Significantly Changing

The mean daily Behaviour change scores are shown in Figure 3d. Visual examinations of the graph show participants' scores starting slightly under 4 out of 4 and slightly decreasing thereafter. The mean participant was becoming slightly less likely to report completely stopping the indicated behaviours over the first 30 days of lockdown. The linear model was the best-fit model (Adjusted R square = 0.17; AIC = −155.79; BIC = −154.39). The average daily decrease was 0.001.

3.3. Outcome of Relationship Tests

A summary of the Granger analyses for each pair of COM-B components is provided here. Tables of the results for all tests are provided in Supplementary Files S1.

The results of the Augmented Dickey–Fuller test for stationary suggest that Capability ($p < 0.05$) and Behaviour ($p < 0.05$) do not have a unit root; i.e., they are stationary. However, the time series of Opportunity ($p = 0.12$) and Motivation ($p = 0.43$) do. Therefore, following the flow chart in Figure 1, the data were transformed into first differences for the cointegration tests.

The results of the Johansen Cointegration tests suggest that there is no cointegration in four pairs: Capability and Motivation ($p = 0.62$), Capability and Behaviour ($p = 0.76$), Opportunity and Behaviour ($p = 0.30$), and Motivation and Behaviour ($p = 0.23$). For the remaining two pairs, there is cointegration: Capability and Opportunity ($p < 0.05$) and Opportunity and Motivation ($p < 0.05$). Following the above algorithm, the vector autoregression is used for pairs that are not cointegrated. The vector error correction model is used for pairs that are cointegrated.

The relationships revealed in the final analysis are pictured in Figure 4. The direction of the errors indicates the direction of influence. A summary of the effects is provided here: Capability forecasts Opportunity (t = −3.13, $p < 0.01$), but not the reverse; Capability forecasts Behaviour ($t = -2.41$, $p < 0.05$), but not the reverse; and Motivation forecasts Opportunity ($t = -3.91$, $p = 0.001$), but not the reverse. No other relationships were significant.

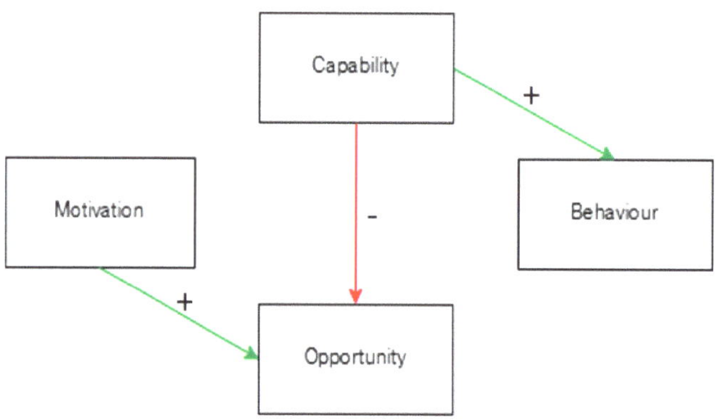

Figure 4. Significant relationships between COM-B components with directionality. Plus signs (green lines) indicate positive relationships, and negative signs (red lines) indicate inverse relationships.

4. Discussion

Across the first lockdown in Great Britain, the current study examines people's Capabilities, Opportunities, Motivations, and Behaviours. Slight decreases in Behaviour change occurred, which could support a descriptive existence of behavioural fatigue. Granger's causality tests suggest that Behaviour change could be forecast by slight changes in Capability at the population level. Rather than viewing behavioural fatigue as inevitable, policymakers could have looked at people's Capabilities to better understand public behaviour and improve public health.

While our trend analyses suggest that slight decreases in Behaviour change occurred, this was not independent of other factors. The present data suggest that Behaviour change could be anticipated by Capability, which is a factor that policy could influence. In this case, communications created about the lockdown rules likely influenced public knowledge that could have influenced adherence (up or down). Other examples exist supporting the notion that policy communications can change behaviour. For example, in August 2020, Parliament announced their "eat out to help out scheme", which aimed to protect jobs in the hospitality sector by encouraging the public to eat out [32]. Despite little changes in the virus threat from July to August (people's Motivation to stay at home), more people went out to eat in August and fewer did after the policy stopped in September. Rather than positing an immutable individual construct that influenced eating-out behaviour, the policy enacted and removed provides a more straightforward explanation for the changes in public behaviour.

Conceptualising behavioural fatigue as an immutable factor supports a narrative emphasising individual responsibility and blame. Such a conceptualisation suggests that public health initiatives fail to work because individuals lack sufficient grit to stick out adverse conditions. Grit is thought of as a personality construct with potential genetic dispositions [33]. Belief in grit could foster fatalistic beliefs that there is little policy can do to change people's behaviour. But this would be a mistake. Even where individual differences exist (even genetic differences), it does not follow that individuals cannot change (at least within some range) [34].

Despite the government and media commonly expressing concerns about people not following lockdown guidance, many people did. King's College London conducted a cluster analysis that grouped 2250 residents into three segments, including those Accepting, Suffering, and Resisting government actions during the pandemic [35]. Even amongst the Resisting, over 70% reported following government guidance to stay 2 meters away from people outside their home and avoiding places where people gather. One area that received lower adherence across all three segments involved self-isolation. Another study conducted during the first lockdown found that residents with less than 100 GBP in savings were three times less likely to report self-isolating than those with 25,000 GBP or more pounds in savings [36]. Thus, factors beyond individual choice likely contribute to following government guidance. Not considering those factors could decrease the public trust on which public policy must rest [37].

4.1. Policy Recommendation

Policymakers could regularly collaborate with data analysts to review and interpret real-time data, ensuring that decisions are informed by quantitative insights and a deep understanding of community contexts. This partnership is crucial, as data do not provide guidance without interpretation. Recommendations regarding how to involve the community in health systems research have been provided elsewhere [38,39]. Where increased adherence coincides with decreases in target public health concerns, such data could also be used to maintain Motivation to follow public health guidance. These Motivational messages could be framed to emphasise that preventive behaviour is within people's control [40].

Additionally, policymakers could critically assess different conceptual frameworks of behaviour change, integrating contemporary models such as the COM-B model, the Heath Beliefs Model, or the theory of planned behaviour [14–16]. Considering each model could facilitate a deeper consideration for the potential consequences of policies aiming to change behaviour in light of economic and social realities. This dynamic approach could better ensure that policymaking is responsive and effective in improving health outcomes.

4.2. Strengths and Limitations

The strengths of the current study include the timing of the surveys and the large number of participants. This is a unique data set collected at a pivotal time that could inform policymaking. That said, the data involve participants' self-reports or perceptions. Other measurements could reveal different relationships. Additionally, the dataset only included the response from the first month of the lockdown period. Further changes may have occurred throughout the pandemic. Demographic information was not available for the research team to analyse and many responders were not included in our analyses.

Inferences can be made about those not included. For instance, nearly half of those omitted reported not using public transit before the lockdown. Therefore, we could infer that those removed are more likely to live in areas without reliable public transit (e.g., more rural locations) and are more likely to own a car. Our findings may not generalise to such people.

In our analyses, changes in Behaviour were not predicted by changes in Motivation or Opportunity. Policy actions taken before the lockdown directly impacted Opportunities but did not change greatly over the 30 days these surveys. For example, the Coronavirus Job Retention Scheme was announced on the 20 March 2024, ten days before the lockdown [41]. This scheme provided grants to employers to pay 80% or up to 2500 GBP of furloughed employee's wages. Employees using that scheme before the lockdown were less likely to experience changes in their Opportunities during the first month of lockdown. Changes in perceived Opportunities were predicted by changes in Motivation, suggesting that Motivation influences how easy people find it to adhere to social distancing rules. More motivated individuals perceive following the rules as easier, which resonates with the evidence [42].

Also not predicted by the original COM-B model, Behaviour did not feedback to predict Capability and Opportunity. As a cross-sectional series of surveys, different individuals completed each survey. While our data show population-level reports of Behaviour change each of the 30 days, we do not have information about individual-level Behaviour change across those 30 days. A repeated measures method could be better suited to assess the feedback loops predicted by the COM-B model. Our retrospective analysis was further limited by the previously collected data, which limits the theories we could consider. We did not have access to data about participant intentions to change their behaviour and so could not evaluate Ajzen's (1991) [15] theory of planned behaviour. Future studies could include items about participants' behavioural intentions.

5. Conclusions

The current retrospective data analysis examined the relationships between people's Capabilities, Opportunities, Motivations, and Behaviour change, i.e., adherence to lockdown guidelines across the first 30 days of the lockdown in Great Britain. Though slight, trend changes were identified in all COM-B components. These changes include a decreasing trend in the levels of Behaviour change. Our relationship analyses suggest that the decreases in Behaviour change were not necessarily inevitable. Changes in Capability could be used by policymakers to forecast Behaviour change. Rather than positing immutable factors to explain why residents do (or do not) adhere to government guidance, policymakers could focus on supporting residents' Capabilities, Opportunities, and Motivations to improve public health.

Supplementary Materials: The following supporting information can be downloaded at: https://www.mdpi.com/article/10.3390/bs14090852/s1, File S1: Analysis of the dynamics of COMB components.

Author Contributions: All authors roles were tantamount to the ultimate publication and may be recognised as first author. Conceptualisation I.V.; Methodology I.V. and K.H.; Formal Analysis K.H.; Resources I.V.; Data Curation S.K.; Writing—Original Draft Preparation K.A.S.; Writing—Review and Editing, all authors coordinated by K.A.S. All authors have read and agreed to the published version of the manuscript.

Funding: This research was supported by the National Recovery and Resilience Plan of the Republic of Bulgaria grant number SUMMIT BG-RRP-2.004-0008-C01.

Institutional Review Board Statement: The study was conducted according to the guidelines of the Declaration of Helsinki and approved by The University of Warwick's Humanities and Social Sciences Research Ethics Committee (ID: 110.20-21, approval date: 23 February 2021).

Informed Consent Statement: Not applicable.

Data Availability Statement: Data would be made available upon the request with corresponding authors.

Conflicts of Interest: The authors declare no conflicts of interest.

References

1. Bharti, N. Linking human behaviors and infectious diseases. *Proc. Natl. Acad. Sci. USA* **2021**, *118*, e2101345118. [CrossRef] [PubMed]
2. West, R.; Michie, S.; Rubin, G.J.; Amlôt, R. Applying principles of behaviour change to reduce SARS-CoV-2 transmission. *Nat. Hum. Behav.* **2020**, *4*, 451–459. [CrossRef] [PubMed]
3. Rose, G. Sick individuals and sick populations. *Int. J. Epidemiol.* **1985**, *14*, 32–38. [CrossRef] [PubMed]
4. Patiño-Lugo, D.F.; Vélez, M.; Velásquez Salazar, P.; Vera-Giraldo, C.Y.; Vélez, V.; Marín, I.C.; Ramírez, P.A.; Quintero, S.P.; Castrillón Martínez, E.; Pineda Higuita, D.A.; et al. Non-pharmaceutical interventions for containment, mitigation and suppression of COVID-19 infection. *Colomb. Med.* **2020**, *51*, e4266. [CrossRef] [PubMed]
5. Cascini, F.; Failla, G.; Gobbi, C.; Pallini, E.; Jin, H.; Wang, L.; Villani, L.; Quentin, W.; Boccia, S.; Ricciardi, W. A cross-country comparison of Covid-19 containment measures and their effects on the epidemic curves. *BMC Public Health* **2022**, *22*, e1765. [CrossRef] [PubMed]
6. Mahase, E. Covid-19: Was the decision to delay the UK's lockdown over fears of "behavioural fatigue" based on evidence? *BMJ* **2020**, *370*, m3166. [CrossRef]
7. Open Letter to the UK Government Regarding COVID-19. Available online: https://sites.google.com/view/covidopenletter/home (accessed on 15 June 2024).
8. Ferguson, N.M.; Laydon, D.; Nedjati-Gilani, G.; Imai, N.; Ainslie, K.; Baguelin, M.; Bhatia, S.; Boonyasiri, A.; Cucunubá, Z.; Cuomo-Dannenburg, G.; et al. *Impact of Non-Pharmaceutical Interventions (NPIs) to Reduce COVID-19 Mortality and Healthcare Demand*; Imperial College COVID-19 Response Team: London, UK, 2020. Available online: https://www.imperial.ac.uk/media/imperial-college/medicine/sph/ide/gida-fellowships/Imperial-College-COVID19-NPI-modelling-16-03-2020.pdf (accessed on 15 July 2024).
9. Prime Minister's Statement on Coronavirus (COVID-19): 23 March 2020. Available online: https://www.gov.uk/government/speeches/pm-address-to-the-nation-on-coronavirus-23-march-2020 (accessed on 15 July 2024).
10. Harvey, N. Behavioral fatigue: Real phenomenon, naïve Construct, or policy contrivance? *Front. Psychol.* **2020**, *11*, e589892. [CrossRef]
11. Michie, S.; West, R.; Harvey, N. The concept of "fatigue" in tackling COVID-19. *BMJ* **2020**, *371*, m4171. [CrossRef]
12. Michie, S.; van Stralen, M.M.; West, R. The behaviour change wheel: A new method for characterising and designing behaviour change interventions. *Implement. Sci.* **2011**, *6*, 42. [CrossRef]
13. Cane, J.; O'Connor, D.; Michie, S. Validation of the theoretical domains framework for use in behaviour change and implementation research. *Implement. Sci.* **2012**, *7*, 37. [CrossRef]
14. Rosenstock, I.M.; Strecher, V.J.; Becker, M.H. Social learning theory and the health belief model. *Health Educ. Behav.* **1988**, *15*, 175–183. [CrossRef] [PubMed]
15. Ajzen, I. The theory of planned behavior. *Organ. Behav. Hum. Decis. Process.* **1991**, *50*, 179–211. [CrossRef]
16. Michie, S.; Atkins, L.; West, R. *The Behaviour Change Wheel: A Guide to Designing Interventions*; Silverback Publishing: London, UK, 2014. Available online: https://www.behaviourchangewheel.com/ (accessed on 1 August 2024).
17. Smith, M. YouGov's Mood Tracker Finds that Britons Are Slowly Finding Happiness Once Again, Although We Are Yet Some Way from a Return to Normal Levels of Joy. Available online: https://yougov.co.uk/society/articles/29322-britains-mood-slowly-starts-recover-covid-19 (accessed on 7 September 2024).
18. Shakespeare, S. Changing Consumer Landscape: Sports, Dieting, and Exercise. Available online: https://yougov.co.uk/sport/articles/29846-changing-consumer-landscape-sports-dieting-and-exe (accessed on 7 September 2024).
19. Curtis, C. One in Five Have Started Breaking Lockdown Rules More Following Cummings Saga. Available online: https://yougov.co.uk/health/articles/30043-one-five-have-started-breaking-lockdown-rules-more (accessed on 7 September 2024).
20. Shakespeare, S. Changing Consumer Landscapes: Charities. Available online: https://yougov.co.uk/economy/articles/30401-changing-consumer-landscapes-charities. (accessed on 7 September 2024).
21. Shakespeare, S. Sports Direct: A COVID-19 Cautionary Tale? Available online: https://yougov.co.uk/consumer/articles/29063-sports-direct-covid-19-cautionary-tale. (accessed on 7 September 2024).
22. Ibbetson, C. Will Primark's Gamble Pay Off? Available online: https://yougov.co.uk/consumer/articles/30167-will-primark-sale-pay-off. (accessed on 7 September 2024).
23. Nolsoe, E. Next's Brand in Healthy Shape as Stores Reopen. Available online: https://yougov.co.uk/consumer/articles/30947-nexts-brand-healthy-shape-stores-reopen. (accessed on 7 September 2024).
24. Humphrys, J. How Should Governments Make Us Do What They Want? Available online: https://yougov.co.uk/politics/articles/30803-how-should-governments-make-us-do-what-they-want (accessed on 7 September 2024).
25. YouGov. Panel Methodology. Available online: https://yougov.co.uk/about/panel-methodology/ (accessed on 15 July 2024).

26. Office for National Statistics. 2011 Census. Available online: https://www.ons.gov.uk/census/2011census (accessed on 15 July 2024).
27. Atanasov, A. *Statistical Methods for Dynamic Series Analysis*; Publishing Complex—UNSS: Sofia, Bulgaria, 2018.
28. Granger, C.W.J. Investigating causal relations by econometric models and cross-spectral methods. *Econometrica* **1969**, 37, 424–438. [CrossRef]
29. Thurman, W.N.; Fisher, M.E. Chickens, Eggs, and Causality, or Which Came First? *Am. J. Agric. Econ.* **1988**, 70, 237–238. [CrossRef]
30. Granger, C. Time Series Analysis, Cointegration, and Applications. *Nobel Lecture*, 8 December 2003; pp. 360–366. Available online: https://www.nobelprize.org/uploads/2018/06/granger-lecture.pdf (accessed on 15 July 2024).
31. Baker, D.; Merkert, R.; Kamruzzaman, M. Regional aviation and economic growth: Cointegration and causality analysis in Australia. *J. Transp. Geogr.* **2015**, 43, 140–150. [CrossRef]
32. UK Parliament. House of Commons Library Eat Out to Help Out Scheme. Available online: https://commonslibrary.parliament.uk/research-briefings/cbp-8978/ (accessed on 15 July 2024).
33. Duckworth, A.L.; Peterson, C.; Matthews, M.D.; Kelly, D.R. Grit: Perseverance and passion for long-term goals. *J. Pers. Soc. Psychol.* **2007**, 92, 1087–1101. [CrossRef]
34. Anders, E.K.; Pool, R. *Peak: Secrets from the New Science of Expertise*; Houghton Mifflin Harcourt: Boston, MA, USA, 2016; pp. 167–168. ISBN 9780544456235. OCLC 913923802.
35. Duffy, B.; Allington, D. *The Accepting, the Suffering, and the Resisting: The Different Reactions to Life Under Lockdown*; Policy Institute, King's College London: London, UK, 2020. Available online: www.kcl.ac.uk/policy-institute/assets/Coronavirus-in-the-UK-cluster-analysis.pdf (accessed on 15 July 2024).
36. Atchison, C.; Bowman, L.R.; Vrinten, C.; Redd, R.; Pristera, P.; Eaton, J.; Ward, H. Early perceptions and behavioural responses during the COVID-19 pandemic: A cross-sectional survey of UK adults. *BMJ Open* **2021**, 11, e043577. [CrossRef]
37. Reicher, S.; Drury, J. Pandemic fatigue? How adherence to covid-19 regulations has been misrepresented and why it matters. *BMJ* **2021**, 372, n137. [CrossRef]
38. Miller, F.A.; Patton, S.J.; Dobrow, M.; Berta, W. Public involvement in health research systems: A governance framework. *Health Res. Policy Syst.* **2018**, 16, e79. [CrossRef]
39. Arumugam, A.; Phillips, L.R.; Moore, A.; Kumaran, S.D.; Sampath, K.K.; Migliorini, F.; Maffulli, N.; Ranganadhababu, B.N.; Hegazy, F.; Botto-van Bemden, A. Patient and public involvement in research: A review of practical resources for young investigators. *BMC Rheumatol.* **2023**, 7, 2. [CrossRef]
40. Ghio, D.; Lawes-Wickwar, S.; Tang, M.Y.; Epton, T.; Howlett, N.; Jenkinson, E.; Stanescu, S.; Westbrook, J.; Kassianos, A.P.; Watson, D.; et al. What influences people's responses to public health messages for managing risks and preventing infectious diseases? A rapid systematic review of the evidence and recommendations. *BMJ Open* **2021**, 11, e048750. [CrossRef] [PubMed]
41. UK Government. Corona Virus Job Retention Scheme. Available online: https://www.gov.uk/government/collections/coronavirus-job-retention-scheme (accessed on 1 August 2023).
42. Almeida-Silva, M.; Andrade, G.; Luis, T.; Santos, M.; Grilo, A. Influence of cognitive factors on adherence to social distancing and the use of masks during the COVID-19 pandemic by young adults: A systematic review. *Soc. Sci.* **2024**, 13, 275. [CrossRef]

behavioral sciences

MDPI

Article

Exploring Job-Related Factors and Exercise Intentions in Relation to Overall Physical Activity and Its Subdivisions

Wei-Hsun Wang [1,2,3,†], Wei-Ting Hsu [4,5,†], Hsin-I Cheng [6], Ren-Hau Li [7,8], Shu-Ling Huang [7,8,*] and Feng-Cheng Tang [1,9,10,*]

1 Department of Post-Baccalaureate Medicine, College of Medicine, National Chung Hsing University, Taichung 402, Taiwan; 132072@cch.org.tw
2 Department of Golden-Ager Industry Management, Chaoyang University of Technology, Taichung 413, Taiwan
3 Department of Orthopedics, Changhua Christian Hospital, Changhua 500, Taiwan
4 Department of Construction Engineering, Chaoyang University of Technology, Taichung 413, Taiwan; wthsu@cyut.edu.tw
5 Department of Leisure Services Management, Chaoyang University of Technology, Taichung 413, Taiwan
6 Child Development Center, Far Eastern Memorial Hospital, New Taipei 220, Taiwan; 410283030@gms.ndhu.edu.tw
7 Department of Psychology, Chung Shan Medical University, Taichung 402, Taiwan; davidrh@csmu.edu.tw
8 Room of Clinical Psychology, Chung Shan Medical University Hospital, Taichung 402, Taiwan
9 Department of Occupational Medicine, Changhua Christian Hospital, Changhua 500, Taiwan
10 Graduate Institute of Clinical Medicine, National Chung Hsing University, Taichung 402, Taiwan
* Correspondence: shuling@csmu.edu.tw (S.-L.H.); 106159@cch.org.tw (F.-C.T.)
† These authors contributed equally to this work.

Abstract: This study examined the relationships between job-related factors and overall physical activity (PA), including its subdivisions: leisure-time PA, transportation PA, and work-related PA. Additionally, this study investigated the associations between exercise intentions and different types of PA. A cross-sectional design was employed, utilizing a questionnaire to collect data on participants' demographics, job-related characteristics, exercise intentions, and levels of PA. A total of 400 full-time workers voluntarily participated in this study. The findings identified women, white-collar workers, those with longer working hours, and individuals with low exercise intentions as high-risk groups for insufficient overall PA in multiple linear regression analysis. After controlling for covariates, occupation was found to be associated with both overall PA ($\beta = 0.146$) and work-related PA ($\beta = 0.236$). Shift workers exhibited higher levels of work-related PA ($\beta = 0.234$). Furthermore, exercise intentions showed associations with overall PA ($\beta = 0.243$), leisure-time PA ($\beta = 0.523$), and transportation PA ($\beta = 0.176$) but did not demonstrate a significant relationship with work-related PA. This study highlights the importance of implementing comprehensive approaches in workplace health promotion programs aimed at enhancing various types of PA. Strategies should focus on improving exercise intentions to boost leisure-time and transportation PA, while work-related PA requires tailored interventions based on job-specific factors.

Keywords: physical activity; workplace health promotion; exercise intention

1. Introduction

Physical activity (PA) encompasses any body movement driven by skeletal muscles that requires energy expenditure. PA is strongly linked with a reduced risk of premature mortality and major non-communicable diseases [1]. The World Health Organization recommends that adults aged 18–64 engage in at least 150–300 min of moderate-intensity aerobic PA per week, or at least 75–150 min of vigorous-intensity aerobic PA, or an equivalent combination of both throughout the week. However, more than a quarter of the global adult population remains inadequately active [2]. In Taiwan, the situation is particularly concerning. Only 25.8% of the adult population in Taiwan manage to achieve the recommended 150 min of moderate-intensity exercise per week [3]. Despite a rise in the proportion of regular exercisers from 18.8% in 2006 to 35.0% in 2023 [3], the prevalence of insufficient PA among individuals aged 18 and above remains alarmingly high at 47.3% [4]. Among these individuals, those aged 30–54 exhibit the lowest activity levels, and they are of prime working age.

The workplace has been acknowledged as a pivotal setting for promoting PA among adults. PA promotion in the workplace holds promise as an integrated initiative that tangibly improves worker health and augments business performance [5,6]. Due to differing work characteristics, blue-collar and white-collar workers display varying levels of PA both at work and during leisure time [7]. Research also highlights that shift work significantly influence PA levels. Time spent engaged in sedentary behavior is lower in shift workers than non-shift workers [8,9]. A nationwide survey reveals that primary reasons for the lack of PA among non-exercising individuals in Taiwan include work-related fatigue (22.5%), laziness (21.4%), and lack of time due to work commitments (21.2%) [3]. However, whether these reasons constitute genuine influencing factors or are mere convenient excuses warrants further elucidation. Research on this topic remains limited in Taiwan, necessitating an exploration of the correlation between job-related factors such as occupational category, whether taking shift work, working hours, work-related burnout, and various forms of PA.

Additionally, research conducted in Taiwan indicates that gender disparities in PA emerge from childhood, with boys engaging in significantly more PA than girls, and this gap widens during adolescence [10]. As individuals enter middle age, this gender gap in PA levels changes, with men becoming less active than women [11]. These findings suggest that gender and age are key factors influencing PA levels. Moreover, although a weak association between PA and body mass index (BMI) is generally found among non-obese individuals, BMI is significantly associated with PA in obese individuals [12,13]. Given the multitude of factors that may influence individual PA levels, demographic variables such as gender, age, and BMI should be considered in studies examining PA.

PA is typically assessed across dimensions including leisure-time PA, work-related PA, transportation PA, and domestic and gardening activities [14]. In the realm of workplace health promotion, attention often centers around the former three dimensions, excluding domestic and gardening activities [9,15,16]. Measurement of PA can be categorized into objective instruments (direct measurement) and subjective questionnaires (indirect measurement), with the specific approach contingent upon particular research objectives [17]. Utilizing objective instruments in the workplace presents challenges. A review paper highlights that self-reported questionnaires predominantly serve as the method for data collection on PA and sedentary behavior at work [18]. Thus, the questionnaires used must reliably reflect energy expenditure.

Implementation intentions serve as a potent strategy for promoting health-related behaviors; exercise intentions, in particular, present a cost-effective means to promote PA and exercise [19,20]. For certain individuals, exercise intentions facilitate the translation of intentions into behavior. Within the context of PA, the Transtheoretical Model provides a framework for conceptualizing and measuring behavior change, in addition to facilitating individualized and adaptable promotion strategies [21]. This model, developed as a comprehensive model of behavior change, integrates intention, behavior, and temporal aspects into a unified approach. This model, which includes five stages, suggests that health behavior change is not an all-or-nothing phenomenon but rather a dynamic process that evolves over time. Individuals undergoing behavior change may cycle through different stages repeatedly. Among these stages, the least amount of change occurs in the precontemplation stage, while the most significant changes take place in the contemplation stage. In this stage, individuals gradually become more aware and engage in continuous self-evaluation, eventually leading them to enter the behavior change phase based on the results of their internal self-assessment [22]. The types of interventions required will thus vary depending on the stage individuals are in. When applied to exercise adoption, these stages of change encompass precontemplation (no intention to exercise), contemplation (intention to exercise within the next six months), preparation (intention to exercise within the next 30 days), action (regular exercise for less than six months), and maintenance (regular exercise for more than six months). Intention plays a pivotal role in delineating the early stages of change. However, relevant research predominantly focuses exclusively on regular exercise or leisure-time PA. Clarification concerning their influences on other types of PA is warranted. In brief, this study aims to explore the relationships between job-related factors and exercise intentions in relation to overall PA and its subdivisions.

2. Materials and Methods

2.1. Participants and Recruitment

This research adopts a cross-sectional design and adheres to the principles outlined in the Declaration of Helsinki. Approval for this study was obtained from the Institutional Review Board of Chung-Shan University Hospital in Taiwan (CSHIRB No: CS18263). Researchers visited workplaces and explained the study's purpose to the occupational health staff. To ensure the representativeness of the sample, one out of every three employees was randomly selected based on their employee numbers. The inclusion criteria for participant recruitment were full-time workers aged 20–65 who were willing to participate. Exclusion criteria included part-time workers, illiterate individuals, and those unwilling to participate. A total of 465 full-time workers were invited to participate in the study. The researchers respected the respondents' autonomy, ensured confidentiality, and obtained informed consent from workers willing to participate. Ultimately, 400 participants agreed to take part in the study and provided complete questionnaire responses. Using the G*Power 3.1.9.7 software to calculate sample size based on the effect size of an R-square of 0.03 with a power of 0.80, a sample size larger than 202 was enough. For additional details regarding the study procedure, please refer to our previous publication [23].

2.2. Measures

The research employed a questionnaire survey method for data collection, encompassing demographic characteristics, job-related factors, exercise intentions, and PA levels. The section on demographic characteristics included inquiries on gender, age, education level, marital status, and BMI. BMI was computed as weight in kilograms divided by height in meters squared (kg/m^2), and BMI status was categorized as underweight ($BMI < 18.5$), ideal weight ($18.5 \leq BMI < 24.0$), overweight ($24.0 \leq BMI < 27.0$), and obese ($BMI \geq 27.0$) following the definition provided by the Health Promotion Administration, Ministry of Health and Welfare in Taiwan [24].

2.2.1. Job-Related Factors

Job-related factors comprised occupation, whether the worker engaged in shift work, working hours, and work-related burnout. Occupation was classified into two categories: white-collar worker (encompassing management, professional, technician, clerical support worker, and service worker) and blue-collar worker (including crafts worker and machine operator) [25].

2.2.2. Burnout

The Copenhagen Burnout Inventory, developed by Kristensen et al. [26], was used to gauge the extent of work-related burnout among participants. This inventory is a valid and reliable questionnaire measuring personal burnout (6 items), work-related burnout (7 items), and client-related burnout (6 items). According to the theoretical framework of this inventory, these subscales can be utilized independently based on the target population. For the current study, the work-related burnout subscale was solely utilized. The internal consistency of this subscale, as measured by Cronbach's alpha, was determined to be 0.934.

Participants rated their responses on a 5-point scale, ranging from 0 (never) to 4 (always), with higher scores indicating heightened levels of burnout.

2.2.3. Exercise Intentions

The levels of exercise intention were assessed utilizing the Transtheoretical Model [6], employing a 5-stage measurement to evaluate exercise behavior. These stages include precontemplation, contemplation, preparation, action, and maintenance. The Transtheoretical Model within the PA context provides a framework for both the conceptualization and measurement of behavior change with a validated construct validity [21]. Evidence suggests that adjacent stages can be effectively distinguished by intention to participate in exercise for adults, although no significant difference was found between action and maintenance [27]. Hence, exercise intentions are categorized as no (precontemplation), mild (contemplation), moderate (preparation), and strong (action and maintenance) levels for this study. Higher scores indicate a higher level of exercise intention [27].

2.2.4. Level of Physical Activity

A self-reported questionnaire, comprising details about leisure-time, transportation, work-related, and overall PA, served as the data collection tool. The PA-related questions were adapted from previous studies conducted in China and in Nordic countries [28–30]. This instrument, previously validated, demonstrates a high correlation with physical fitness measured through energy expenditure [31,32].

Leisure-time PA was categorized as follows: (1) low: indicating almost complete inactivity or engaging in minor PA, albeit not at a moderate or high intensity; (2) moderate: involving some moderate-intensity PA for more than 4 h per week, such as walking, cycling, or light gardening; and (3) high: inclusive of vigorous PA for more than 3 h per week, such as running, jogging, skiing, swimming, or heavy gardening.

Transportation PA was categorized as follows: (1) low: using motorized transportation; (2) moderate: walking or bicycling for 1–29 min; and (3) high: walking or bicycling for 30 min or more.

Work-related PA was categorized as follows: (1) low: physically very easy work with seated office tasks (e.g., secretarial work); (2) moderate: work involving standing and walking (e.g., store assistant, light industrial work); and (3) high: work involving walking and lifting, or heavy manual labor (e.g., industrial work, farm work).

All three subdivisions of PA were consolidated and reclassified into three categories to determine the overall PA level: (1) low: participants reported low levels of leisure-time, transportation, and work-related PA; (2) moderate: participants reported moderate to high levels of PA in only one of the three subdivisions; and (3) high: participants reported moderate to high levels of PA in two or all three subdivisions.

2.3. Statistical Analysis

The Chi-square test was adopted to compare the differences in overall PA levels by demographic characteristics and job-related variables. Cramér's V was employed to assess the effect size. Pearson's correlation was used to analyze the relationships between the continuous variables. Mean, standard deviation, skewness, and kurtosis were calculated for the continuous variables to evaluate normality. The demographic characteristics showing significant differences in overall PA were controlled for in multiple linear regressions. Accordingly, gender and education level were controlled for in multiple linear regressions. The categorical variables, including gender, whether taking shift work, and occupational category, were transformed into dummy variables beforehand. Female, without shift work, and white-collar worker were coded as referents. Multiple linear regression analysis was adopted to investigate the relationships between job-related factors and PA levels, incorporating overall PA and its subdivisions. The roles of exercise intentions on PAs were explored as well. All statistical procedures were performed using SPSS-20.0 software for

Microsoft Windows (IBM Corp., Armonk, NY, USA); a p-value less than 0.05 was considered statistically significant.

3. Results

Out of the 465 distributed questionnaires, 400 were successfully collected, yielding an 86.0% response rate. Among the participants, 89.8% were male, and 10.3% were female. The average age was 37.7 years (SD = 6.1). The majority of the participants were married (65.5%), held a bachelor's degree (76.8%), identified as white-collar workers (80.8%), and did not engage in shift work (71.8%). Approximately one-third of the participants had an ideal weight (34.3%), while 31.8% were overweight, and 32.3% were classified as obese. The prevalence of overall PA levels was as follows: 5.0% for low level, 26.3% for moderate level, and 68.8% for high level. Table 1 details the overall PA levels concerning demographic characteristics and job-related variables. Gender, education level, occupational category, and shift work demonstrated significant differences in overall PA levels.

Table 1. The comparisons of the level of overall physical activity by demographic variables and job-related factors.

Variables	Total (n = 400)	Low Level (n = 20, 5.0%)	Moderate Level (n = 105, 26.3%)	High Level (n = 275, 68.8%)	χ^2	p	Effect Size
	n (%)	n (%) [a]	n (%) [a]	n (%) [a]			
Gender					47.1	<0.001	0.343
female	41 (10.3)	0 (0.0)	29 (70.7)	12 (29.3)			
male	359 (89.8)	20 (5.6)	76 (21.2)	263 (73.3)			
Marital status					1.0	0.601	0.050
not-married	138 (34.5)	5 (3.6)	35 (25.4)	98 (71.0)			
married	262 (65.5)	15 (5.7)	70 (26.7)	177 (67.6)			
Education					12.8	0.012	0.127
senior high	63 (15.8)	4 (6.3)	10 (15.9)	49 (77.8)			
graduate	307 (76.8)	12 (3.9)	83 (27.0)	212 (69.1)			
postgraduate	30 (7.5)	4 (13.3)	12 (40.0)	14 (46.7)			
BMI					8.6	0.198	0.104
underweight	6 (1.5)	0 (0.0)	3 (50.0)	3 (50.0)			
ideal weight	136 (34.3)	6 (4.4)	46 (33.8)	84 (61.8)			
overweight	126 (31.8)	8 (6.3)	27 (21.4)	91 (72.2)			
obesity	128 (32.3)	6 (4.7)	29 (22.7)	93 (72.7)			
Occupation					14.9	0.001	0.193
white-collar	323 (80.8)	19 (5.9)	96 (29.7)	208 (64.4)			
blue-collar	77 (19.3)	1 (1.3)	9 (11.7)	67 (87.0)			
Shift work					15.8	<0.001	0.199
without	287 (71.8)	14 (4.9)	91 (31.7)	182 (63.4)			
with	113 (28.3)	6 (5.3)	14 (12.4)	93 (82.3)			

[a] Calculated as a percentage of valid counts within each row's cells. Effect size is Cramér's V.

Table 2 presents the bivariate correlations and descriptive statistics for the research variables. All skewness and kurtosis coefficients were between −1.56 and 1.20, showing that they were close to a normal distribution. Age was positively associated with working hours (r = 0.113, $p < 0.05$) and negatively associated with work-related PA (r = −0.151, $p < 0.01$). Working hours exhibited a positive association with work-related burnout (r = 0.154, $p < 0.01$) and a negative association with overall PA (r = −0.117, $p < 0.05$). Exercise intention displayed positive associations with overall PA (r = 0.211, $p < 0.01$), leisure-time PA (r = 0.529, $p < 0.01$), and transportation PA (r = 0.179, $p < 0.01$). Regarding specific PAs, overall PA showed positive associations with leisure-time PA (r = 0.471, $p < 0.01$), transportation PA (r = 0.457, $p < 0.01$), and work-related PA (r = 0.452, $p < 0.01$). Leisure-time PA also exhibited a positive relationship with transportation PA (r = 0.118, $p < 0.05$). However, work-related PA did not show significant associations with leisure-time PA or transportation PA.

Table 2. The correlations of research variables.

Variables	1	2	3	4	5	6	7	8
1 Age	–							
2 Working hours	0.113 *	–						
3 Work-related burnout	−0.068	0.154 **	–					
4 Exercise intentions	−0.005	0.012	−0.052	–				
5 Overall PA	−0.067	−0.117 *	−0.045	0.211 **	–			
6 Leisure-time PA	−0.056	−0.009	−0.067	0.529 **	0.471 **	–		
7 Transportation PA	−0.014	−0.019	−0.018	0.179 **	0.457 **	0.118 *	–	
8 Work-related PA	−0.151 **	−0.063	−0.005	−0.085	0.452 **	0.003	−0.007	–
Mean	37.72	44.00	41.16	2.65	2.64	1.75	1.94	1.74
Standard deviation	6.14	4.27	14.34	0.96	0.58	0.89	0.59	0.70
Skewness	−0.16	0.73	0.19	−0.19	−1.34	0.51	0.02	0.41
Kurtosis	−0.04	1.20	0.60	−0.90	0.81	−1.56	−0.17	−0.93

* $p < 0.05$; ** $p < 0.01$; standard error of skewness is 0.122, and the standard error of kurtosis is 0.243.

Table 3 summarizes multiple linear regressions predicting PAs based on job-related factors and exercise intentions. For overall PA (F = 9.706, $p < 0.001$; adjusted $R^2 = 0.132$), with gender and education level controlled, occupational category (β = 0.146, $p < 0.01$), working hours (β = −0.119, $p < 0.05$), and exercise intentions (β = 0.243, $p < 0.001$) were significant factors. The other multiple linear regressions were also controlled with covariates. For leisure-time PA (F = 24.300, $p < 0.001$; adjusted $R^2 = 0.290$), only exercise intentions (β = 0.523, $p < 0.001$) demonstrated significance. Similarly, for transportation PA (F = 2.874, $p < 0.01$; adjusted $R^2 = 0.032$), only exercise intentions (β = 0.176, $p < 0.001$) displayed significance. For work-related PA (F = 22.733, $p < 0.001$; adjusted $R^2 = 0.277$), occupational category (β = 0.236, $p < 0.001$) and shift work (β = 0.234, $p < 0.001$) were significant.

Table 3. Summary of multiple linear regression predicting overall PA and its subdivisions.

Variables	Overall PA			Leisure-Time PA			Transportation PA			Work-Related PA		
	B	SE	β	B	SE	β	B	SE	β	B	SE	β
Constant	2.597	0.378		0.059	0.531		2.286	0.412		1.098	0.423	
Gender	0.334	0.093	0.176 ***	0.401	0.131	0.136 **	−0.115	0.101	−0.059	0.563	0.104	0.243 ***
Education	−0.084	0.059	−0.069	0.148	0.083	0.079	−0.111	0.064	−0.089	−0.157	0.066	−0.106 *
Occupation	0.212	0.072	0.146 **	0.074	0.101	0.033	0.072	0.078	0.048	0.419	0.080	0.236 ***
Shift work	0.083	0.065	0.065	−0.057	0.092	−0.029	−0.115	0.071	−0.087	0.364	0.073	0.234 ***
Working hours	−0.016	0.007	−0.119 *	−0.007	0.009	−0.033	−0.003	0.007	−0.022	−0.006	0.007	−0.039
Work-related burnout	−0.001	0.002	−0.033	−0.002	0.003	−0.040	0.000	0.002	−0.008	−0.001	0.002	−0.027
Exercise intentions	0.146	0.028	0.243 ***	0.489	0.040	0.523 ***	0.109	0.031	0.176 ***	−0.013	0.032	−0.017
Adjusted R^2		0.132			0.290			0.032			0.277	
F		9.706	***		24.300	***		2.874	**		22.733	***

B denotes unstandardized regression coefficient; SE denotes standard error; β denotes standardized regression coefficient. Female, white-collar worker, and without shift work were coded as referents. * $p < 0.05$; ** $p < 0.01$; *** $p < 0.001$.

4. Discussion

The aim of this study was to investigate the relationship between job-related factors and exercise intentions concerning overall PA and its three subdivisions: leisure-time PA, transportation PA, and work-related PA. The findings identify specific demographic and job-related factors, highlighting women, white-collar workers, individuals with extended working hours, and those with diminished exercise intentions as high-risk groups for inadequate overall PA. Notably, exercise intentions showed significant correlations with leisure-time PA and transportation PA. Conversely, work-related PA was associated with shift work and occupational categories. The present study emphasizes the necessity of employing tailored approaches in workplace health promotion initiatives, thereby acknowledging the diverse influences on various forms of PA.

This study demonstrates that exercise intention significantly influences overall PA, leisure-time PA, and transportation PA. Particularly, exercise intention reflects an individual's willingness and proactive engagement, exerting a more pronounced impact on leisure-time PA. The concept of intention plays a central role in theories explaining health behaviors, including PA engagement [33,34]. Despite a considerable intention–behavior gap in PA [35], intention remains a significant correlate of PA behavior [20,36,37]. The intricate interplay between exercise intentions and various dimensions of PA underscores the importance of addressing intention as a critical factor in shaping health behaviors, especially in the context of full-time employment. Strategic interventions aimed at enhancing exercise self-esteem and alleviating exercise barriers are pivotal for fostering sustainable exercise habits among workers [23].

The observed correlation between exercise intention and transportation PA, while significant, displays a slight diminution, possibly attributed to the accessibility of public transportation and time constraints. The workplace setting of this study, located in a rural area with participants managing familial responsibilities, suggests potential limitations in enhancing transportation-related PA. Recognizing the impact of neighborhood physical environmental variables on transportation PA [38], workplace interventions, such as adjusting parking distances or transportation boarding areas, may contribute to augmenting transportation PA. Health and transportation researchers have examined PA from different perspectives for a long time. In the 2000s, they began encountering studies from the transportation field [39]. PA and active transport, usually termed "non-motorized transport", need more collaboration. In the future, it will be necessary to explore the essential factors influencing transportation PA for workplaces with convenient public transportation in urban areas.

As expected, exercise intention was not significantly associated with work-related PA, suggesting that factors influencing PA during work hours may not solely depend on an individual's exercise intention. Job-related variables emerged as more prominent determinants of work-related PA, with blue-collar and shift workers exhibiting significantly higher levels compared to their white-collar counterparts and non-shift workers. Previous studies show similar findings [9,16]. Even using objective measurement, workers with shift work were found to be less sedentary than those with non-shift work [8,40]. Shift work is associated with various health problems, such as cardiovascular disease and metabolic syndrome [16,41]. Shift workers, therefore, require a better healthy lifestyle and to engage in health behaviors in order to decrease health hazards. However, shift workers are found to have insufficient sleep, poor sleep quality, and poor nutritional intake [15]. A prospective cohort study confirmed that irrespective of the level of work-related PA, a consistently lower risk with increasing leisure-time PA was found for both cardiovascular and all-cause mortality among workers [42]. Fortunately, shift work was not significantly related to leisure-time PA and transportation PA in the current study. Increasing these two types of PA might, therefore, be another approach to promote shift workers' health.

A review article found that PA levels at work are generally low, while sedentary behavior is high. This was largely a function of occupation; white-collar workers exhibited more sedentary behavior than blue-collar workers [18]. Our study shows similar findings, with white-collar workers reporting lower levels of overall PA and work-related PA. Regarding overall PA, this aligns with the extant literature, indicating a propensity for higher overall PA levels among those engaged in manual labor [43]. Other research also finds that full-day sedentarism is more likely to occur among white-collar workers and in those with higher levels of education [44,45]. Moreover, the negative association between long work hours and overall PA underscores the potential risk posed by extended working hours, particularly among white-collar workers engaged in overtime. This situation emphasizes the need for targeted interventions to address the specific challenges faced by this demographic in maintaining sufficient levels of overall PA. Additionally, although work-related fatigue and lack of time due to work commitments have been reported as reasons for Taiwanese workers not engaging in exercise [3], working hours and work-related burnout were not significantly associated with any subdivision of PA. Addressing how to debunk these misconceptions and improve workers' intentions may present a challenge.

The present study was conducted with a rigorous approach; nonetheless, it is essential to acknowledge certain limitations. The study's participants were exclusively sourced from the manufacturing industry, and the sample size was relatively small. This might impact the generalizability of the study findings. Additionally, the assessment of PA relied on self-reported measures, introducing the possibility of overestimation or underestimation. Moreover, the voluntary participation of workers may have led to selective bias, potentially impacting the generalizability of the study's results. Consequently, caution is advised when extrapolating and applying the findings of this study.

5. Conclusions

Unlike most previous studies that focus on leisure-time PA, this study offers a comprehensive analysis of overall PA and its subdivisions. The findings reveal the complex relationships between job-related factors, exercise intentions, and various types of PA. Tailored workplace health promotion programs should address the distinct influences on leisure-time PA, transportation PA, and work-related PA. Exercise intention was the key factor significantly associated with overall, leisure-time, and transportation PA. Interestingly, long working hours and burnout were not linked to any PA subdivisions. These findings highlight the importance of enhancing workers' exercise intentions to promote both leisure-time and transportation PA. Future research should assess the effectiveness of workplace programs in improving exercise intentions. Work-related PA was largely influenced by occupational factors, necessitating job-specific strategies. White-collar workers, who often have sedentary jobs, may benefit from structured exercise breaks and ergonomic adjustments. Meanwhile, shift workers, despite exhibiting higher levels of work-related PA, could benefit from initiatives that promote transportation and leisure-time PA, such as encouraging cycling or walking as modes of transportation or flexible exercise options like 24 h gym access or digital platforms. Tailoring interventions to specific occupational groups remains essential for improving all types of PA.

Author Contributions: Conceptualization, W.-H.W., W.-T.H. and F.-C.T.; data curation, H.-I.C.; formal analysis, R.-H.L.; investigation, H.-I.C.; methodology, S.-L.H.; resources, F.-C.T.; supervision, S.-L.H. and F.-C.T.; writing—original draft, W.-H.W. and S.-L.H.; writing—review and editing, W.-T.H. and F.-C.T. All authors have read and agreed to the published version of the manuscript.

Funding: This research received no external funding.

Institutional Review Board Statement: The study was conducted in accordance with the Declaration of Helsinki and approved by the Institutional Review Board of Chung Shan Medical University Hospital (CSHIRB No: CS18263, date of approval: 12 March 2019).

Informed Consent Statement: Informed consent was obtained from all subjects involved in the study.

Data Availability Statement: The research data will be available upon request to the corresponding author.

Acknowledgments: All participants in this study are gratefully acknowledged.

Conflicts of Interest: The authors declare no conflicts of interest.

References

1. World Health Organization. *Preventing Noncommunicable Diseases in the Workplace through Diet and Physical Activity: WHO/World Economic Forum Report of a Joint Event*; World Health Organization: Geneva, Switzerland, 2008.
2. World Health Organization. WHO Guidelines on Physical Activity and Sedentary Behavior. Available online: https://apps.who.int/iris/handle/10665/336656 (accessed on 15 March 2024).
3. Sports Administration, Ministry of Education. *2023 Sports Status Survey Report*; Shih Hsin University: Taipei, Taiwan, 2023.
4. Health Promotion Administration, Ministry of Health and Welfare, Taiwan. *Taiwan's Obesity Prevention and Management Strategy*; Health Promotion Administration, Ministry of Health and Welfare: Taipei, Taiwan, 2018.
5. Batt, M.E. Physical activity interventions in the workplace: The rationale and future direction for workplace wellness. *Br. J. Sports Med.* **2009**, *43*, 47–48. [CrossRef] [PubMed]

6. Pronk, N.P.; Kottke, T.E. Physical activity promotion as a strategic corporate priority to improve worker health and business performance. *Prev. Med.* **2009**, *49*, 316–321. [CrossRef] [PubMed]
7. Azevedo, L.M.; Chiavegato, L.D.; Carvalho, C.R.F.; Braz, J.R.; Nunes Cabral, C.M.; Padula, R.S. Are blue-collar workers more physically active than white-collar at work? *Arch. Environ. Occup. Health* **2021**, *76*, 338–347. [CrossRef] [PubMed]
8. Loprinzi, P.D. The effects of shift work on free-living physical activity and sedentary behavior. *Prev. Med.* **2015**, *76*, 43–47. [CrossRef]
9. Monnaatsie, M.; Biddle, S.J.; Khan, S.; Kolbe-Alexander, T. Physical activity and sedentary behaviour in shift and non-shift workers: A systematic review and meta-analysis. *Prev. Med. Rep.* **2021**, *24*, 101597. [CrossRef]
10. Wu, H.-T.; Liao, C.-M. Participation in Physical Activities for 9 to 15 year-old Taiwan Students' Gender and Age Differences in Motives. *Phys. Educ. J.* **2011**, *44*, 407–422. [CrossRef]
11. Hsu, C.-L.; Chen, H.-H.; Mo, J.-U. Relationships among Physical Activity Levels, Functional Fitness Test and Sleep Quality for the Middle-age and Elderly Adults. *Natl. Pingtung Univ. J.* **2012**, *15*, 128–143.
12. Hemmingsson, E.; Ekelund, U. Is the association between physical activity and body mass index obesity dependent? *Int. J. Obes.* **2007**, *31*, 663–668. [CrossRef]
13. Cooper, A.R.; Page, A.; Fox, K.R.; Misson, J. Physical activity patterns in normal, overweight and obese individuals using minute-by-minute accelerometry. *Eur. J. Clin. Nutr.* **2000**, *54*, 887–894. [CrossRef]
14. World Health Organization. Guidelines for Data Processing and Analysis of the International Physical Activity Questionnaire (IPAQ). Available online: https://drive.google.com/file/d/1gehdq1-04eSWfbxscwtzXa1MUlD8Mffa/view (accessed on 15 March 2024).
15. Crowther, M.E.; Ferguson, S.A.; Reynolds, A.C. Longitudinal studies of sleep, physical activity and nutritional intake in shift workers: A scoping review. *Sleep Med. Rev.* **2022**, *63*, 101612. [CrossRef]
16. Esquirol, Y.; Bongard, V.; Mabile, L.; Jonnier, B.; Soulat, J.M.; Perret, B. Shift work and metabolic syndrome: Respective impacts of job strain, physical activity, and dietary rhythms. *Chronobiol. Int.* **2009**, *26*, 544–559. [CrossRef] [PubMed]
17. Dishman, R.K.; Washburn, R.A.; Schoeller, D.A. Measurement of physical activity. *Quest* **2001**, *53*, 295–309. [CrossRef]
18. Castillo-Retamal, M.; Hinckson, E.A. Measuring physical activity and sedentary behaviour at work: A review. *Work* **2011**, *40*, 345–357. [CrossRef] [PubMed]
19. Bélanger-Gravel, A.; Godin, G.; Amireault, S. A meta-analytic review of the effect of implementation intentions on physical activity. *Health Psychol. Rev.* **2013**, *7*, 23–54. [CrossRef]
20. Kompf, J. Implementation intentions for exercise and physical activity: Who do they work for? A systematic review. *J. Phys. Act. Health* **2020**, *17*, 349–359. [CrossRef]
21. Nigg, C.R.; Geller, K.S.; Motl, R.W.; Horwath, C.C.; Wertin, K.K.; Dishman, R.K. A research agenda to examine the efficacy and relevance of the transtheoretical model for physical activity behavior. *Psychol. Sport Exerc.* **2011**, *12*, 7–12. [CrossRef]
22. Prochaska, J.O.; DiClemente, C.C.; Norcross, J.C. In search of how people change: Applications to addictive behaviors. *Am. Psychol.* **1992**, *47*, 1102–1114. [CrossRef]
23. Cheng, H.-I.; Hsu, W.-T.; Wang, W.-H.; Li, R.-H.; Tang, F.-C.; Huang, S.-L. Health Behavior Models and Regular Exercise Levels Among Workers in Taiwan. *J. Multidiscip. Healthc.* **2023**, *16*, 4149–4159. [CrossRef]
24. Health Promotion Administration, Ministry of Health and Welfare, Taiwan. The Measurement of Body Mass Index. Available online: http://health99.hpa.gov.tw/OnlinkHealth/Onlink_BMI.aspx (accessed on 15 March 2024).
25. National Statistics, R.O.C. (Taiwan). Standard Occupational Classification. Available online: http://eng.stat.gov.tw/ct.asp?xItem=5015&ctNode=1528&mp=5 (accessed on 15 March 2024).
26. Kristensen, T.S.; Borritz, M.; Villadsen, E.; Christensen, K.B. The Copenhagen Burnout Inventory: A new tool for the assessment of burnout. *Work Stress* **2005**, *19*, 192–207. [CrossRef]
27. Schumann, A.; Estabrooks, P.; Nigg, C.; Hill, J. Validation of the stages of change with mild, moderate, and strenuous physical activity behavior, intentions, and self-efficacy. *Int. J. Sports Med.* **2003**, *24*, 363–365. [CrossRef]
28. Hu, G.; Pekkarinen, H.; Hänninen, O.; Yu, Z.; Guo, Z.; Tian, H. Commuting, leisure-time physical activity, and cardiovascular risk factors in China. *Med. Sci. Sports Exerc.* **2002**, *34*, 234–238. [CrossRef] [PubMed]
29. Hu, G.; Qiao, Q.; Silventoinen, K.; Eriksson, J.G.; Jousilahti, P.; Lindström, J.; Valle, T.T.; Nissinen, A.; Tuomilehto, J. Occupational, commuting, and leisure-time physical activity in relation to risk for Type 2 diabetes in middle-aged Finnish men and women. *Diabetologia* **2003**, *46*, 322–329. [CrossRef] [PubMed]
30. Tuomilehto, J.; Hu, G.; Bidel, S.; Lindström, J.; Jousilahti, P. Coffee consumption and risk of type 2 diabetes mellitus among middle-aged Finnish men and women. *JAMA* **2004**, *291*, 1213–1219. [CrossRef] [PubMed]
31. Albanes, D.; Conway, J.M.; Taylor, P.R.; Moe, P.W.; Judd, J. Validation and comparison of eight physical activity questionnaires. *Epidemiology* **1990**, *1*, 65–71. [CrossRef]
32. Sallis, J.F.; Haskell, W.L.; Wood, P.D.; Fortmann, S.P.; Rogers, T.; Blair, S.N.; Paffenbarger, R.S., Jr. Physical activity assessment methodology in the Five-City Project. *Am. J. Epidemiol.* **1985**, *121*, 91–106. [CrossRef]
33. Couraeya, K.S.; McAuley, E. Predicting physical activity from intention: Conceptual and methodological issues. *J. Sport Exerc. Psychol.* **1993**, *15*, 50–62. [CrossRef]
34. Schwarzer, R. Modeling health behavior change: How to predict and modify the adoption and maintenance of health behaviors. *Appl. Psychol.* **2008**, *57*, 1–29. [CrossRef]

35. Rhodes, R.E.; de Bruijn, G.J. How big is the physical activity intention–behaviour gap? A meta-analysis using the action control framework. *Br. J. Health Psychol.* **2013**, *18*, 296–309. [CrossRef]
36. McEachan, R.R.C.; Conner, M.; Taylor, N.J.; Lawton, R.J. Prospective prediction of health-related behaviours with the theory of planned behaviour: A meta-analysis. *Health Psychol. Rev.* **2011**, *5*, 97–144. [CrossRef]
37. Rhodes, R.E.; Cox, A.; Sayar, R. What predicts the physical activity intention–behavior gap? A systematic review. *Ann. Behav. Med.* **2022**, *56*, 1–20. [CrossRef]
38. Troped, P.J.; Saunders, R.P.; Pate, R.R.; Reininger, B.; Addy, C.L. Correlates of recreational and transportation physical activity among adults in a New England community. *Prev. Med.* **2003**, *37*, 304–310. [CrossRef] [PubMed]
39. Sallis, J.F.; Frank, L.D.; Saelens, B.E.; Kraft, M.K. Active transportation and physical activity: Opportunities for collaboration on transportation and public health research. *Transp. Res. Part A Policy Pract.* **2004**, *38*, 249–268. [CrossRef]
40. Loef, B.; Van Der Beek, A.J.; Holtermann, A.; Hulsegge, G.; Van Baarle, D.; Proper, K.I. Objectively measured physical activity of hospital shift workers. *Scand. J. Work. Environ. Health* **2018**, *44*, 265–273. [CrossRef] [PubMed]
41. Torquati, L.; Mielke, G.I.; Brown, W.J.; Kolbe-Alexander, T. Shift work and the risk of cardiovascular disease. A systematic review and meta-analysis including dose–response relationship. *Scand. J. Work. Environ. Health* **2018**, *44*, 229–238. [CrossRef] [PubMed]
42. Holtermann, A.; Marott, J.L.; Gyntelberg, F.; Søgaard, K.; Suadicani, P.; Mortensen, O.S.; Prescott, E.; Schnohr, P. Does the benefit on survival from leisure time physical activity depend on physical activity at work? A prospective cohort study. *PLoS ONE* **2013**, *8*, e54548. [CrossRef]
43. Kirk, M.A.; Rhodes, R.E. Occupation correlates of adults' participation in leisure-time physical activity: A systematic review. *Am. J. Prev. Med.* **2011**, *40*, 476–485. [CrossRef]
44. Gal, D.L.; Santos, A.-C.; Barros, H. Leisure-time versus full-day energy expenditure: A cross-sectional study of sedentarism in a Portuguese urban population. *BMC Public Health* **2005**, *5*, 1–7. [CrossRef]
45. McCormack, G.; Giles-Corti, B.; Milligan, R. Demographic and individual correlates of achieving 10,000 steps/day: Use of pedometers in a population-based study. *Health Promot. J. Aust.* **2006**, *17*, 43–47. [CrossRef]

behavioral sciences

MDPI

Article

The Discursive Configuration of the Therapeutic Community for Substance Users: Positioning and Ethnopsychological Processes Concerning Entry

Antonio Iudici [1,*], Tobia Berardelli [1], Davide Fenini [2], Emiliano Subissi [2] and Jessica Neri [1,2]

[1] Department of Philosophy, Education, Sociology and Applied Psychology of Padua (FISPPA), University of Padua, 35139 Padua, Italy; t.berardelli@scuolainterazionista.it (T.B.); j.neri@scuolainterazionista.it (J.N.)

[2] Institute of Psychology and Psychotherapy, Scuola Interazionista, 35100 Padua, Italy; d.fenini@scuolainterazionista.it (D.F.); e.subissi@scuolainterazionista.it (E.S.)

* Correspondence: antonio.iudici@unipd.it

Abstract: Therapeutic communities face high drop-out rates and general distrust of their effectiveness among substance users. Actively involving users early in treatment promotes greater compliance with the treatment and is predictive of better outcomes. However, users often occupy a passive and subordinate role, exacerbated by the lack of research that explores their perspectives, beliefs, and experiences. This study examined the discourses of 57 consumers who were part of a community for less than 15 days, investigating the meanings attributed to service entry and treatment. A protocol of four written open-ended questions was employed and analysed through discourse analysis and positioning theory. The results indicate that participants configure the community as a place symbolically and spatially distinct from the rest of the world, where they isolate themselves to seek support during times of extreme difficulty. However, what they are seeking is a solution to acute distress caused by substance use, intertwined with social, economic, and relational issues. The concept of treatment is built on the image of the substance user as an individual making a weak request for help, attributing the problem solely to drugs and exhibiting reduced agency in addressing their issues. The collected texts provide a better understanding of the experiences of new users, highlighting the importance of co-constructing personalised projects that empower consumers to feel actively involved in their own change, exploring their theories and definitions of self to structure pathways based strictly on their needs.

Keywords: users' perspective; discourse analysis; interactionism; residential community; health promotion

1. Introduction

Interventions related to substance abuse are complex and involve various disciplinary fields, including medical–pharmacological, psychological, social, and occasionally, psychiatric [1]. The study of the physiological effects of psychoactive substance consumption has expanded the tools and intervention possibilities from a biochemical standpoint. Such possibilities include the implementation of pharmacological support for detoxification, tolerance, and dependence [2], as well as the study of comorbidity situations when substance use is associated with other disorders that exacerbate the course of both [3].

The results achieved in this field have shifted the research focus on substance use towards quantitative data [4,5], with a prevalence of approaches that reduce mental conditions of the brain's physical structure and functioning [6–9], favouring a reductionist conception of the overlap between substance use and the neurophysiological effects of consumption. Indeed, individuals who use substances have often been studied as ill patients before being considered as persons [10]. Consequently, the focus of studies and interventions has been on 'substance use' as a pathology and 'drug users' as individuals with disorders. Psychological research has predominantly sought elements of distress or cognitive factors that could explain relapses and therapeutic failures [11]. Across these research domains, there has been an overall interest in addressing people seeking treatment for substance use primarily as passive subjects with a lack of self-determination and diminished cognitive capacities [12]. This approach has led to the reduced involvement of individuals who use substances in analysing their responsibilities, experiences, beliefs, and methods of addressing social reintegration and treatment [4,8,13,14].

Conversely, some authors argue that understanding how consumption occurs and replicates necessitates studying the cultural and social narratives present in specific contexts, delving into how these narratives are practised and interactively re-signified [15,16]. For instance, Copes' meta-analysis [17] illustrates how substance use places individuals in a position of extreme identity vulnerability, emphasising the need to focus on symbolic and existential aspects, as well as biomedical ones. The literature review revealed that individuals with substance use disorders approached treatment and residential communities in a subordinate role, predominantly delegating their rehabilitative pathway to the professionals within these facilities [4,18,19].

This perception of consumption as an inability to cope with use suggests that individuals are at the mercy of drugs for life [20]. Some authors argue that this passivity and sense of incapacity may partly explain the significant level of the inefficacy or discontinuation of rehabilitative treatment [21,22]. Indeed, it has been found that 50% of individuals admitted to communities did not complete the first 10 months of a programme, and 45% of consumers remained unaware of the available services [23,24].

Several studies have highlighted how the intake phase is particularly crucial for the programme's trajectory [5]. Specifically, this phase is significant for forming the so-called 'therapeutic alliance' [25] and for defining a solid, enduring path. Some authors argue that treatment is more effective based on the duration of stay [5] and user involvement [26]. Others have underscored the importance of establishing a co-operative relationship in treatment [27], involving the consumer and their expectations [28,29]. Some authors emphasise the importance of collaboration between service providers and users in the initial stages of the pathway, particularly the need to tailor treatment to the user's characteristics [30–32]. Some authors [24,33,34] argue that the way individuals who use substances access services is much more varied than the stereotypical conceptions of 'motivation' and 'personal choice'. This study aims to analyse the narratives and interactive modalities involved in entering the therapeutic community (TC) and utilising interventions by capturing the discourses that lead substance users to seek help in communities and understanding their approach to treatment. A TC is a service in which individuals with addictive (and other) problems live together in an organised and structured manner to promote change and facilitate a drug-free life in society [35].

Based on the research and considerations presented, this study begins with specific questions: What is the basis for substance users to request help? What kind of assistance do they anticipate from the community?

This study, therefore, focuses on the moment of access to residential services, delving into how consumers assign meaning to the service itself. This investigation can provide a deeper understanding of the discursive construction of therapeutic communities and the identities of individuals who use substances, specifically the socio-cultural and contextual elements that contribute to shaping the phenomenon and its potential trajectories of change. Analysing the interactive dynamics of accessing the residential community can illuminate the complexities of the help-seeking process. It can uncover barriers or facilitators of engaging with services, as well as highlighting opportunities for improving the delivery of care.

2. Materials and Methods

2.1. Theoretical Background

This study adopts the interactionist paradigm as its theoretical framework [36–39]. In this paradigm, the individual is conceptualised as an active agent constantly negotiating their reality based on the meanings they attribute to it, which are generated interactively within socio-cultural matrices [40–43].

The self is seen as having a dialogical character [44,45], positioning it as an intersection between multiple levels. Identity is thus viewed as a dialogical process that allows for the interaction of intrapersonal (self-attribution) and interpersonal (other attribution) elements within the cultural matrix of reference, converging into an organising structure of self-knowledge [46–48]. Therefore, attention is placed on analysing discursive and interactive processes that contribute to the configuration of the phenomena under investigation [41,49]. Regarding this, entry into a community, like any institutionalised or therapeutic context, is considered significant when analysing the discursive processes used by those who populate it [50,51] and their pragmatic implications.

2.2. Aims

This study aims to investigate how individuals who use legal and illegal psychoactive substances shape the residential community and their activities during the entry phase into a TC. Specifically, considering the potential biographical transition represented by entering into such a service, attention has been focused on the following areas of investigation:

- Analysis of the discursive configuration regarding the entry of substance users into the service;
- Analysis of the discursive configuration regarding expectations and activities within the community.

These areas of investigation allow for an in-depth exploration of the theories, beliefs, and expectations of individuals entering TCs regarding the entry and utilisation of interventions promoted within these contexts.

2.3. Participants

The research was conducted in northern Italy, specifically in the regions of Veneto and Lombardia. These regions were chosen because they host the highest number of therapeutic communities in Italy. The study included 57 individuals who had accessed four therapeutic–rehabilitative residential communities for drug addiction within the previous 15 days.

For participant recruitment, an initial mapping of local services was conducted based on the provision of programmes for managing and treating substance-related issues. These facilities were contacted, and the research objectives were shared with the responsible personnel. Potential participants were then approached and invited to collaborate, with the research objectives and methods explained to them. Regarding entry requirements, all participants were poly-consumers, predominantly alcohol and drug users. All participants had previously attended at least one other community in their lives. This requirement was established to detect established theories about therapeutic communities. The questionnaire was shared with them shortly before entering the new community. Individuals who used only one substance or were entering a community for the first time were excluded from the research. Participants were divided into (a) substance users who had a regular entry, that is, based on a referral from the Services for First Integration (Ser.D), and (b) individuals using substances accessing the community as an alternative to prison. Under Italian law [52], some detained persons can follow a community-based treatment pathway (alternative measure programme). Each participant was provided with a module to give their informed consent. Each participant was asked to complete a written questionnaire. Our study has been approved by the University of Padua's Ethics Committee for Research (protocol code: 3653).

Table 1 presents the demographic data of the participants. It is noteworthy that most participants are male, and the average age is 37.7 years, which aligns with the national average data reported by the Department of Anti-Drug Policies [53].

Table 1. Demographic data.

Gender	N	%
Male	41	71.9
Female	16	28.1
Age range		
18–30	20	35.1
31–50	26	45.6
51–70	11	19.3
Age average	37.7	/
Typology of entry		
Regular entry	42	73.7
Alternative measure programme	15	26.3

2.4. Data Collection

According to the theoretical background, a qualitative approach was adopted to understand the complexity of the experiences provided by the participants, limiting the risk of reducing them to quantitative categories. The research is understood as a relational, collaborative practice and dialogical process [54,55], with the object of analysis considered co-constructed by the researchers and the interlocutors.

The research instrument consists of a written protocol of six open-ended questions (Table 2).

Table 2. Research protocol.

Research Area: Discursive Configuration Regarding Entry into the Therapeutic Community
1. How did you come to the decision to enter a therapeutic community (TC)?
2. What is your image of a therapeutic community?
3. What goals do you intend to achieve in this process?
4. How do you imagine a therapeutic community works?
5. How do you think the TC could facilitate you in achieving your goals?
6. What situations would you recommend to someone seeking help from a TC?

The questions were designed to elicit responses adhering to specific themes while allowing for a breadth of content and form [56]. The choice of open-ended questions was crucial within the qualitative research paradigm [57,58], particularly in collecting written text [59–63]. The question prompts were constructed concerning the research objective and its unique areas of investigation to delineate the scope of potential discourses. At the same time, the open-ended questions allowed ample room for participants to freely express themselves and manage their responses and relationships with the researcher present.

The questions were presented to participants individually, clarifying the methods and objectives of the research, ensuring anonymity, and assuring that the produced texts would not be disclosed to service personnel. The researcher was available to clarify any questions during the completion process. Responses were provided in written form autonomously, taking between 25 and 60 min.

The responses were transcribed verbatim and reviewed with the participants before delivery to ensure understanding of the written text [64,65]. In two cases of limited literacy, the participants dictated their answers to the researcher, who transcribed and read the answers immediately. The completion occurred within 15 days of entering the community. The texts were then translated into English.

2.5. Data Analysis

The texts were analysed using discourse analysis [66,67]. This method aims to capture the narratives (or discursive positioning) present in the written text, analysing simple content and the discursive processes through which specific theories and ideologies are perpetuated in the text. The framework of positioning [68–70] was utilised to underscore the dynamic aspects through which the discursive shaping of identity occurred, such as that of substance users.

Adopting a particular positioning allows one to perceive the world from that standpoint, interpreting it through the lens of the relevant images, metaphors, and concepts within the discursive frameworks in which one is situated [68]. Moreover, positioning manifests the illocutionary and intentional force of the speaker, utilising language to position oneself and others within a framework of rights and obligations, potentially affecting certain outcomes [71]. Special attention was devoted to analysing the socio-cultural and ethnopsychological elements of the narratives, as they are significant and central in the discursive construction of the investigated reality.

The analysis of discourse and positioning made it possible to explore how participants articulated their narratives and positions concerning the area of investigation: entry into the community. The analysis of discursive processes enables the identification of the most pertinent discourses and positions, elucidating their practical implications within the life stories and pathways of intervention for the participants.

The analytical procedure involved a comprehensive examination of the texts written by the participants, conducted separately for the two primary thematic areas explored in this study. This re-evaluation process occurred at various points in time and involved the collaboration of three different researchers to pinpoint any discrepancies in the analysis.

Upon identifying the fundamental discursive patterns related to positioning, we organised the findings into groups to enhance clarity and facilitate the interpretation of the results. Both the identified positions and their articulations, aligned with the analytical methodology, are recognised as discursive processes that significantly contribute to the emergence of the phenomenon under investigation [72].

3. Results

The responses collected through the protocols make it possible to analyse what people who use substances, also as citizens, think about the services offered by the TC through their activities.

How is the therapeutic community (TC) configured?

We can detect four different representations of the TC through discourse analysis Table 3).

Table 3. Result diagram.

Results: How the Therapeutic Community (TC) Is Configured
1. The TC as a Refuge
2. The TC as the Final Liberation
3. The TC as a Place for the Acquisition of New Values
4. The TC as a Symbol of Redemption towards Familiar Figures

3.1. The TC as a Refuge

The first representation we can consider is that of the TC as a refuge. Within this category of responses, the TC is seen as a space of welcoming and sustenance, shelter, and containment, and only afterwards can it take on a role referring to objectives related to therapeutic changes.

One participant affirms that *'If you are addicted and lonely, many times you don't know where to hit your head, and you see yourself with no way out'* (P8).

From these premises, some participants narrate the entrance with a rhetoric constructed based on losing control, seeing the TC as an alternative to irreversible situations. *'In recent times, drinking was a daily act, so, remembering my past, I decided to ask for help before sinking into the abyss...and here I am...'* (P17). This request is based, as we can see, on generic references, such as the request for a harbouring place or the reference to the fear of sinking into the abyss.

Within this configuration, the TC is represented as a place to turn to: *'When a person is by now in the state of destroying himself physically and psychologically'* (P13), when no alternative possibilities are identified, *'I could no longer live'* (P29).

P20 reports that 'For the umpteenth time, I lost everything: my job, my girlfriend, my family, my dignity, my respect for myself. On top of all this, I was about to lose my life, I saved myself by a miracle'.

The answers underline the fact that the choice to enter the TC is linked to a contingent and momentary experience of discomfort rather than to the progressive development of a plan of change and that the choice is restricted to a generic request for assistance. A representation of the TC is based on the perceived need to distance oneself from a situation of difficulty (I couldn't bear it anymore) without any reference to a need for personal change.

Defining themselves as unable to manage consumption and to distance themselves from the contexts that facilitate it, several participants portray themselves as in need of generic help based on the exigencies of physical containment, symbolic and physical dislocation from the drugs, and support regarding problems such as loss of work, loss of housing, loss of emotional and family relationships, or health problems. P1 says that the *'TC is recommended for those who, after several attempts, have failed to stop permanent use, even more so if they struggle to break ties with old acquaintances and are unable to manage to rebuild their lives from a new beginning'*.

The institutionalised and residential nature of the TC is considered functional in detaching it from a context deemed uncontrollable, particularly due to issues of social exclusion, economic difficulties, or the inability to modulate consumption. *'A help that I find fundamental already comes from the environment itself. Getting away from home, work, and the stress of everyday life is very much helping me to focus on myself and allows me, on the one hand, not to feel the weight of all these things, but at the same time to be able to concentrate on my own in a safe place'* (P11).

One participant reports that *'The community is useful when you would like to stop but you can't, and instead, you continue in the same direction, the substance is totally in control of your willpower'* (P17), while another says that *'When you see a person or a friend who is in a state of social dis-ease, living in absolute degradation, using and abusing, living a life in disarray...I would recommend going to a community to give meaning to life'* (P19).

There is also mention of the possibility, through entrance into the TC, of distancing oneself from the constraints of a stereotyped and stigmatised identity: *'Now I hope people will evaluate me for what I am... but I doubt it; there is so much ignorance in the world' (P4). 'It is not easy to accept being labelled by society... because, let's not fool ourselves, people look at you differently' (P3).*

Within this configuration, the community represents a safe refuge for the 'drug addict' who, in the very need of this refuge, feels the need not to be stigmatised.

3.2. The TC as the Final Liberation

A second category of responses configures the TC as the final liberation. Within this configuration, the consumption of psychotropic substances is represented as an addiction, maybe not explicitly a 'disease', from which one must be freed permanently.

One respondent says that 'After ten years of continuous use and after becoming a father, I decided to try this path to finally get rid of the addiction...to definitely stop use' (P29), and similarly, another respondent affirms that 'If a person uses, it is right that at some point in his life, he decides to get treatment and get definitively out of this tunnel' (P14).

The TC is thus configured as a place for ceasing consumption, with abstinence becoming a primary objective. Abstinence assumes the role of a unique and definitive reference for change. The goal of abstinence is considered not pursuable independently; the theory 'I can't stop' prevails. Therefore, the necessary contribution to the transformation is delegated to third parties: *'When you want to quit on your own, it is almost never possible to do so... entering a path with addiction experts to find myself and realise that there are better things to do' (P6).* Thus, the main index of liberation is the achievement of abstinence, configuring the treatment in terms of 'momentary success' (abstinence maintained to date) or 'failure' (stopping abstinence).

Some problems are objectified, reified, and inscribed in aut-aut dynamics that do not anticipate space for mediation. Some participants use the expression 'I've decided to enter the community to get out of it' (P26); another says that *'I said stop to drugs; now I have to get out of it, to get rid of them' (P36).* Service is thus represented as resolutive and salvific, aimed at people who say '*Enough*'.

Finally, among the answers emerges an objectification of 'addiction', considered an ontologically determined reality. The object of treatment is therefore not the person in his or her entirety, but only certain circumscribed aspects linked to consumption, conceiving the person as subordinate to his or her addiction: *'You find yourself no longer in control of your life, and you find yourself at the mercy of a substance in the middle of an addiction'* (P48).

3.3. The TC as a Place for the Acquisition of New Values

A third category of answers configures the TC as a place for acquiring new values, a configuration within which the dimension of moral judgement regarding past misconduct and the search for new values that can represent a reference for the future are central. Service is thus described as an educational and maturing place where people can understand themselves and learn other ('healthy' or 'normal') values to pivot a new life.

In this regard, one participant says that 'I have to understand the mistakes I have made in life, not to make them in the future' (P9). The abandonment of a 'negative or wrong mentality' is wished for (P24), affirming that 'My goal is to change my mentality, my outlook on life, and my lifestyle' (P6).

Entering the TC becomes a potential existential reset. One participant speaks of it as *'a painful decision to enter the road or the path that can map out who I am and who I want to be' (P3),* reiterating the idea that the TC can generate a concrete shift in one's biography, in deep and identity aspects, and thus hold it responsible for a radical axiological transformation.

Contextually, many participants consider the community a place for the acquisition of new values, and they use modes of confrontation and comparison between the present and the past. The past is narrated through theories regarding vice and moral corruption, reiterating a mortification and dramatisation of themselves and their biography. Abusive conduct is represented as detrimental to a 'true identity'; in the TC, they search for the re-emergence of an authentic self.

In this regard, one respondent affirms that he needs to *'understand who we are beyond use'* (P42), while another participant claims to want 'to understand what led to the use of drugs' (P22). Another participant reports that *'I couldn't understand who I became anymore...seeing the years go by and remain inside the vicious circle I had created for myself...'* (P8).

In this configuration, consumption is often used as the cause of a ruinous drift, not the conditions/actions that contributed to generating it and making it critical. If *'addiction makes you deaf by taking possession of you' (P2),* one participant affirms that *'The goal is to return to be the person I used to be, honest, sincere, loyal' (P46),* and another says that *'I hope to go back to the guy I used to be before I was addicted' (P55).* Within this configuration, if we remove the 'addiction', we have the chance to go back to what we were before, without considering that this option also implies a return to the conditions in which consumption began and the consequences that today trigger the demand for change.

The generated position is that of an aspiration—and therefore a prior acceptance—for a change that is expressed through the 'reflection' and the understanding of specific consumption-related aspects: *'I hope to take away this damn vice, and at the end of this path, I will start to cultivate new goals'* (P49). One participant hopes to *'return to living a healthy life without substance by understanding what leads me to always make the same mistakes, slip-ups, etc.'* (P11), emphasising the dimension of returning to a previous life that was subsequently spoiled by substance use.

3.4. The TC as a Symbol of Redemption towards Familiar Figures

For a proportion of newcomers, the abandonment by significant figures in their lives, particularly the family, is considered the main evidence of existential failure. Entry into the TC is, therefore, reported as an extreme attempt at reconnection, reconquest, and social redemption. One participant says that *'I want to prove to myself and others that I have really cleaned myself up truly'* (P41). Another person affirms that *'The thing that made me decide was the fact that I was hurting myself and all the people who love me. I felt lonely; I had lost the will to live, and my only goal was to get through the day'* (P38).

Another participant reports that 'Since drugs marginalised me from everything and everyone, the desire to enter TC came from the need for social redemption to show people that I have changed and thus have a decent job and, above all, the satisfaction of the people who love me' (P54). The choice to approach the service is spoken of as following a dynamic of encouragement or actual persuasion. This is sometimes explicit, as reported by one respondent, *'I was driven by the continuous perseverance of people close to me because most probably if they had not been there now, I would still be on the street getting high' (P37)*, while in other cases, it manifests itself with the loss of recognition and spatial–emotional proximity to family members.

The identity of an 'addict' is strategically assumed, showing awareness of one's own discomfort and willingness to ask for help, to the point of sticking to the identity of a 'sick person'. This process seems consistent with the attempt to show oneself as changed, eventually determined to take responsibility and face problems. Entry into the TC is thus charged with a high symbolic value, representing in and of itself a change already in progress. The prevailing instance is providing evidence of the change, demonstrating it to themselves and others.

4. Discussion

As discussed above, for some participants, the value of the service lies solely in its ability to provide sustenance and relief from acute distress. While this is sometimes seen as functional in creating a safe space to initiate pathways of help, what emerges from the participants' narratives is the absence of explicit planning. Entry into a community is described as a purely biographical coincidence, supported by a passive welfare-seeking issue. Frank and Walters [34] also noted that entry into TCs is often the result of an interactive and social process rather than an individual decision stemming from a reflective and introspective journey.

Peer and family pressure, along with aspects of criminalisation and the stigmatisation of consumption, appear central to promoting the decision to seek a service. The self-definitions collected through the research protocols highlight how participants tend to dramatise their condition and adopt a self-victimising rhetoric. Often, after the initial feelings of well-being due to abstinence from use (*'I have stopped using here'*, P12), individuals who use substances tend to attribute responsibility for their behaviour to 'drug addiction', thereby depriving themselves of agency, medicalising their situation, and delegating their actions to specialists.

Another noteworthy aspect is how TCs assume the character of a 'Hail Mary pass', permeated by an implicit institutional resignation [32], with the evaluation of their efficacy often reduced to their competence in facilitating abstinence. This seems to result from multiple processes linked to socially available discourses regarding consumption, previous failed experiences of abstinence, attempts to construct a non-dependent identity, and the moral order within which these discourses are generated [32,65]. Within this framework, the call to action for TCs is configured along the bipolarity of being powerless–responsible, such that it becomes the result of contact with an inherently uncontrollable substance or reckless and deliberate conduct, as also reported by Harré and Van Langenhove [69].

The theory of 'substance use as an organic disease' and the simultaneous exclusive search for a 'pharmacological cure' trigger a dichotomous logic based on healthy/sick and, consequently, cured/not cured individuals. One implication of this is to reify addiction as a circumscribed pathological core. The second is to consider this core as detached from the individual using the substance and their history, as also argued by Tibirica et al. [73], who pointed out this harmful dichotomy.

The aim (sometimes implicit and sometimes explicit) of the request for intervention is the interruption of substance consumption, thus triggering the reference to abstinence as the sole criterion. This assumption implies that a possible 'relapse' is considered a failure of the programme, dramatising the problem and leading the individual to justify substance use again. Consequently, contact with the substance triggers the resumption of use, diminishing the role of personal choice and responsibility concerning the initial contact. If substance consumption is the issue to be avoided, the opportunity to articulate one's hesitations about quitting becomes critical. This leads to the paradox whereby, in the TC, the issue of substance consumption becomes silenced, with consumers utilising discourses of sobriety as mere adaptation and pursuit of secondary goals.

Despite its evolution into a service with less binding access thresholds, TCs remain pathways that imply a break with previous behaviours and contexts. This is perceived by participants as both an added value and a significant sacrifice. The nature of the (almost) total institution is assessed as necessary and welcome to generate that biographical shock useful for starting anew, with the TC experience serving as a junction between a before and an after.

If the protected and isolated nature of the TC can be salvific in moments of extreme crisis, it is essential to consider the capacity to construct other identities within a service that binds individuals to a separate context, both spatially and symbolically. This contradicts the principles of community care [74].

We have seen how, for participants, the choice to enter the TC often represents 'the last resort'. It is only considered in the face of 'losing everything' or 'hitting *rock bottom' ('if the person does not touch bottom, it is like dealing with walls', P30),* prompting questions about the type of consumers the service can intercept, the prevention practices in action, and how the TC presents itself to those it might benefit [75].

A further implication of the detected service configurations is that entry into TCs is used strategically for communicative purposes, attempting to promote in the eyes of others (and thus in their own) evidence of change aimed at secondary goals. This offers a potentially generative ground to establish some desirable repercussions of a life away from substances. At the same time, it entails the need to quickly encourage individuals to co-generate a project that, otherwise, risks being reduced to the objective of mere permanence in the service.

Moreover, individuals are relational beings who need to be considered to avoid implementing interventions detached from the real contexts they inhabit, reflecting on the sense of identity that substance consumption has socially. Rather than being 'for others', overshadowed by the substances, entry seems functional to reconfigure oneself 'in the eyes of others', alleviating feelings of guilt, inadequacy, and the concrete and material repercussions dictated by disavowal.

Overall, TCs are described as distant from the rest of the world, resulting from a symbolic gap that delineates an inside and an outside. Starting from this assumption, it is even more pertinent to consider which identity configurations are being generated. Which aspects of the newcomer's self cross the threshold of the service, and which become the focus of attention? If the TC is a space apart from the world, what possibilities does it have of generating changes that resonate beyond its confines?

5. Conclusions

Based on the texts collected, it was possible to detect how TCs accommodated discomforts that extended beyond a clinical and specialist domain, as substance consumption—at least that intercepted by the services—is often intertwined with critical issues of economic, work, social, and relational aspects. This underscores the need to develop reflection on the role of TCs, both present and future, within a broad and interconnected system of services [21].

Overall, participants positioned themselves as passive recipients of treatment decided by others, and their approach to the service appears to respond to contextual, and often emergency, needs, rather than personal projects developed over time. This demand is predominantly based on the consequences of consumption and calls for both causes and consequences to be eliminated.

Intervention focused solely on consumption or achieving abstinence cannot be considered exhaustive and risks validating the notion that the problem lies with the substance or the implications concerning abstinence such as diminished feelings of responsibility for use and a loss of agency. Building on this research, we consider it useful to develop tools and methodologies not aimed at confirming this belief but rather favouring the individual's ownership of their path based on requests and questions defined in intentional terms. Thus, access to the service is a decisive event with high symbolic and pragmatic value, requiring accompaniment and support to co-construct the meaning of the pathway and its function in the individual's life within a framework of co-responsibility.

The shared construction of goals and pathways in the community can be a potentially innovative first step for individuals entering the community. This approach markedly differs from the passive, substance-dependent, and service-dependent attitudes observed in participants during our research. Involvement can trigger a sense of responsibility towards one's own path and health care [76] and encourage the activation of social inclusion processes, as confirmed by other studies [51], which showed that storytelling in drug treatment is an interactive achievement.

Finally, it can foster the legitimisation of treatment as a shared and personalised pathway, thereby increasing the likelihood of a positive outcome. This was noted by other authors [10,28] who emphasised the importance of involving substance users in services and the necessity of reducing barriers to involvement.

In this way, users will be better equipped to anticipate the challenges they may encounter during the process, facilitating their management from the outset. The shared construction requires and simultaneously generates a reduction in the rigidity of the relationship between substance users and community workers (healthcare professionals providing treatment at the facility), positively transforming the helping relationship.

Regarding the limitations of this study, the written form of the answers presented some challenges. First, we encountered difficulty in writing the texts for users (a minority) with minimal literacy levels. Since this remains a reality in TCs, it is important to include elements of flexibility that can simultaneously promote the sharing of significant elements while maintaining methodological consistency.

There were also several responses marked with a peremptory 'I don't know', which, while potentially useful from an operational perspective as indicative of how individuals legitimised the service and the requests received, could have been further explored to examine the underlying contents and processes.

Author Contributions: A.I.: conceptualisation, methodology, data curation, writing; T.B.: conceptualisation, investigation, methodology, writing; D.F.: conceptualisation, writing, supervision; E.S.: analysis, writing; J.N.: supervision, writing. All authors have read and agreed to the published version of the manuscript.

Funding: This research received no external funding.

Institutional Review Board Statement: This study was conducted in accordance with the Declaration of Helsinki and approved by the Ethics Committee of the University of Padua (protocol code: 3653 and date of approval: 10 June 2020).

Informed Consent Statement: Informed consent was obtained from all subjects involved in this study.

Data Availability Statement: The dataset presented is not available for privacy reasons.

Conflicts of Interest: The authors declare no conflicts of interest.

References

1. Jason, L.A.; Luna, R.D.; Alvarez, J.; Stevens, E. Collectivism and individualism in Latino recovery homes. *J. Ethn. Subst. Abus.* **2018**, *17*, 223–236. [CrossRef] [PubMed]
2. Maruf, M.M.; Khan, M.Z.R.; Jahan, N. Pattern of substance use: Study in a de-addiction clinic. *Oman Med. J.* **2016**, *31*, 327–331. [CrossRef] [PubMed]
3. Han, B.; Compton, W.M.; Blanco, C.; Colpe, L.J. Prevalence, treatment, and unmet treatment needs of US adults with mental health and substance use disorders. *Health Aff.* **2017**, *36*, 1739–1747. [CrossRef] [PubMed]
4. Neale, J.; Sheard, L.; Tompkins, C. Factors that help injecting drug users to access and benefit from services: A qualitative study. *Subst. Abus. Treat. Prev. Policy* **2007**, *2*, 31. [CrossRef]
5. Chen, G.; Elisha, E.; Timor, U.; Ronel, N. Why do adolescents drop out of a therapeutic community for people with drug addiction? *J. Child Adolesc. Subst. Abus.* **2016**, *25*, 65–77. [CrossRef]
6. Iudici, A.; Castelnuovo, G.; Faccio, E. New drugs and polydrug use: Implications for clinical psychology. *Front. Psychol.* **2015**, *6*, 267. [CrossRef]
7. Chatwin, C.; Porteous, D. Insiders? The Experiences and Perspectives of Long-Term, Regular Cannabis Users. *Contemp. Drug Probl.* **2013**, *40*, 235–257. [CrossRef]
8. Rhodes, T.; Stimson, G.V.; Moore, D.; Bourgois, P. Qualitative social research in addictions publishing: Creating an enabling journal environment. *Int. J. Drug Policy* **2010**, *21*, 441–444. [CrossRef]
9. Rhodes, T.; Moore, D. On the qualitative in drugs research: Part one. *Addict. Res. Theory* **2001**, *9*, 279–297. [CrossRef]
10. Tait, L.; Lester, H. Encouraging user involvement in mental health services. *Adv. Psychiatr. Treat.* **2004**, *11*, 168–175. [CrossRef]
11. Priester, M.A.; Browne, T.; Iachini, A.; Clone, S.; DeHart, D.; Seay, K.D. Treatment access barriers and disparities among individuals with co-occurring mental health and substance use disorders: An integrative literature review. *J. Subst. Abus. Treat.* **2016**, *61*, 47–59. [CrossRef] [PubMed]
12. Tutenges, S.; Kolind, T.; Uhl, A. Explorations into drug users' perspectives. *Drugs Educ. Prev. Policy* **2015**, *22*, 173–174. [CrossRef]
13. Eslami-Jahromi, M.; Keshvardoost, S.; Ershad-Sarabi, R.; Bahaadinbeigy, K. Information Needs of Addicted Individuals: A Qualitative Case Study. *Addict. Health* **2021**, *13*, 138–147. [CrossRef] [PubMed]
14. Miles, M.B.; Huberman, A.M. *Qualitative Data Analysis: An Expanded Source Book*, 2nd ed.; Sage Publications: Washington, DC, USA, 1994.
15. Loseke, D.R. The study of identity as cultural, institutional, organizational, and personal: Theoretical and Empirical Integrations. *Sociol. Q.* **2007**, *48*, 661–688. [CrossRef]
16. Turchi, G. *"Addiction": Generate the Change between Paradigm Shift and Pragmatic Effects*; Upsel Domeneghini Editore: Padua, Italy, 2002.
17. Copes, H. A narrative approach to studying symbolic boundaries among drug users: A qualitative meta-synthesis. *Crime Media Cult.* **2016**, *12*, 193–213. [CrossRef]
18. Järvinen, M.; Andersen, D. The Making of the chronic addict. *Subst. Use Misuse* **2009**, *44*, 865–885. [CrossRef]
19. Iudici, A. Identity and Deviance: How the Architecture of Services Shapes Self-Awareness. *Sci. Dell'interazione* **2011**, *2*, 68–84.
20. Zamperini, A. The Social Construction of the Drug Addict. In *Drugs. Toxicophilia and Addiction*; Salvini, A., Ed.; De Agostini Scuola: Segrate, Italy, 2002; pp. 20–31.
21. Grosso, L. Community, low threshold and harm reduction. In *The Therapeutic Community in the Society of Addictions*; Palumbo, M., Dondi, M., Torrigiani, C., Eds.; Erickson: Trento, Italy, 2012; pp. 165–182.
22. Iudici, A.; Fenini, D.; Baciga, D.; Volponi, G. The role of the admission phase in the Italian treatment setting: A research on individuating shared practices in psychotropic substance users' communities. *J. Ethn. Subst. Abus.* **2020**, *21*, 127–148. [CrossRef]
23. Fenini, D.; Briatore, P. Services for Drug Addiction: Methodologies, Characteristics, and Developments. In *"Addiction". Generate the Change between Paradigm Shift and Pragmatic Effects*; Turchi, G., Ed.; Upsel Domeneghini Editore: Padua, Italy, 2002; pp. 191–213.
24. Gilchrist, G.; Moskalewicz, J.; Nutt, R.; Love, J.; Germeni, E.; Valkova, I.; Kantchelov, A.; Stoykova, T.; Bujalski, M.; Poplas-Susic, T.; et al. Understanding access to drug and alcohol treatment services in Europe: A multi-country service users' perspective. *Drugs: Educ. Prev. Policy* **2014**, *21*, 120–130. [CrossRef]
25. Janeiro, L.; Ribeiro, E.; Faisca, L.; Lopez Miguel, M.J. Therapeutic alliance dimensions and dropout in a therapeutic community: "Bond with me and I will stay". *Ther. Communities Int. J. Ther. Communities* **2018**, *39*, 73–82. [CrossRef]

26. Lovejoy, M.; Rosenblum, A.; Magura, S.; Foote, J.; Handelsman, L.; Stimmel, B. Patients' Perspective on the Process of Change in Substance Abuse Treatment. *J. Subst. Abus. Treat.* **1995**, *12*, 269–282. [CrossRef] [PubMed]
27. Deane, F.; Wootton, D.; Hsu, C.I.; Kelly, P. Predicting dropout in the first 3 months of 12-step residential drug and alcohol treatment in an Australian sample. *J. Stud. Alcohol Drugs* **2012**, *73*, 216–225. [CrossRef]
28. Morris, Z.S.; Gannon, M. Drug misuse treatment services in Scotland: Predicting outcomes. *Int. J. Qual. Health Care* **2008**, *20*, 271–276. [CrossRef] [PubMed]
29. Burrell, M.J. Personal meaning, drug use, and addiction: An evolutionary constructivist perspective. *J. Constr. Psychol.* **2010**, *12*, 41–63. [CrossRef]
30. McIntosh, J.; McKeganey, N. Addicts' narratives of recovery from drug use: Constructing a non-addict identity. *Soc. Sci. Med.* **2000**, *50*, 1501–1510. [CrossRef]
31. Dingle, G.A.; Cruwys, T.; Frings, D. Social Identities as Pathways into and out of Addiction. *Front. Psychol.* **2015**, *6*, 1795. [CrossRef]
32. Selseng, L.B.; Ulvik, O.S. Talking about change—Positioning and interpretative repertoires in stories about substance abuse and change. *Qual. Soc. Work* **2016**, *7*, 216–235. [CrossRef]
33. Guelfi, G.P. Therapeutic community: New challenges for renewal in continuity. In *The Therapeutic Community in the Society of Addictions*; Palumbo, M., Dondi, M., Torrigiani, C., Eds.; Erickson: Trento, Italy, 2012; pp. 133–148.
34. Frank, D.; Walters, S.M. "I'm going to stop myself before someone stops me": Complicating narratives of volitional substance use treatment. *Front. Sociol.* **2021**, *6*, 619677. [CrossRef]
35. Broekaert, E.; Vandevelde, S.; Soyez, V.; Yates, R.; Slater, A. The third generation of therapeutic communities: The early development of the TC for addictions in Europe. *Eur. Addict. Res.* **2005**, *12*, 1–11. [CrossRef]
36. Mead, G.H. *Mind, Self, and Society*; University of Chicago Press: Chicago, IL, USA, 1934.
37. Blumer, H. *Symbolic Interactionism: Perspective and Method*; University of California Press: Berkeley, CA, USA, 1986.
38. Salvini, A.; Dondoni, M. *Clinical Psychology of Interaction*; Giunti Editore: Florence, Italy, 2011; pp. 238–264.
39. Iudici, A.; Turchi, G.P.; Faccio, E. Some considerations about auditory verbal hallucinations in the clinical field. *Psychiatr. Psychol. Klin.* **2020**, *20*, 77–79. [CrossRef]
40. Neri, J.; Iudici, A. The Use of "Science" and "Scientific Language" in the DSM-5: Theoretical, Clinical, and Operative Implications for Health Professionals. *Int. J. Interdiscip. Soc. Community Stud.* **2023**, *18*, 83–95. [CrossRef]
41. Iudici, A.; Fabbri, M. The Construction of "Discomfort Psychological": An exploration of Italians teachers' reports. *Qual. Rep.* **2017**, *22*, 2281–2295. [CrossRef]
42. Pagliaro, G.; Dighera, B. Words and Stories in Psychotherapy: Change Through Discursive Practice. In *The discursive mind*; Harrè, R., Gillet, G., Eds.; Raffaello Cortina Editore: Milano, Italy, 1996.
43. Turchi, G.; Baciga, D. Symbolic Interactionism: The Contribution of A. Salvini. In *"Addiction". Generate the Change between Paradigm Shift and Pragmatic Effects*; Upsel Domeneghini Editore: Padua, Italy, 2002.
44. Salgado, J.; Ferreira, T.; Fraccascia, F. The Dialogical Self as a Triadic System: The I as a Part of the We. In *Ricerche di Psicologia*; Franco Angeli: Milan, Italy, 2005; Volume 3, pp. 13–31. [CrossRef]
45. Iudici, A.; Renzi, C. The configuration of job placement for people with disabilities in the current economic contingencies in Italy: Social and clinical implications for health. *Disabil. Health J.* **2015**, *8*, 586–593. [CrossRef] [PubMed]
46. Iudici, A.; Masiello, P.; Faccio, E.; Turchi, G. Tackling prejudice and discrimination towards families with same-sex parents: An exploratory study in Italy. *Sex. Cult.* **2020**, *24*, 1544–1561. [CrossRef]
47. Salvini, A. *Topics in Psychology*; Upsel Domeneghini: Padova, Italy, 1998.
48. Turchi, G.; Maiuro, T. The epistemological reflection as a criterion of scientificity in clinical psychology. In *Clinical Psychology: Dialogues and Comparisons*; Molinari, E., Labella, A., Eds.; Springer: Milano, Italy, 2007; pp. 41–50.
49. Romania, V. *Roles, Identities, Interactions. An Interactionist Approach*; Liguori Editore: Napoli, Italy, 2012.
50. Mantovani, G. *Discourse Analysis and Social Context*; Il Mulino: Bologna, Italy, 2008.
51. Andersen, D. Stories of change in drug treatment: A narrative analysis of 'whats' and 'hows' in institutional storytelling. *Sociol. Health Illn.* **2015**, *37*, 1–15. [CrossRef]
52. Iudici, A.; Maiocchi, A. Community justice and juvenile offender: The management of an individual case with criminal slope with community involvement. *Mediterr. J. Soc. Sci.* **2014**, *5*, 2015–2027. [CrossRef]
53. Department of Anti-Drug Policies. *Annual Report to Parliament on the Phenomenon of Drug Addiction in Italy*; Presidenza del Consiglio dei Ministri: Rome, Italy, 2021.
54. Cardano, M. *Qualitative Research*; Il Mulino: Bologna, Italy, 2011.
55. Gergen, K.J.; Josselson, R.; Freeman, M. The Promises of Qualitative Inquiry. *Am. Psychol.* **2015**, *70*, 1–9. [CrossRef]
56. Baciga, D.; Fenini, D. The Question as an Intervention Tool in Psychotherapy. *Sci. Dell'interazione* **2019**, *1–2*, 62–85.
57. Flick, U. *Qualitative Research Designs. Designing Qualitative Research*; Sage Publications: Thousand Oaks, CA, USA, 2007.
58. Denzin, N.K.; Lincoln, Y.S. *Strategies of Qualitative Inquiry*, 2nd ed.; Sage Publications: Thousand Oaks, CA, USA, 2008.
59. Charmaz, K. Grounded theory: Objectivist and constructivist methods. In *Strategies for Qualitative Inquiry*, 2nd ed.; Denzin, N.K., Lincoln, Y.S., Eds.; Sage Publications: Thousand Oaks, CA, USA, 2003; pp. 249–291.
60. Iudici, A.; Gagliardo Corsi, A.; Turchi, G. Evaluating a case of parent separation in social services through a text analysis: Clinical and health implications. *J. Soc. Serv. Res.* **2018**, *46*, 1–11. [CrossRef]

61. Iudici, A.; Corsi, A.G. Evaluation in the field of social services for minors: Measuring the efficacy of interventions in the Italian Service for Health Protection and Promotion. *Eval. Program Plan.* **2017**, *61*, 160–168. [CrossRef]
62. Turchi, G.P.; Salvalaggio, I.; Croce, C.; Dalla Riva, M.S.; Orrù, L.; Iudici, A. The Health of Healthcare Professionals in Italian Oncology: An Analysis of Narrations through the MADIT Methodology. *Behav. Sci.* **2022**, *12*, 134. [CrossRef] [PubMed]
63. Turchi, G.P.; Dalla Riva, M.S.; Orrù, L.; Pinto, E. How to intervene in the health management of the oncological patient and of their caregiver? A narrative review in the psycho-oncology field. *Behav. Sci.* **2021**, *11*, 99. [CrossRef] [PubMed]
64. Goodman, S. How to conduct a psychological discourse analysis. *Crit. Approaches Discourse Anal. Across Discip.* **2017**, *9*, 142–153.
65. Van Langenhove, L. Varieties of Moral orders and the dual structure of society: A perspective from positioning theory. *Front. Sociol.* **2017**, *2*, 9. [CrossRef]
66. Wetherell, M.; Potter, J. Discourse analysis and the identification of interpretative repertoires. In *Analysing Everyday Explanation: A Casebook of Methods*; Antaki, C., Ed.; Sage Publications: Thousand Oaks, CA, USA, 1988; pp. 168–183.
67. Wetherell, M. Positioning and interpretative repertoires: Conversation analysis and poststructuralism in dialogue. *Discourse Soc.* **1998**, *9*, 387–412. [CrossRef]
68. Davies, B.; Harrè, R. Positioning: The Discursive Production of Selves. *J. Theory Soc. Behav.* **1990**, *20*, 43–63. [CrossRef]
69. Harrè, R.; Van Langenhove, L. Varieties of positioning. *J. Theory Soc. Behav.* **1991**, *21*, 393–407. [CrossRef]
70. Harrè, R.; Moghaddam, F. Positioning theory. In *The Discursive Turn in Social Psychology*; Bozatzis, N., Dragona, T., Eds.; Taos Institute Publications: Chagrin Falls, OH, USA, 2014; pp. 129–138.
71. Stephens, C.; Carryer, J.; Budge, C. To have or to take: Discourse, positioning, and narrative identity in women's accounts of HRT. *Health* **2004**, *8*, 329–350. [CrossRef]
72. Bondarouk, T.; Ruël, H.J.M. Discourse analysis: Making complex methodology simple. In Proceedings of the 12th European Conference on Information Systems (ECIS), Turku, Finland, 14–16 June 2004.
73. Tibirica, V.A.; Luchini, E.P.M.; Almeida, C.S. Drug users' perspective on their treatment and the psychosocial care network. *SMAD Rev. Eletrônica Saúde Ment. Álcool E Drog.* **2019**, *15*, 1–9. [CrossRef]
74. Palumbo, M.; Dondi, M.; Torrigiani, C. *The Therapeutic Community in the Society of Addictions*; Erickson: Trento, Italy, 2012.
75. Chen, G. Building Recovery Capital: The Role of "Hitting Bottom" in Desistance and Recovery from Substance Abuse and Crime. *J. Psychoact. Drugs* **2018**, *50*, 420–429. [CrossRef]
76. Turchi, G.P.; Orrù, L.; Iudici, A.; Pinto, E. A contribution towards health. *J. Eval. Clin. Pract.* **2022**, *28*, 717. [CrossRef] [PubMed]

behavioral sciences

MDPI

Article

The Road to Recovery: A Two-Year Longitudinal Analysis of Mental Health Among University Students During and After the COVID-19 Pandemic

Rosie E. Allen [1,*], Kevin D. Hochard [2], Chathurika Kannangara [1] and Jerome Carson [1]

[1] School of Psychology, Faculty of Health and Wellbeing, University of Bolton, Deane Road, Bolton BL3 5AB, UK; c.kannangara@bolton.ac.uk (C.K.); j.carson@bolton.ac.uk (J.C.)
[2] Division of Psychology, University of Chester, Parkgate Road, Chester CH1 4BJ, UK; k.hochard@chester.ac.uk
* Correspondence: r.allen@bolton.ac.uk

Abstract: Longitudinal research into the impact of COVID-19 on university students' mental health beyond the pandemic is lacking. This study aims to address the gap in the literature by tracking the mental health of university students over a two-year period, spanning the COVID-19 pandemic and its aftermath. A two-year longitudinal study surveyed a sample of university students (n = 302) three times between May 2020 and May 2022. Students' psychological distress, generalised anxiety, flourishing, and personal wellbeing were assessed at each time point. It was found that students' psychological distress levels spiked in May 2021 (T1) during the first year of the pandemic but reverted back to similar levels seen in May 2020 (T0) at the two-year follow-up (T2). While generalised anxiety gradually improved, both students' psychological distress and generalised anxiety remained considerably worse than pre-pandemic norms obtained in other studies. Students' flourishing scores remained very low, while their life satisfaction and state happiness improved slightly between May 2021 (T1) and May 2022 (T2). These findings clearly demonstrate that students' mental health is still in crisis, even after the COVID-19 pandemic. More needs to be done to support students beyond the pandemic generally, including this particularly unique cohort of students who endured unprecedented challenges for prolonged periods, and who are now transitioning into the working world. Practical implications and recommendations are discussed.

Keywords: mental health; psychological wellbeing; university students; anxiety; psychological distress; flourishing; higher education; longitudinal research; COVID-19

1. Introduction

Pandemics have widespread impacts on global health, economies, and societies, and are expected to become more frequent in the future. In order to better understand how recovery can be effectively managed, the latest COVID-19 pandemic can be used as a model to assess strategies and outcomes in the aftermath of such crises.

University students were one of the most vulnerable groups to the consequences of the COVID-19 pandemic [1,2]. Social restrictions meant that students were deprived of their usual social support networks which are crucial for buffering the adversities associated with transitioning into and managing university life [3]. The transition to remote learning and the lack of campus activities meant that students had limited interaction with peers and lost face-to-face contact with lecturers, heightening feelings of loneliness and exacerbating distress [4–8]. Unpredictability and a lack of clarity around assessment formats and academic expectations contributed to increased stress and anxiety [9,10]. These factors have created unique challenges that have significantly affected the mental health of university students, and as a result, research into the mental health impacts of the pandemic on university students was declared a top priority [11]. A substantial body of evidence has demonstrated the severe mental health impacts of the pandemic on university students, with increased stress, anxiety, and depression, along with the exacerbation of pre-existing mental health conditions [12–18]. For instance, a recent systematic review and meta-analysis [19] showed a pooled proportion of generalised anxiety across 36 studies at a prevalence of 41%, suggesting that students are experiencing high rates of anxiety. Increasing poor mental health generated a significantly higher demand for mental health services [20], which meant many students did not receive timely access to support, and this caused further distress [21–23].

The re-introduction of a typical campus environment in the post-pandemic period meant students could reconnect with peers and academic staff, providing crucial physical and emotional support. As academic life stabilised, students began to restore a sense of control and predictability in their lives, which positively impacted their mental health [24,25]. Subsequently, some recent research has shown that the mental health of university students has started to improve [26]. For instance, Lemyre et al. (2024) carried out a longitudinal study of around 150 students across four universities in England, capturing data in April 2021 and November 2021. They found that initial wellbeing was negatively impacted and that there was a significant improvement in students' wellbeing between April and November 2021 [26].

Nonetheless, longitudinal research on the impact of the COVID-19 pandemic on university student mental health post-pandemic is significantly lacking. There still remains a crucial need to understand the trajectory of mental health impacts, providing a timeline of students' wellbeing during and after the pandemic. Therefore, more comprehensive research is needed to provide deeper insights into the lasting effects of the pandemic on students' mental wellbeing. It is important for universities, policymakers and mental health professionals to have a greater understanding of the complexities of students' mental health trajectories to inform support strategies and address the evolving needs of students. Therefore, the main aim of this study was to address the gap in the literature by assessing the mental health of university students during and after the COVID-19 pandemic. By tracking their mental health over a two-year period—collecting data in May 2020 (T0), May 2021 (T1), and May 2022 (T2)—this study aimed to assess whether there were significant improvements in the wellbeing of university students after the COVID-19 pandemic (T2). Considering the unprecedented nature of the COVID-19 pandemic and its multifaceted impact on university students [12–18], the authors hypothesised that there would be a significant improvement in the overall mental health of university students in the post-pandemic period across measures of mental illness and of positive mental wellbeing. This would align with what recent studies have found, indicating an improvement in university students' wellbeing in the later phases, and coming out of the pandemic [24–26]. Specifically, it was hypothesised that psychological distress would increase initially (T0 to T1), reflecting heightened stress during the first years of the pandemic, before decreasing by the end of the two-year period (T2) as students adjusted to post-pandemic life. Generalised anxiety was hypothesised to gradually decrease over time (T0 to T2) as uncertainties related to the pandemic diminished and students began returning to normal. Flourishing and wellbeing scores were also hypothesised to show minimal or no improvement by T1, given the ongoing pandemic, with a more noticeable increase by T2 as conditions normalised following the end of the pandemic.

2. Materials and Methods

2.1. Design

This was a longitudinal study that adopted a repeated measures online survey design, aiming to track the mental health of university students from the early stages of the COVID-19 pandemic to the post-pandemic era. Data were collected online at three time points. First, between 14 and 16 May 2020 (T0), where those completing T0 (n = 1578) were invited to complete a follow-up one year later (T1) between 14 May and 4 June 2021 (n = 554). Those who completed the one-year follow-up (T1) were invited to complete the survey again another year later (T2), between 10 June and 24 June 2022 (n = 302). Data were collected through Prolific, which is an online crowdsourcing platform that was specifically designed for use in a research context [27]. Certain features available to researchers such as pre-screening and 'allowlisting' participants permit the collection of longitudinal data [28]. A timeline can be seen in Supplementary Materials, which offers context to the data collection periods in reference to what was happening in the UK for the general public, and university students specifically, around each time the data were collected.

2.2. Participants

In order to be deemed eligible to participate, Prolific users needed to be university students, currently residing and studying in the UK. A total of 1578 students completed the survey at T0 (May 2020), 554 completed the survey at T1 (May 2021), and a total of 302 university students in the UK completed the two-year follow-up (T2) survey online (May 2022). The attrition rate after two years was high, at 80.8%, and will be discussed further in the limitations. Table 1 presents the demographic characteristics of the participant sample at T0 (May 2020). At T0, participants were mostly female (76.5%), with a mean age of 24.6. Of the 302 participants at T2, 89 were recent graduates and were no longer studying at university. We asked the 89 recent graduates what they were doing now they had left university. Mostly, they were in full-time employment (n = 63) or part-time employment (n = 8). Some were unemployed and looking for work (n = 9), unemployed but not looking for work (n = 4), or self-employed (n = 5).

Table 1. Demographic characteristics of the sample in May 2020 (T0).

Demographic Characteristic		Number of Participants (n)	Percentage of Sample (%)
Gender	Female	231	76.5
	Male	69	22.8
	Non-Binary	2	0.7
Age	18–19	62	20.6
	20–21	100	33.1
	22–24	49	16.2
	25–30	37	12.3
	31–40	35	11.7
	41+	19	6.1
Year of Study	Foundation	44	14.6
	First Year	92	30.5
	Second Year	71	23.5
	Third Year	50	16.6
	Fourth Year	33	10.9
	Masters	10	3.3
	PhD	2	0.6

2.3. Measures

At each phase of data collection, participants were asked to complete a series of mental health-related standardised measures.

2.3.1. Psychological Distress (CORE-10)

Clinical Outcomes in Routine Evaluation (CORE-10) is a 10-item measure of psychological distress [29]. This scale is rated on a 5-point frequency of occurrence basis (0–4), from "not at all" to "most or all of the time" in response to items such as "I have felt tense or anxious". Participants are asked to rate their response to the items based on how they have been over the last week. Items 2 and 3 are positively worded and are therefore reverse-coded before a total CORE-10 score is calculated, where a higher score is reflective of higher psychological distress. The reliability and validity of this scale have been extensively tested and confirmed [30–32]. Internal reliability analysis using the data from the present study (T0) revealed a Cronbach's alpha estimate of 0.84.

2.3.2. Generalised Anxiety (GAD-7)

The generalised anxiety disorder (GAD-7) scale is a 7-item measure of generalised anxiety disorder and is often used as a screening tool and symptom severity measure for clinically significant anxiety disorders in outpatient settings [33]. This scale is rated on a 4-point (0–3) frequency of occurrence basis, from "not at all" to "nearly every day", in response to items such as "Worrying too much about different things". All items are negatively worded and are added together to calculate a total GAD-7 score. Participants are asked to rate their responses based on how they felt over the past 2 weeks. The GAD-7 scale has been shown to have good reliability and validity [15,34,35]. Internal reliability analysis using the data from the present study (T0) revealed a Cronbach's alpha estimate of 0.90.

2.3.3. Flourishing (PERMA-Profiler)

The PERMA-Profiler is a 23-item measure of flourishing [36]. Five PERMA subscales denote the overall flourishing score: positive emotions (3 items), engagement (3 items), relationships (3 items), meaning (3 items), and accomplishments (3 items). This scale also includes eight filler items aimed to control response bias that cover physical health (3 items), negative emotions (3 items), loneliness (1 item), and overall happiness (1 item). Participants rate their responses along an 11-point rating scale, which includes positively and negatively worded items. All items, when reverse coded, are scored from 0, which represents "never", "terrible", and "not at all", to 10, which represents "always", "excellent", and "completely", depending on the item. For example, Item 5 asks "How often do you feel joyful?" with anchors of 0 ("Never") and 10 ("Always"). This scale has good reliability and validity and has been successfully used by other researchers [37,38]. For the overall flourishing score, internal reliability analysis using the data from the present study (T0) revealed a Cronbach's alpha estimate of 0.93.

2.3.4. Personal Wellbeing (ONS-4)

This is a short, 4-item measure of personal wellbeing, adapted from the ONS Annual Population Survey [39,40]. Each item of the ONS-4 focuses on a specific concept: life satisfaction, worthwhile life, happiness, and anxiety. Two items (Life satisfaction and worthwhile life) are general questions about participants' feelings on those aspects of their lives. For example, one item focused on life satisfaction asks "Overall, how satisfied are you with your life nowadays?" The other two items (happiness and anxiety) specifically ask participants how happy/anxious they felt yesterday. The ONS-4 is scored in the form of a rating scale from 0 ("Not at all") to 10 ("Completely"), where each item is considered independently.

2.4. Procedure

The survey was compiled on Qualtrics and uploaded to Prolific, an online platform designed to recruit participants for online research. Participants were invited at T0 if they were studying at university at the time. Participation in this research was voluntary, and after participants read the study information and gave written informed consent to take part, they were asked to provide basic demographic information including age and gender. Participants were then asked to complete a series of questionnaires: CORE-10, PERMA-Profiler, GAD-7, and ONS-4. Participants were paid GBP 1.25 for each time they completed the survey, taking approximately 10 min. Participants who were lost to follow-up phases of the research were traced and contacted once via Prolific to offer the study information and an invitation to take part [41]. Ethical approval for the study was obtained from the University of Bolton Ethics Committee in line with British Psychological Society guidelines.

2.5. Statistical Analysis

In this research, we used the platform Prolific, which provides each participant with a unique and consistent participant ID. This ID remains unchanged each time a participant completes a survey on the platform, making it possible to track responses over multiple time points. By using this consistent identifier, we were able to accurately match participants' responses across all time points, ensuring reliable longitudinal data-pairing for our analysis. Sum scores were computed for the CORE-10, GAD-7, and PERMA measures with mean imputation for up to 10% missing data per instrument [42]. The repeated measures outcomes were restructured from a wide format to a long format and followed the nested structure whereby each participant (n = 302) provided data for 3 time points. All analyses were performed using the open software Jamovi (version 2.1.3) [43].

Mixed-effect models accounting for fixed and random effects were performed in the General Analyses for Linear Models in Jamovi (GAMLj), package version 2.4.8 [44]. These analyses accounted for both the overall trends over time and the individual variations.

Seven models (one per outcome) were computed, which included the repeated measure (T0, T1, and T2) as our fixed-factor predictor (time) and included correlated participant-level random intercepts, using a restricted maximum-likelihood estimate (REML) with the bobyqa optimizer, as this function produces less biased estimates of the variance components and is widely employed in Generalised Linear Mixed Models (GLMMs) [45].

Little's missing completely at random (MCAR) test, with Expectation Maximisation, was used to assess whether missing data on the outcome variables were missing completely at random (MCAR) [46]. Further to this, a chi-squared test was performed to determine gender differences in dropout, and an independent samples Kruskal–Wallis test was carried out to look for age differences in dropout. Finally, independent samples t-tests were conducted to determine whether mental health at T0 differed for those who dropped out compared to those who were retained.

3. Results

Means and standard deviations for study variables across each of the time points are reported in Table 2. Mixed-effect models for flourishing, distress, and generalised anxiety are reported in Table A1 while ONS outcomes of life satisfaction, life worthwhile, happiness, and anxiety are reported in Table A2.

Table 2. Mean and standard deviation of UK students at each time point for psychological distress, generalised anxiety, flourishing, and personal wellbeing.

	T0 (n = 302)		**T1 (n = 297)**		**T2 (n = 299)**	
	Mean	**SD**	**Mean**	**SD**	**Mean**	**SD**
Flourishing	95.60	23.73	92.29	26.37	92.96	27.03
Distress	13.69	7.26	15.30	5.64	13.76	5.72
Generalised Anxiety	7.44	5.30	7.06	5.03	6.25	5.06
Personal Wellbeing						
Life Satisfaction	5.76	2.34	5.96	2.30	6.04	2.38
Life Worthwhile	6.05	2.44	6.00	2.44	6.16	2.45
Happiness Yesterday	5.81	2.51	6.05	2.48	6.27	2.44
Anxiety Yesterday	5.56	2.95	4.44	2.96	3.89	2.87

The mixed-effect models reported displayed approximately normally distributed, homoscedastic residuals. For all models, a small marginal R^2 relative to the condition R^2 suggests a large impact of individual differences and a small effect of the fixed factor. The ICC for the models showed that the clustering for participants was substantial.

With respect to flourishing, we observed a small yet significant negative effect of time, with reductions from T0 to T1 and from T0 to T2. Distress increased significantly from T0 to T1 but was not significantly different from T0 to T2. Generalised anxiety at T1 did not significantly differ from T0 but did significantly reduce from T0 to T2. Similarly, both life satisfaction and happiness displayed no difference from T0 to T1 but increased from T0 to T2. Life worthwhile did not demonstrate any significant change over time from T0. However, anxiety demonstrated significant reductions from T0 to T1 and T2.

Retention and Dropout

At T0 (May 2020), there were 1578 responses. At the two-year (T2) follow-up (May 2022), there were 302 responses. Overall retention after 2 years was 80.8%.

A chi-squared test revealed that females were more likely to be retained, and males were more likely to drop out, $\chi^2(1, n = 302) = 299$, $p < 0.001$ As age was not normally distributed, an independent samples Kruskal–Wallis test was carried out to test whether the age of participants at T0 was associated with dropout from the 2-year follow-up. The findings showed that age was significantly associated with retention, $H(2002) = 6.45$, $p < 0.05$, where older students at T0 were more likely to be retained at T2.

However, independent samples t-tests were conducted to determine whether mental health outcomes at T0 (May 2020) differed for those who dropped out compared to those who were retained at T2 (May 2022). The findings indicated that there were no significant differences at T0 between participants who stayed for the entirety of the research ($n = 302$) and participants who dropped out ($n = 1276$) for psychological distress ($p = 0.603$), anxiety ($p = 0.789$), flourishing ($p = 0.506$), life satisfaction ($p = 0.302$), worthwhileness ($p = 0.551$), happiness felt yesterday ($p = 0.637$), or anxiety felt yesterday ($p = 0.321$). These findings suggest that those who stayed in the research and those who dropped out were similar in terms of mental wellbeing at T0 (May 2020). Therefore, females and older participants were more likely to be retained. However, retention was not related to the mental health of participants at T0.

This pattern is supported by Little's missing completely at random (MCAR) test conducted using Expectation Maximisation on our outcome variables, including CORE-10, PERMA-Profiler, GAD-7, and four ONS items ($\chi^2(343) = 255.55$, $p = 1.000$), which indicated that the data were missing completely at random (MCAR). Therefore, no further adjustments for missing data are necessary.

4. Discussion

The findings indicate that psychological distress levels increased between May 2020 and May 2021, likely due to the continuous effects of lockdowns, academic disruptions, and uncertainty [47,48]. The increase in students' psychological distress scores in May 2021 (T1) could have been impacted based on the nature of the questioning in the CORE-10 measure, which asks participants to rate their responses based on their feelings over the last week. For instance, at this time, in-person lectures had recently been re-introduced with periodic testing and mandatory mask-wearing (see Supplementary Materials), which could have heightened levels of anxiety related to their personal health and changing academic routines. It is also important to note that in the UK, May generally tends to be a period in the lead-up to exams at university, and so this could be a contributing factor, as students adjust to evolving forms of assessment in the changing climate. By the second year (May 2022), psychological distress levels decreased, returning to similar levels to that at T0 (May 2020), aligning with recent research in a non-student sample [49]. This might be due to the fact that two years into the pandemic, these cumulative effects, particularly around fear and uncertainty, had started to diminish [50], and people had adapted to changing academic and living conditions [51]. It is also possible that greater familiarity with pandemic-related changes, and reduced perceived risks following public health measures, such as the vaccination rollout, might have encouraged a sense of control in people's lives and contributed towards the reduction in distress in May 2022 (T2) [52]. At this time, all legal restrictions, including the requirement to wear a mask, had recently been lifted (see Supplementary Materials) and may have resulted in a reduction in their levels of psychological distress.

Current findings also revealed that generalised anxiety levels remained stable during the first year (T0–T1), but that they started to improve by May 2022 (T2), gaining support from recent research [53]. Similarly, anxiety yesterday (as measured by ONS4) demonstrated significant reductions from T0 to T1 and further to T2, indicating that both state and trait levels of anxiety were improved by May 2022 (T2). Anxiety levels were highest in May

2020, at a time when the COVID-19 pandemic was in its early stages with greater levels of fear and uncertainty [54,55]. As time went on, it is likely that students were becoming more familiar with the new living conditions, academic adjustments, and social restrictions, leading to a gradual reduction in their generalised anxiety levels [53,56], as shown by the reductions in students' scores at T1 and T2. Specifically, during May 2021, students, like the general population, were undergoing a period of relaxing of social restrictions, where the nation was at Step 3 of the roadmap that was devised by the British government to bring us out of lockdown indefinitely. Students during this period were allowed to gather in groups of six indoors and fifty outdoors, and indoor venues such as pubs and cinemas had recently re-opened which may have helped to facilitate leisure and social activities and alleviate some anxiety (see Supplementary Materials). By May 2022, students' social and academic environments had returned to a typical pre-pandemic experience as all legal restrictions had been lifted a few months prior (see Supplementary Materials). After such long periods in which this was restricted, increasing possibilities for social interaction were likely to contribute towards reduced anxiety in university students, due to the strong association between positive social contact and decreased anxiety [57,58]. This coincides with Relational Regulation Theory [59] which posits that an individual's relationships with other people can help to regulate their emotions and help them cope with stressful events.

Nevertheless, even in May 2022 (T2), when we saw some significant improvements, students' generalised anxiety remained significantly higher than scores that were captured by other researchers (M = 4.75) before the COVID-19 pandemic [60]. On top of this, their psychological distress was still around 3x higher than normative scores of 4.7 that were captured by other researchers before the pandemic [29], reinforcing the long-lasting impact of the pandemic on students' mental health [61,62]. It is likely that the prolonged stress from the pandemic, including academic and social challenges, financial instability, and uncertainty about the future, were collectively contributing towards sustained psychological distress and anxiety in students, even post-COVID-19, as reflected in sustained psychological distress at T2. Further, a study carried out by King's College London using the data collected from the Student Academic Experiences Survey revealed that over 15% of UK students were still reporting a mental health problem in 2023 [62].

The findings demonstrate that students' flourishing decreased over the two-year period, likely reflecting the prolonged stress and disruption caused by the pandemic [63]. More specifically, we know that students' distress and anxiety remained elevated in this post-pandemic era when drawing comparisons to normative scores from studies that were carried out pre-pandemic [29,60]. These prolonged mental health problems are likely hindering students' abilities to experience positive emotions. Dealing with academic adjustments, ongoing uncertainty, and poor mental health is likely to impact students' ability to engage in their usual academic and social activities [64]. At a point when students and recent graduates may have been struggling with re-transitioning to typical social and academic life, including a reported rise in social anxiety post-pandemic [65], this may negatively impact students' relationships and social fulfilment. Finally, not only did students face cancelled and delayed graduation ceremonies, but the prominent lack of practical learning opportunities during the pandemic [66] may negatively impact their skills and competence [67], which is likely to affect their sense of accomplishment [11]. Therefore, it is plausible that students have been unable to meet the criteria and demands to achieve flourishing mental health [68], as students' ability to experience positive emotions, engagement, relationships, meaning in life, and accomplishments may have been severely limited, if not withheld entirely, during the COVID-19 pandemic. It is important to note, however, that flourishing scores remained particularly low even after the COVID-19 pandemic when students were more likely to have regained access to their preferred academic and social routines and support systems. This could potentially highlight the lasting impact of having sustained restrictions and access to the things that bring them joy, security, and support. Additionally, as a consequence of the pandemic, students may re-evaluate their priorities and feel a sense of uncertainty about the future and their career prospects [1,47], which could influence their perceptions of meaning in their lives.

While both life satisfaction and happiness yesterday showed no difference between T0 and T1, both had improved by T2. Interestingly, students' scores of happiness yesterday appeared higher ($M = 6.27$) in May 2022 (T2) than the pre-pandemic norm of 5.5 as captured by the Office for National Statistics (ONS) in 2018 [40]. As a state measure of happiness, that is, capturing students' immediate emotional states at a specific moment in time [69,70], their happiness felt yesterday at the time of data collection in May 2022 may have been particularly sensitive to environmental and societal changes occurring. For instance, the lifting of legal restrictions and the return to normal social and university life may have boosted their immediate emotional wellbeing, resulting in higher happiness yesterday scores.

Current findings revealed that life worthwhileness did not demonstrate any significant change over time from T0 (May 2020) to T2 (May 2022). The psychological construct of life being worthwhile may, naturally, be more stable over time and less sensitive to temporary changes or external challenges [71]. While other measures, such as happiness yesterday and anxiety yesterday, demonstrated significant changes over the duration of the pandemic, the fundamental aspects of what makes life worthwhile for students may have remained stable. For instance, despite the transition to distance learning, continuity of learning meant that students could still pursue their ongoing academic and personal goals, as their long-term goals of academic success and career progress were likely to remain constant.

4.1. Limitations

Self-report measures were used, which are often confounded with social desirability [72], to which individuals of certain demographic or cultural backgrounds are more likely to provide socially desirable answers [73]. Nevertheless, psychological research is dominated by self-report measures, and standardised measures were used that have had extensive reliability and validity testing. Also, a large proportion of the research samples were female. However, this was expected due to the unequal gender balance apparent in higher education [74] and the increased likelihood of females participating in online research [75]. The length of longitudinal research is associated with higher dropout rates [76], and 'attrition bias' refers to the systematic differences between those who are retained and those who drop out of research [77]. In the current study, the attrition rate after two years was 80.8%, which is out of the range of the commonly reported (30–70%) attrition rate in longitudinal epidemiological studies [78]. This could potentially be related to increased binge drinking [79,80], increased job loss and employment instability [8], and reduced access to typical social support systems [81] that were reported during the COVID-19 pandemic, which are all associated with higher dropout rates [79,82]. Additionally, previous research has shown that mental health problems predict non-response in longitudinal research [83], especially in university students [84]. Indeed, high levels of psychological distress [80,85], anxiety, and depression [86] can predict attrition. In the current study, psychological distress and generalised anxiety scores were considerably high across all time points and were shown to be worse than the pre-pandemic norm, so attrition was likely to be impacted. In this study, females and older students were more likely to be retained, which may influence the generalisability of findings. This research is limited to drawing inferences and conclusions from data captured during and after the COVID-19 pandemic (May 2020–May 2022) and does not allow for pre-pandemic comparisons with this sample.

4.2. Practical Implications and Recommendations

After more than four years since the beginning of the pandemic, it is crucial to understand how the mental wellbeing of university students fluctuated throughout the pandemic, and how they are faring in a post-pandemic context. We have only recently started to understand the long-term psychological impacts of COVID-19 on university students. The current longitudinal study provided the ability to provide a picture of university students' mental health throughout an unprecedented global health pandemic. These findings show that students are still particularly vulnerable and need continued support extending beyond the pandemic. These findings can provide several practical implications and recommendations for further research, with regard to addressing the mental health of university students post-pandemic. While there have been some signs of improvement, students' psychological distress and generalised anxiety are still elevated and remain considerably worse than pre-pandemic norms. Also, student flourishing continued to gradually decline over the course of the pandemic, remaining low even after personal and academic life began to return to that of a pre-pandemic state.

Policy Implications

Clearly, universities need to adapt and improve the mental health services they have available to students to help them cope with the lasting impacts. The university setting plays an important role in shaping the future of its students and is the perfect platform for health and mental health promotion. Further investments are needed to screen and monitor students' health and wellbeing to help with the identification of students who could benefit from health and wellbeing services. More inventive ways of supporting and protecting students' wellbeing are needed moving forward to redefine mental health services, including rethinking how policies can support this. For example, greater efforts to consult with students themselves to co-produce in-person and digital programmes that could complement the curriculum, improve engagement with and the relevance of services, and alleviate the strain on overwhelmed mental health services.

Policymakers should consider the effectiveness of Positive Psychology Interventions (PPIs) in mitigating mental health problems and protecting university students' wellbeing, whereby such approaches are integrated into mental health support services. Worsley et al. (2022) recently conducted a systematic literature review of other reviews, focusing on interventions designed to support the mental health and wellbeing of university students. The authors reviewed 27 reviews and concluded that the strongest or most effective interventions to improve student mental health were mindfulness-based interventions and cognitive–behavioural interventions [87]. Future research should continue to evaluate the effectiveness of different mental health interventions in this context, to help refine and adapt existing interventions, as well as develop new evidence-based practices that are specifically targeted to the needs of this unique group.

This is a cohort of students who had particularly unique personal and academic experiences, which are not only important to consider during the pandemic, but these impacts are likely to continue to be felt long after the pandemic. After all, nearly a third of the current sample at the two-year follow-up were recent graduates, and they too were still experiencing considerably poor mental health. These recent graduates did not have the experiences that past generations of students would have had, and this will have impacted their competence and confidence in being successful in securing graduate employment [88]. Therefore, we need to consider the longer-term impacts beyond university, advocating for continued graduate support and further research into how their experiences during that time might have impacted their life, personally, but also professionally, after university.

5. Conclusions

Improvements in psychological distress, both state and trait anxiety, and overall personal wellbeing suggest a positive trend towards mental health recovery post-pandemic in this unique cohort of university students. However, mental health scores are still poor, remaining considerably worse than the pre-pandemic norm. These findings demonstrate the desperate need for continued attention in addressing students' mental health challenges beyond the pandemic. The need for more mental health support for university students remains the same now as it was during the COVID-19 pandemic. It also calls for continued support for this disproportionately impacted cohort in the post-pandemic era as they transition into the graduate job market. The current findings will contribute towards a greater awareness of the short- and long-term psychological impacts on student mental health, helping to inform and shape future general mental health support strategies, as well as specifically reducing risks in the event of a future global health pandemic.

Supplementary Materials: The following supporting information can be downloaded at https://www.mdpi.com/article/10.3390/bs14121146/s1: Figure S1: COVID-19 Timeline in the UK: Context for Data Collection.

Author Contributions: Conceptualization, C.K., R.E.A. and J.C.; methodology, R.E.A. and K.D.H.; formal analysis, K.D.H. and R.E.A.; investigation, K.D.H. and R.E.A.; data curation, R.E.A. and K.D.H.; writing—original draft preparation, R.E.A. and K.D.H.; writing—review and editing, C.K. and J.C.; supervision, C.K. and J.C.; project administration, R.E.A.; funding acquisition, C.K. All authors have read and agreed to the published version of the manuscript.

Funding: The authors gratefully acknowledge funding from the University of Bolton.

Institutional Review Board Statement: The study was conducted in accordance with the Declaration of Helsinki, and approved by the University of Bolton (1 May 2020).

Informed Consent Statement: Informed consent was obtained from all subjects involved in the study.

Data Availability Statement: The original data presented in the study are openly available in FigShare at https://doi.org/10.6084/m9.figshare.26262254 (accessed on 24 November 2024).

Conflicts of Interest: The authors declare no conflicts of interest.

Appendix A

Table A1. Mixed-effect models of time on flourishing, psychological distress, and generalised anxiety.

Fixed Effects	Flourishing (PERMA)					Distress (CORE-10)					Generalised Anxiety (GAD-7)				
		95% CI					95% CI					95% CI			
	Est	LL	UL	*t*	*p*	Est	LL	UL	*t*	*p*	Est	LL	UL	*t*	*p*
Intercept	93.59	90.99	96.20	70.44	<0.001	14.24	13.66	14.83	47.79	<0.001	6.92	6.42	7.42	27.34	<0.001
T1–T0	−3.34	−5.62	−1.07	−2.88	0.004	1.62	0.93	2.32	4.57	<0.001	−0.37	−0.90	0.15	−1.39	0.164
T2–T0	−2.69	−4.96	−0.41	−2.32	0.021	0.11	−0.59	0.80	0.30	0.764	−1.19	−1.71	−0.66	−4.44	<0.001
Random Effects (Intercept)			Model Fit					Model Fit					Model Fit		
	σ^2	ICC	AIC	R^2 marginal	R^2 conditional	σ^2	ICC	AIC	R^2 marginal	R^2 conditional	σ^2	ICC	AIC	R^2 marginal	R^2 conditional
Participant	462.24	0.70	7919.90	<0.01	0.70	20.34	0.52	5576.88	0.01	0.53	15.64	0.59	5174.96	0.01	0.60

Note: Est: Estimates; LL: Lower Limit; UL: Upper Limit; σ^2: residual variance; ICC: intraclass correlation coefficient; AIC: Akaike information criterion; R^2 marginal: variance explained by the fixed effects over the total (expected) variance of the dependent variable; R^2 conditional: variance explained by the fixed and random effects over the total (expected) variance of the dependent variable.

Table A2. Mixed-effect models of time on personal wellbeing (ONS).

Fixed Effects	Life Satisfaction					Life Worthwhile					Happiness					Anxiety				
		95% CI					95% CI					95% CI					95% CI			
	Est	LL	UL	*t*	*p*	Est	LL	UL	*t*	*p*	Est	LL	UL	*t*	*p*	Est	LL	UL	*t*	*p*
Intercept	5.92	5.69	6.14	51.13	<0.001	6.07	5.83	6.31	49.23	<0.001	6.04	5.82	6.26	54.03	<0.001	4.63	4.44	4.82	47.31	<0.001
T1–T0	0.19	−0.05	0.43	1.59	0.113	−0.06	−0.29	0.18	−0.48	0.629	0.23	−0.07	0.54	1.49	0.136	−1.12	−1.59	−0.65	−4.66	<0.001
T2–T0	0.27	0.03	0.51	2.21	0.028	0.10	−0.14	0.33	0.83	0.409	0.46	0.15	0.76	2.96	0.003	−1.67	−2.14	−1.20	−6.97	<0.001
Random Effects (Intercept)			Model Fit					Model Fit					Model Fit					Model Fit		
	σ^2	ICC	AIC	R^2 marginal	R^2 conditional	σ^2	ICC	AIC	R^2 marginal	R^2 conditional	σ^2	ICC	AIC	R^2 marginal	R^2 conditional	σ^2	ICC	AIC	R^2 marginal	R^2 conditional
Participant	3.27	0.60	3765.46	0.00	0.60	3.84	0.64	3778.08	0.00	0.64	2.55	0.42	4031.51	0.01	0.42	0.00	0.00	4470.42	0.05	0.05

Note: Est: Estimates; LL: Lower Limit; UL: Upper Limit; σ^2: residual variance; ICC: intraclass correlation coefficient; AIC: Akaike information criterion; R^2 marginal: variance explained by the fixed effects over the total (expected) variance of the dependent variable; R^2 conditional: variance explained by the fixed and random effects over the total (expected) variance of the dependent variable.

References

1. Aristovnik, A.; Keržič, D.; Ravšelj, D.; Tomaževič, N.; Umek, L. Impacts of the COVID-19 pandemic on life of higher education students: A global perspective. *Sustainability* **2020**, *12*, 8438. [CrossRef]
2. Blustein, D.L.; Guarino, P.A. Work and unemployment in the time of COVID-19: The existential experience of loss and fear. *J. Humanist. Psychol.* **2020**, *60*, 702–709. [CrossRef]
3. Hwang, T.J.; Rabheru, K.; Peisah, C.; Reichman, W.; Ikeda, M. Loneliness and social isolation during the COVID-19 pandemic. *Int. Psychogeriatr.* **2020**, *32*, 1217–1220. [CrossRef] [PubMed]
4. Labrague, L.J.; De los Santos, J.A.A.; Falguera, C. Social and emotional loneliness among college students during the COVID-19 pandemic: The predictive role of coping behaviours, social support, and personal resilience. *Perspect. Psychiatr. Care* **2021**, *57*, 1578–1584. [CrossRef] [PubMed]
5. Lee, C.M.; Cadigan, J.M.; Rhew, I.C. Increases in loneliness among young adults during the COVID-19 pandemic and association with increases in mental health problems. *J. Adolesc. Health* **2020**, *67*, 714–717. [CrossRef] [PubMed]
6. Alhamed, A.A. The link among academic stress, sleep disturbances, depressive symptoms, academic performance, and the moderating role of resourcefulness in health professions students during COVID-19 pandemic. *J. Prof. Nurs.* **2023**, *46*, 83–91. [CrossRef]
7. Azmi, F.M.; Khan, H.N.; Azmi, A.M. The impact of virtual learning on students' educational behavior and pervasiveness of depression among university students due to the COVID-19 pandemic. *Glob. Health* **2022**, *18*, 70. [CrossRef]
8. Barada, V.; Doolan, K.; Burić, I.; Krolo, K.; Tonković, Ž.; Student Life During the COVID-19 Pandemic Lockdown: Europe-Wide Insights. University of Zadar. 2020. Available online: http://ehea.info/Upload/BFUG_DE_UK_73_11_6_students_Covid_19_survey_results.pdf (accessed on 15 August 2023).
9. Ben Salah, A.; DeAngelis, B.N.; Al'Absi, M. Uncertainty and psychological distress during COVID-19: What about protective factors? *Curr. Psychol.* **2022**, *42*, 21470–21477. [CrossRef]
10. Huang, Q.; Wang, X.; Ge, Y.; Cai, D. Relationship between self-efficacy, social rhythm, and mental health among college students: A 3-year longitudinal study. *Curr. Psychol.* **2021**, *42*, 9053–9062. [CrossRef]
11. Burns, D.; Dagnall, N.; Holt, M. Assessing the impact of the COVID-19 pandemic on student wellbeing at universities in the United Kingdom: A conceptual analysis. *Front. Educ.* **2020**, *5*, 582882. [CrossRef]
12. Allen, R.; Kannangara, C.; Carson, J. Long-term mental health impacts of the Covid-19 Pandemic on university students in the UK: A longitudinal analysis over 12 months. *Br. J. Educ. Stud.* **2023**, *71*, 585–608. [CrossRef]
13. Catling, J.C.; Bayley, A.; Begum, Z.; Wardzinski, C.; Wood, A. Effects of the COVID-19 lockdown on mental health in a UK student sample. *BMC Psychol.* **2022**, *10*, 118. [CrossRef] [PubMed]
14. Heumann, E.; Helmer, S.M.; Busse, H.; Negash, S.; Horn, J.; Pischke, C.R.; Niephaus, Y.; Stock, C. Depressive and anxiety symptoms among university students during the later stages of the COVID-19 pandemic in Germany-Results from the COVID 19 German Student Well-being Study (C19 GSWS). *Front. Public Health* **2024**, *12*, 1459501. [CrossRef] [PubMed]
15. Kannangara, C.; Allen, R.; Vyas, M.; Carson, J. Every cloud has a silver lining: Short-term psychological effects of COVID-19 on British university students. *Br. J. Educ. Stud.* **2021**, *71*, 29–50. [CrossRef]
16. Kavanagh, B.E.; O'donohue, J.S.; Ashton, M.M.; Lotfaliany, M.; McCallum, M.; Wrobel, A.L.; Croce, S.; Berk, M.; Saunders, L.; Lai, J.; et al. Coping with COVID-19: Exploring coping strategies, distress, and post-traumatic growth during the COVID-19 pandemic in Australia. *Front. Psychiatry* **2022**, *13*, 1025767. [CrossRef]
17. Li, Y.; Wang, A.; Wu, Y.; Han, N.; Huang, H. Impact of the COVID-19 Pandemic on the mental health of college students: A systematic review and meta-analysis. *Front. Psychol.* **2021**, *12*, 669119. [CrossRef]
18. Paton, L.W.; Tiffin, P.A.; Barkham, M.; Bewick, B.M.; Broglia, E.; Edwards, L.; Knowles, L.; McMillan, D.; Heron, P.N. Mental health trajectories in university students across the COVID-19 pandemic: Findings from the Student Wellbeing at Northern England Universities prospective cohort study. *Front. Public Health* **2023**, *11*, 1188690. [CrossRef]
19. Liyanage, S.; Saqib, K.; Khan, A.F.; Thobani, T.R.; Tang, W.C.; Chiarot, C.B.; AlShurman, B.A.; Butt, Z.A. Prevalence of anxiety in university students during the COVID-19 Pandemic: A systematic review. *Int. J. Environ. Res. Public Health* **2021**, *19*, 62. [CrossRef] [PubMed]
20. Lisiecka, A.; Chimicz, D.; Lewicka-Zelent, A. Mental health support in Higher Education during the COVID-19 Pandemic: A case study and recommendations for practice. *Int. J. Environ. Res. Public Health* **2023**, *20*, 4969. [CrossRef]
21. Moghimi, E.; Stephenson, C.; Gutierrez, G.; Jagayat, J.; Layzell, G.; Patel, C.; McCart, A.; Gibney, C.; Langstaff, C.; Ayonrinde, O.; et al. Mental health challenges, treatment experiences, and care needs of post-secondary students: A cross-sectional mixed-methods study. *BMC Public Health* **2023**, *23*, 655. [CrossRef]
22. Park, S.Y.; Andalibi, N.; Zou, Y.; Ambulkar, S.; Huh-Yoo, J. Understanding students' mental wellbeing challenges on a university campus: Interview study. *JMIR Form. Res.* **2020**, *4*, e15962. [CrossRef] [PubMed]
23. Salimi, N.; Gere, B.; Talley, W.; Iriogbe, B. College students mental health challenges: Concerns and considerations in the COVID-19 pandemic. *J. Coll. Stud. Psychother.* **2021**, *37*, 39–51. [CrossRef]
24. Brailovskaia, J.; Margraf, J. Less sense of control, more anxiety, and addictive social media use: Cohort trends in German university freshmen between 2019 and 2021. *Curr. Res. Behav. Sci.* **2023**, *4*, 100088. [CrossRef]
25. He, M.; Zhan, X.; Liu, C.; Li, L.; Zhao, X.; Ren, L.; Li, K.; Luo, X. The relationship between self-control and mental health problems among Chinese university students. *Front. Public Health* **2023**, *11*, 1224427. [CrossRef]

26. Lemyre, A.; Chrisinger, B.W.; Palmer-Cooper, E.; Messina, J.P. Mental wellbeing among higher education students in England during the pandemic: A longitudinal study of COVID-19 experiences, social connectedness and greenspace use. *Br. Educ. Res. J.* **2024**, *50*, 1281–1307. [CrossRef]
27. Kothe, E.J.; Ling, M. Retention of Participants Recruited to a Multi-Year Longitudinal Study via Prolific. *PsyArXiv* **2019**. [CrossRef]
28. Palan, S.; Schitter, C. Prolific. ac—A subject pool for online experiments. *J. Behav. Exp. Financ.* **2018**, *17*, 22–27. [CrossRef]
29. Barkham, M.; Bewick, B.; Mullin, T.; Gilbody, S.; Connell, J.; Cahill, J.; Evans, C. The CORE-10: A short measure of psychological distress for routine use in the psychological therapies. *Couns. Psychother. Res.* **2013**, *13*, 3–13. [CrossRef]
30. Allen, R.; Kannangara, C.; Vyas, M.; Carson, J. European university students' mental health during COVID-19: Exploring attitudes towards COVID-19 and governmental response. *Curr. Psychol.* **2023**, *42*, 20165–20178. [CrossRef]
31. Coates, R.; Ayers, S.; de Visser, R.; Thornton, A. Evaluation of the CORE-10 to assess psychological distress in pregnancy. *J. Reprod. Infant Psychol.* **2020**, *38*, 311–323. [CrossRef]
32. La Tona, A.; Tagini, S.; Brugnera, A.; Poletti, B.; Aiello, E.N.; Lo Coco, G.; Del Piccolo, L.; Compare, A. Italian validation of the Clinical Outcomes in Routine Evaluation-10 (CORE-10): A short measure for routine outcome monitoring in clinical practice. *Res. Psychother* **2023**, *26*, 671. [CrossRef] [PubMed]
33. Spitzer, R.L.; Kroenke, K.; Williams, J.B.; Löwe, B. A brief measure for assessing generalized anxiety disorder: The GAD-7. *Arch. Intern. Med.* **2006**, *166*, 1092–1097. [CrossRef] [PubMed]
34. Dhira, T.A.; Rahman, M.A.; Sarker, A.R.; Mehareen, J. Validity and reliability of the Generalized Anxiety Disorder-7 (GAD-7) among university students of Bangladesh. *PLoS ONE* **2021**, *16*, e0261590. [CrossRef]
35. Tiirikainen, K.; Haravuori, H.; Ranta, K.; Kaltiala-Heino, R.; Marttunen, M. Psychometric properties of the 7-item Generalized Anxiety Disorder Scale (GAD-7) in a large representative sample of Finnish adolescents. *Psychiatry Res.* **2019**, *272*, 30–35. [CrossRef]
36. Butler, J.; Kern, M. The PERMA-Profiler: A brief multidimensional measure of flourishing. *Int. J. Wellbeing* **2016**, *6*, 1–48. [CrossRef]
37. Ascenso, S.; Perkins, R.; Williamson, A. Resounding meaning: A PERMA wellbeing profile of classical musicians. *Front. Psychol.* **2018**, *9*, 1895. [CrossRef]
38. Wammerl, M.; Jaunig, J.; Mairunteregger, T.; Streit, P. The German version of the PERMA-Profiler: Evidence for construct and convergent validity of the PERMA theory of wellbeing in German speaking countries. *J. Wellbeing Assess.* **2019**, *3*, 75–96. [CrossRef]
39. Michaelson, J.; Mahony, S.; Schifferes, J. *Measuring Wellbeing: A Guide for Practitioners*; New Economics Foundation: London, UK, 2012.
40. Office for National Statistics. Personal Wellbeing User Guidance. Available online: https://www.ons.gov.uk/peoplepopulationandcommunity/wellbeing/methodologies/personalwellbeingsurveyuserguide (accessed on 16 January 2024).
41. Teague, S.; Youssef, G.J.; Macdonald, J.A.; Sciberras, E.; Shatte, A.; Fuller-Tyszkiewicz, M.; Greenwood, C.; McIntosh, J.; Olsson, C.A.; Hutchinson, D.; et al. Retention strategies in longitudinal cohort studies: A systematic review and meta-analysis. *BMC Med. Res. Methodol.* **2018**, *18*, 151. [CrossRef]
42. Tsikriktsis, N. A Review of Techniques for Treating Missing Data in OM Survey Research. *J. Oper. Manag.* **2005**, *24*, 53–62. [CrossRef]
43. *Jamovi*, Version 2.1.3.; Computer Software; The Jamovi Project: 2022. Available online: https://www.jamovi.org (accessed on 15 August 2024).
44. Gallucci, M. GAMLj Suite for Jamovi. 2020. Available online: https://github.com/gamlj/gamlj (accessed on 15 August 2024).
45. Maestrini, L.; Hui, F.K.; Welsh, A.H. Restricted maximum likelihood estimation in generalized linear mixed models. *arXiv* **2024**, arXiv:2402.12719.
46. Little, R.J. A test of missing completely at random for multivariate data with missing values. *J. Am. Stat. Assoc.* **1988**, *83*, 1198–1202. [CrossRef]
47. Browning, M.H.E.M.; Larson, L.R.; Sharaievska, I.; Rigolon, A.; McAnirlin, O.; Mullenbach, L.; Cloutier, S.; Vu, T.M.; Thomsen, J.; Reigner, N.; et al. Psychological impacts from COVID-19 among university students: Risk factors across seven states in the United States. *PLoS ONE* **2021**, *16*, e0245327. [CrossRef] [PubMed]
48. Hughes, J.W.; Vander Horst, A.; Gibson, G.C.; Cleveland, K.A.; Wawrosch, C.; Hunt, C.; Granot, M.; Woolverton, C.J. Psychological distress of college students during the COVID-19 pandemic. *J. Am. Coll. Health* **2023**, *71*, 981–983. [CrossRef] [PubMed]
49. Reutter, M.; Hutterer, K.; Gründahl, M.; Gall, D.; Dannlowski, U.; Domschke, K.; Leehr, E.J.; Lonsdorf, T.B.; Lueken, U.; Reif, A.; et al. Mental health improvement after the COVID-19 pandemic in individuals with psychological distress. *Sci. Rep.* **2024**, *14*, 5685. [CrossRef] [PubMed]
50. Quigley, M.; Whiteford, S.; Cameron, G.; Zuj, D.V.; Dymond, S. Longitudinal assessment of COVID-19 fear and psychological wellbeing in the United Kingdom. *J. Health Psychol.* **2023**, *28*, 726–738. [CrossRef]
51. Dehghani, M.; Hakimi, H.; Talebi, M.; Rezaee, H.; Mousazadeh, N.; Ahmadinia, H.; Almasi, S. The relationship between fear of Covid-19 and obsessive-compulsive disorder. *BMC Psychol.* **2023**, *11*, 133. [CrossRef]
52. Perez-Arce, F.; Angrisani, M.; Bennett, D.; Darling, J.; Kapteyn, A.; Thomas, K. COVID-19 vaccines and mental distress. *PLoS ONE* **2021**, *16*, e0256406. [CrossRef]

53. Amendola, S.; von Wyl, A.; Volken, T.; Zysset, A.; Huber, M.; Dratva, J. A longitudinal study on generalized anxiety among university students during the first wave of the COVID-19 pandemic in Switzerland. *Front. Psychol.* **2021**, *12*, 643171. [CrossRef]
54. Chen, T.; Lucock, M. The mental health of university students during the COVID-19 pandemic: An online survey in the UK. *PLoS ONE* **2022**, *17*, e0262562. [CrossRef]
55. Son, C.; Hegde, S.; Smith, A.; Wang, X.; Sasangohar, F. Effects of COVID-19 on college students' mental health in the United States: Interview survey study. *J. Med. Internet Res.* **2020**, *22*, e21279. [CrossRef]
56. Bao, Y.; Sun, Y.; Meng, S.; Shi, J.; Lu, L. 2019-nCoV epidemic: Address mental health care to empower society. *Lancet* **2020**, *395*, e37–e38. [CrossRef] [PubMed]
57. Huang, A.; Liu, L.; Wang, X.; Chen, J.; Liang, S.; Peng, X.; Li, J.; Luo, C.; Fan, F.; Zhao, J. Intolerance of uncertainty and anxiety among college students during the re-emergence of COVID-19: Mediation effects of cognitive emotion regulation and moderation effects of family function. *J. Affect. Disord.* **2023**, *327*, 378–384. [CrossRef] [PubMed]
58. Margraf, J.; Zhang, X.C.; Lavallee, K.L.; Schneider, S. Longitudinal prediction of positive and negative mental health in Germany, Russia, and China. *PLoS ONE* **2020**, *15*, e0234997. [CrossRef] [PubMed]
59. Lakey, B.; Orehek, E. Relational regulation theory: A new approach to explain the link between perceived social support and mental health. *Psychol. Rev.* **2011**, *118*, 482–495. [CrossRef]
60. Jordan, P.; Shedden-Mora, M.C.; Löwe, B.; van Wouwe, J.P. Psychometric analysis of the Generalized Anxiety Disorder scale (GAD-7) in primary care using modern item response theory. *PLoS ONE* **2017**, *12*, e0182162. [CrossRef]
61. Kohls, E.; Guenthner, L.; Baldofski, S.; Brock, T.; Schuhr, J.; Rummel-Kluge, C. Two years COVID-19 pandemic: Development of university students' mental health 2020–2022. *Front. Psychiatry* **2023**, *14*, 1122256. [CrossRef]
62. Sanders, M. *Student Mental Health in 2023. Who Is Struggling and How the Situation is Changing*; King's College London: London, UK, 2023. Available online: https://www.kcl.ac.uk/policy-institute/assets/student-mental-health-in-2023.pdf (accessed on 15 August 2024).
63. Graham, M.A.; Eloff, I. Comparing mental health, wellbeing and flourishing in undergraduate students pre-and during the COVID-19 pandemic. *Int. J. Environ. Res. Public Health* **2022**, *19*, 7438. [CrossRef]
64. Csikszentmihalyi, M. *Finding Flow: The Psychology of Engagement with Everyday Life*; Hachette UK: London, UK, 2020.
65. Kindred, R.; Bates, G.W. The influence of the COVID-19 Pandemic on social anxiety: A systematic review. *Int. J. Environ. Res. Public Health* **2023**, *20*, 2362. [CrossRef]
66. Idris, F.; Zulkipli, I.N.; Abdul-Mumin, K.H.; Ahmad, S.R.; Mitha, S.; Rahman, H.A.; Rajabalaya, R.; David, S.R.; Naing, L. Academic experiences, physical and mental health impact of COVID-19 pandemic on students and lecturers in health care education. *BMC Med. Educ.* **2021**, *21*, 542. [CrossRef] [PubMed]
67. Puljak, L.; Čivljak, M.; Haramina, A.; Mališa, S.; Čavić, D.; Klinec, D.; Aranza, D.; Mesarić, J.; Skitarelić, N.; Zoranić, S.; et al. Attitudes and concerns of undergraduate university health sciences students in Croatia regarding complete switch to e-learning during COVID-19 pandemic: A survey. *BMC Med. Educ.* **2020**, *20*, 416. [CrossRef]
68. Seligman, M.E. *Flourish: A Visionary New Understanding of Happiness and Wellbeing*; Simon and Schuster: New York, NY, USA, 2012.
69. Stones, M.J.; Hadjistavropoulos, T.; Tuuko, H.; Kozma, A. Happiness has traitlike and statelike properties: A reply to Veenhoven. *Soc. Indic. Res.* **1995**, *36*, 129–144. [CrossRef]
70. Veenhoven, R. Two state-trait discussions on happiness: A reply to Stones et al. *Soc. Indic. Res.* **1998**, *43*, 211–225. [CrossRef]
71. Baumeister, R.F.; Vohs, K.D.; Aaker, J.L.; Garbinsky, E.N. Some key differences between a happy life and a meaningful life. In *Positive Psychology in Search for Meaning*; Leontiev, D., Ed.; Routledge: Abingdon, UK, 2016; pp. 49–60. [CrossRef]
72. Larson, R.B. Controlling social desirability bias. *Int. J. Mark. Res.* **2019**, *61*, 534–547. [CrossRef]
73. Johnson, T.P.; Van de Vijver, F.J. Social desirability in cross-cultural research. *Cross-Cult. Surv. Methods* **2003**, *325*, 195–204.
74. A Systematic Review and Meta-Analysis of Longitudinal Studies of the Antecedents and Consequences of Wellbeing Among University Students. Available online: https://internationaljournalofwellbeing.org/index.php/ijow/article/view/1897/1075 (accessed on 15 August 2024).
75. Mulder, J.; de Bruijne, M. Willingness of online respondents to participate in alternative modes of data collection. *Surv. Pract.* **2019**, *12*, 8356. [CrossRef]
76. Schaffer, H.R. *Social Development*; Blackwell Publishing: Hoboken, NJ, USA, 1996.
77. Nunan, D.; Aronson, J.; Bankhead, C. Catalogue of bias: Attrition bias. *BMJ Evid.-Based Med.* **2018**, *23*, 21–22. [CrossRef]
78. Gustavson, K.; von Soest, T.; Karevold, E.; Røysamb, E. Attrition and generalizability in longitudinal studies: Findings from a 15-year population-based study and a Monte Carlo simulation study. *BMC Public Health* **2012**, *12*, 918. [CrossRef]
79. Morton, F.; Tighe, B. Prevalence of, and factors influencing, binge drinking in young adult university under-graduate students. *J. Hum. Nutr. Diet.* **2011**, *24*, 296–267. [CrossRef]
80. Torvik, F.A.; Rognmo, K.; Tambs, K. Alcohol use and mental distress as predictors of non-response in a general population health survey: The HUNT study. *Soc. Psychiatry Psychiatr. Epidemiol.* **2012**, *47*, 805–816. [CrossRef]
81. Elmer, T.; Mepham, K.; Stadtfeld, C. Students under lockdown: Comparisons of students' social networks and mental health before and during the COVID-19 crisis in Switzerland. *PLoS ONE* **2020**, *15*, e0236337. [CrossRef]
82. Abdullah, N.; Kamaruddin, M.A.; Goh, Y.-X.; Othman, R.; Dauni, A.; Jalal, N.A.; Yusuf, N.A.M.; Kamat, S.A.; Basri, N.H.; Jamal, R. Participant's attrition in a longitudinal study: The Malaysian cohort study experience. *Int. J. Environ. Res. Public Health* **2021**, *18*, 7216. [CrossRef] [PubMed]

83. Tambs, K.; Rønning, T.; Prescott, C.A.; Kendler, K.S.; Reichborn-Kjennerud, T.; Torgersen, S.; Harris, J.R. The Norwegian Institute of Public Health twin study of mental health: Examining recruitment and attrition bias. *Twin Res. Hum. Genet.* **2009**, *12*, 158–168. [CrossRef] [PubMed]
84. Murai, H.; Nakayama, T. A one-year follow-up study on predictors of temporary leaves and drop-outs among students at a women's junior college. *J. Epidemiol.* **2008**, *18*, 26–36. [CrossRef] [PubMed]
85. Allott, K.; Chanen, A.; Yuen, H.P. Attrition bias in longitudinal research involving adolescent psychiatric outpatients. *J. Nerv. Ment. Dis.* **2006**, *194*, 958–961. [CrossRef]
86. Bjerkeset, O.; Nordahl, H.M.; Larsson, S.; Dahl, A.A.; Linaker, O. A 4-year follow-up study of syndromal and sub-syndromal anxiety and depression symptoms in the general population: The HUNT study. *Soc. Psychiatry Psychiatr. Epidemiol.* **2008**, *43*, 192–199. [CrossRef] [PubMed]
87. Worsley, J.D.; Pennington, A.; Corcoran, R. Supporting mental health and wellbeing of university and college students: A systematic review of review-level evidence of interventions. *PLoS ONE* **2022**, *17*, e0266725. [CrossRef]
88. Moores, E.; Reddy, P. No regrets? Measuring the career benefits of a psychology placement year. *Assess. Eval. High. Educ.* **2012**, *37*, 535–554. [CrossRef]

behavioral sciences

MDPI

Article

The Role of Guilt Feelings in the Development of the Burnout Process: The Influence on Psychosomatic Problems

Pedro Gil-LaOrden [1,*], Mary Sandra Carlotto [2] and Pedro R. Gil-Monte [1]

1 Unidad de Investigación Psicosocial de la Conducta Organizacional (UNIPSICO), Faculty of Psychology, Universitat de València, Av. Blasco Ibáñez 21, 46010 Valencia, Spain; pedro.gil-monte@uv.es
2 Postgraduate Program in Social, Work and Organizational Psychology, Universidade de Brasília, Campus Universitário Darci Ribeiro, ICC Sul, Brasília 70900-910, Brazil; mary.carlotto@unb.br
* Correspondence: pegilaor@alumni.uv.es

Abstract: Burnout is a psychological consequence of prolonged work-related stress. Previous studies have concluded that guilt feelings could explain the development of the burnout process and its relationship with other health disorders. The aim of this study was to evaluate the mediating role of guilt feelings in the relationship between burnout and psychosomatic problems. The sample comprised 714 Brazilian teachers (82.10% women). Burnout was assessed using the Spanish Burnout Inventory (SBI). The hypotheses were evaluated together using a path model to test the mediating role of guilt feelings in the development of burnout and its relationship with psychosomatic problems. Two models were constructed: the hypothesized model (i.e., indolence → guilt → psychosomatic problems) vs. the alternative model (i.e., indolence → psychosomatic problems → guilt). According to the results, the hypothesized model obtained a satisfactory fit to the data, whereas the alternative model's fit was found to be inadequate. We concluded that the hypothesized model was a good representation of the relationship among burnout, guilt feelings and psychosomatic problems. We recommend taking into consideration feelings of guilt to improve the diagnosis of burnout.

Keywords: burnout; feelings of guilt; psychosomatic problems; Spanish Burnout Inventory; occupational stress; teachers

1. Introduction

According to the World Health Organization [1], burnout is a consequence of chronic work-related stress that has not been successfully managed. It has been included in the International Classification of Diseases and Related Health Problems (ICD-11), and classified as a factor influencing health status or contact with health services (QD85). It is considered as a circumstance rather than a disease and it is not considered a medical condition. It refers specifically to phenomena in the labor context and should not be applied to experiences in other life domains. Therefore, burnout should be considered a health disorder, but not a psychiatric syndrome or a mental illness. It is characterized by three dimensions: (1) feelings of energy depletion; (2) feelings of negativism related to one's job; and (3) a sense of ineffectiveness and low accomplishment (ICD-11). This definition currently finds considerable consensus in the field and is most frequently used to evaluate burnout. It takes as its reference the psychometric model of the Maslach Burnout Inventory (MBI) [2].

In addition, several studies have suggested the existence of profiles and alternative theoretical frameworks for burnout [3–7], and latent profiles for burnout dimensions [8–13]. Studies on latent profiles are not based on a theoretical model, but rather on a psychometric model. Most of these studies used the theoretical definition provided by the WHO [1] and the MBI to differentiate burnout profiles [11,12,14]. For example, Leiter and Maslach [11], working with the MBI, identified five burnout profiles, labeled as burnout, disengaged, overextended, ineffective, and engagement. However, other studies have obtained four profiles [15,16]. Some studies have used alternative profiles to those of the MBI for assessing burnout, but these lacked a theoretical model that explains the syndrome's development process [10,13,17,18].

1.1. Theoretical Background

Gil-Monte [19] defined burnout as a syndrome resulting from chronic occupational stress of an interpersonal nature, which appears in professionals in service organizations. It is characterized by loss of enthusiasm towards the job, psychological exhaustion, indolence, and, in some cases, feelings of guilt may appear and lead to more serious health consequences. Three of them are partially similar to the definition of burnout given by the World Health Organization in the ICD-11: psychological exhaustion is similar to emotional exhaustion, indolence overlaps with depersonalization and cynicism, and low enthusiasm towards the job partially overlaps with lack of accomplishment. Feelings of guilt is a new dimension to burnout syndrome [20]. These symptoms constitute the four dimensions of the Spanish Burnout Inventory (SBI) [19].

According to Gil-Monte [19], burnout progresses in parallel from low enthusiasm towards the job and psychological exhaustion to indolence. Indolence is viewed as a dysfunctional rather than an effective coping strategy, which is employed after the reappraisal stage. This approach considered the model of attitudes developed by Eagly and Chaiken [21], and it took into consideration the mediating role of emotional and cognitive experiences in the relationship between perceived job stress and attitudinal outcomes.

Guilt is a social emotion characterized by an unpleasant feeling arising when we perceive that our actions have violated a moral or ethical standard and involves a negative self-assessment of our behavior [22]. It is a prosocial emotion, which motivates behavior adapted to social and cultural rules. It has a potentially positive function within social interactions by stimulating pro-social behaviors and promoting positive actions towards those who have been wronged to amend any damage caused [23].

Guilt has been incorporated by the model of Gil-Monte to explain two profiles of burnout. In both profiles, indolence is considered as a coping strategy used to alleviate cognitive (i.e., lower enthusiasm towards the job) and emotional (i.e., psychological exhaustion) deterioration. But this coping strategy yields different outcomes for different professionals. While some professionals effectively manage strain levels using the attitudes and behaviors of indolence (Profile 1), others find it uncomfortable, leading to increased guilt feelings and more severe burnout (Profile 2).

Profile 1 characterizes professionals who do not develop high levels of guilt. They experience moderate job-related stress, resulting in noticeable discomfort that, while not debilitating, does impact work performance to some degree. This profile is marked by low enthusiasm towards the job, coupled with high levels of psychological exhaustion and indolence. On the contrary, professionals who develop Profile 2 feel more intense burnout symptoms and health disorders [24]. They perceive the use of indolence as a non-adaptative coping strategy. When these professionals see themselves as becoming dehumanized, they experience high levels of guilt and reaffirm their commitment to other people (e.g., students and their parents) and professional involvement as a way of mitigating their feelings of guilt, mending past transgressions and any damage caused [25–27]. However, negative working conditions do not change (e.g., negative workplace relationships), their results do not improve, and job stress levels do not decrease, giving rise to more indolence (a negative coping strategy) and more intense feelings of chronic guilt [28–30]. Profile 2 suggests a mediator role for feelings of guilt in the relationship between burnout and more severe health disorders such as depression [4] because they work as a "trigger variable" in the progress of burnout. These profiles have been validated through cluster analysis [9] and predictive validity studies [24].

Self-efficacy has been identified as a relevant variable for professional development and well-being in the teaching profession, and for explaining the increasing teacher shortages observed in recent years [31]. Perceived self-efficacy refers to "beliefs in one's capabilities to organize and execute the courses of action required to produce given attainments" [32]. An efficacy expectation refers to an individual's belief in their ability to perform the necessary actions to achieve the desired results. Teacher self-efficacy refers to the teacher's belief in their capabilities to effectively cope with the responsibilities, duties, and obstacles associated with the professional role, including didactical tasks and addressing disciplinary problems in the classroom [33,34].

Self-efficacy has been identified as a relevant resource in preventing burnout [35–37] in educational settings. The relationship among these variables was found to be negative [38,39]. The results of previous studies have indicated that self-efficacy is primarily positively associated with personal accomplishment, and the relationship is weaker and negatively associated with the emotional component of burnout [40–44].

On the other hand, social support has been identified as a relevant psychosocial resource at work to prevent burnout [36,45–47]. Previous studies in the literature have shown a positive relationship between social support and the cognitive dimension of burnout –i.e., personal accomplishment or enthusiasm towards the job– and a negative relationship with the emotional dimension—i.e., psychological exhaustion [48–51].

Previous studies have identified health disorders that are positively associated with burnout among teachers. Chronic burnout is a serious health disorder, leading to mental health problems [52], anxiety [53,54], sleep disturbances [55,56], cardiovascular disease, musculoskeletal disorders, respiratory problems, gastroenteritis, and migraines [57].

1.2. Teachers' Burnout

Studies in education have concluded that burnout in non-university teachers is a serious problem around the world [48,58–60]. Teaching has become a high-risk profession for this syndrome due to the challenging working conditions in education. The demanding nature of the job, which involves constant interaction with people, exposes teachers to an increased risk of developing burnout. Teaching involves dealing with disruptive or difficult students, satisfying high expectations from parents and administrators, coping with excessive workloads, having high levels of commitment to the job, and facing the fact that most educational centers do not take into consideration the work–life balance of their teachers [61]. Moreover, principals focus on external inspections, accountability, and a blame culture, which increases job stress and burnout [62].

According to estimations by Marsollier et al. [59], the prevalence of burnout in Latin American teachers was higher than 30%, for high and very high (critical) levels. Carlotto and Câmara [48] found that the prevalence of critical burnout among Brazilian teachers was 25.80%, which indicated a high prevalence of burnout in Latin American and Brazilian teachers.

1.3. The Present Study

Based on the previous results, the aim of this study was to evaluate the mediator role of guilt feelings in the process of burnout and the relationship between burnout and psychosomatic problems, and to test the cross-national validation of the model of burnout developed by Gil-Monte [19]. The hypotheses were evaluated together using a path model to test the mediator role of guilt (as a symptom of burnout) in the process of burnout, and its relationship with levels of psychosomatic problems (Figure 1). We expected that indolence would be positively related to guilt (Hypothesis 7), and that guilt would be positively related to psychosomatic problems (Hypothesis 8).

Similarly, the possible reversed effect was also investigated, that is, whether psychosomatic problems mediate the relationship between indolence and guilt (alternative model). Psychosomatic problems could increase the difficulty of development in a demanding role, which ultimately increases the feelings of guilt. People with chronic psychosomatic problems may experience feelings of guilt, stemming from the physical and psychosocial symptoms of their illness. These feelings can arise from various factors, including the inability to perform daily activities independently and the impact on their work relationships [63]. Teachers can feel guilt related to a subjectively perceived responsibility, for inaction and not achieving their goals, and for not fulfilling a responsibility because of their own diseases or traumatic experiences [25].

Two path models were utilized to analyze the relationships among the variables. The order of the guilt–psychosomatic problems relationship established the distinction between the models. According to the hypothesized model, the feelings of guilt will occur prior to the psychosomatic problems (i.e., indolence → guilt → psychosomatic problems), while the alternative model states that the psychosomatic problems will occur prior to the feelings of guilt (i.e., indolence → psychosomatic problems → guilt).

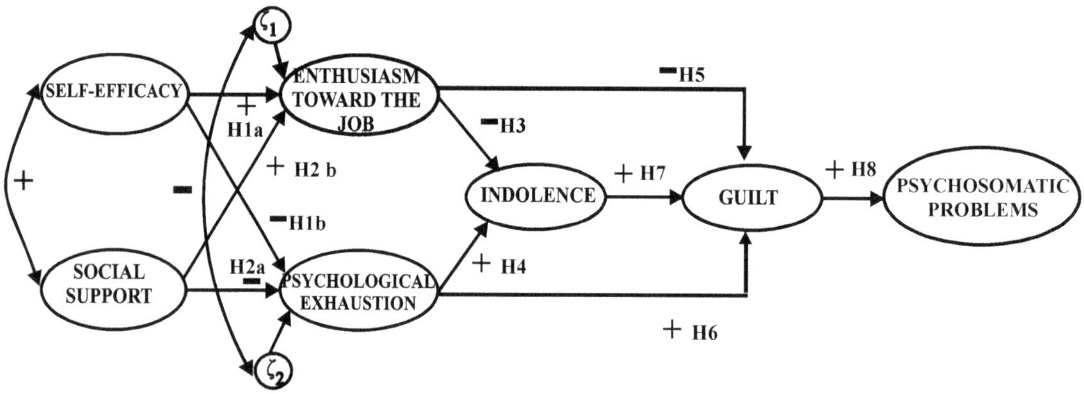

Figure 1. Hypothesized model.

2. Materials and Methods

2.1. Participants

The sample included 714 non-university teachers from the south of Brazil (men, 115; women, 586) (82.10% women). The mean age was 39.32 years (SD = 10.01, age range = 19–67 years). Regarding the type of contract, 66.80% of the sample (n = 477) were tenured teachers, and 30.10% (n = 215) were temporary teachers. The mean years of seniority in the profession of all the participants was 13.80 years (SD = 9.30, seniority range = 1–48 years), working in public institutions (63.50%) and working exclusively in teaching (62.1%).

2.2. Instruments

Sociodemographic data. All respondents were given a standard set of sociodemographic variables to obtain information about gender, age, contract type, and professional seniority.

Self-efficacy was measured using an adaptation of the *General Self-efficacy Scale* [64]. The adapted scale consisted of 8 items, similar to those of the original version but referring to work environment (e.g., When I am confronted with a problem in my job, I can usually find several solutions) ($\alpha = 0.87$). The scale is a self-assessment tool designed to evaluate optimistic self-beliefs in coping with challenging demands at work.

Social support was evaluated using the scale from the *UNIPSICO questionnaire* [65]. This scale consists of 6 items that measure the emotional and the instrumental support from colleagues, direct supervisor, and principal (e.g., How often do your co-workers help you when problems arise at work? Do you feel appreciated by your direct supervisor at work?) ($\alpha = 0.85$).

Burnout was measured using the *Spanish Burnout Inventory (SBI)* [19]. This questionnaire is a 20-item scale, divided into four subscales: *Enthusiasm towards the job*, which refers to an individual's desire to reach work-related goals because it is a source of personal accomplishment (5 items, e.g., I think my job gives me positive experiences) ($\alpha = 0.83$); *Psychological exhaustion*, which is the appearance of emotional and physical exhaustion, resulting from the demands of interacting with people experiencing problems (4 items, e.g., I feel I am overwhelmed by work) (α = 0.80); *Indolence*, which refers to the appearance of negative attitudes and behaviors of indifference and cynicism towards the organization's clients (6 items, e.g., I treat some people in my work with indifference) (α = 0.80); and, *Guilt*, which manifests as feelings of remorse about negative workplace attitudes and behaviors, particularly towards the people with whom the professionals establish work relationships (5 items, e.g., I feel bad about some of the things I have said at work) (α = 0.81). Low levels of enthusiasm towards the job, with high levels of psychological exhaustion and indolence, as well as guilt, indicate high levels of burnout. The version adapted for the Brazilian Portuguese language was applied [66,67].

Psychosomatic problems were evaluated by the psychosomatic disorders scale of the *UNIPSICO questionnaire* [24]. Items on this scale include different work-related psychosomatic problems (9 items, e.g., headaches, sleep quality, and anxiety, e.g., Do you have a headache?) (α = 0.90).

All scales were translated into Brazilian Portuguese using the back translation procedure [66]. Participants answered the items on all the scales on a 5-point frequency scale ranging from "Never" (0) to "Very frequently: Every day" (4).

2.3. Data Collection

The study respected the fundamental principles of the Declaration of Helsinki [68] and was approved by the Institutional Review Board of Pontifical Catholic University of Rio Grande do Sul, with particular emphasis on the confidentiality and non-discrimination of participants. Resolution 196 of the National Health Council (NHC) guided the ethical procedures. The participation in the study was voluntary and anonymous. Prior to the start of the assessment, the school principal was contacted to obtain the authorization to carry out the study and design the data collection. Teachers were informed about the purpose of the study, and it was clarified that their participation would not result in any individual or organizational assessment consequences. The questionnaire was distributed to teachers at the beginning of their work day, and they were asked to submit the completed questionnaire by placing it in a box in the teachers' room at the end of the day. Teachers expressed their agreement in a free and informed consent form before completing the questionnaire.

2.4. Data Analysis

To calculate the descriptive statistics, reliability and Pearson correlations the SPSS program (version 28.0) were used. To test the models, a structural equation analysis was carried out using the AMOS 25.0 program. The maximum likelihood estimation method was applied to test the models. Because the χ^2 test is sensitive to sample size, alternative fir indices were proposed. The *Goodness of Fit Index* (GFI) is a measure of the relative degree of variance and covariance accounted by the model. The *Adjusted Goodness of Fit Index (AGFI)* is a correction of the GFI based upon degrees of freedom. The *Non-Normed Fit Index* (NNFI) and the *Comparative Fit Index* (CFI) compared the relative fit of the hypothesized model with that of a baseline, or null, model. They should be greater than 0.90 [69]. However, some studies [70] have recommended a cutoff value of 0.95 as rule of thumb for GFI, AGFI [71] (p. 107), NNFI [72], and CFI [72,73]. The *Root Mean Square Error of Approximation* (RMSEA) quantified the error of the approximate fit, and the *Standardized Root Mean Squared Residual* (SRMR) was the square-root of the difference between the sample covariance matrix residuals and the proposed model. For both indices, values less than 0.05 indicated a close model fit, and values less than 0.08 suggested a reasonable model-data fit [74–76]. Values greater than 0.10 indicated poor fit [75]. For testing mediation and indirect effects, bootstrapping was carried out, with the number of bootstrap samples set at 5000 and 95% confidence intervals [77].

3. Results

Descriptive statistical analyses and internal consistency values are shown in Table 1. All scales showed good reliability values, with Cronbach's higher than 0.70. Regarding the skewness and kurtosis values, the variables fitted the normal distribution because all values ranged between +1 and −1.

Table 1. Descriptive statistics for scales in this study and Cronbach's alpha values.

	M	SD	Min	Max	Skewness	Kurtosis	Alpha
1. Self-efficacy	2.92	0.59	1.00	4.00	−0.38	0.22	0.87
2. Social support	2.48	0.85	0.00	4.00	−0.13	−0.61	0.85
3. Enthusiasm towards job	3.01	0.80	0.20	4.00	−0.69	−0.21	0.83
4. Psychological exhaustion	1.63	0.89	0.00	4.00	0.43	−0.17	0.80
5. Indolence	1.01	0.74	0.00	4.00	0.95	0.78	0.80
6. Guilt	1.11	0.77	0.00	4.00	0.66	0.30	0.81
7. Psychosomatic problems	1.38	0.93	0.00	4.00	0.60	−0.23	0.90

Table 2 shows the Pearson correlations among the variables included in this study. All correlations followed the hypothesized direction, and they were significant at $p < 0.01$ or lower, except for social support and guilt correlation, which was not significant. For self-efficacy and social support, higher levels were related to lower burnout, and higher levels of burnout were related to higher levels of psychosomatic problems.

Table 2. Pearson correlations among the study variables.

	1	2	3	4	5	6	7
1. Self-efficacy	1						
2. Social support	0.25	1					
3. Enthusiasm towards job	0.40	0.39	1				
4. Psychological exhaustion	−0.26	−0.24	−0.42	1			
5. Indolence	−0.26	−0.14	−0.41	0.57	1		
6. Guilt	−0.13	−0.00	−0.15	0.40	0.54	1	
7. Psychosomatic problems	−0.15	−0.12	−0.20	0.51	0.34	0.30	1

Note. Values > $|0.12|$ were significant at $p < 0.001$, and values $\leq |0.12|$ were significant at $p < 0.01$, except social support and guilt correlation, which was not significant.

The hypothesized model resulted in a significant Chi[2] value ($\chi^2_{(9)} = 168.645$, $p < 0.001$), suggesting an inadequate model fit. While the GFI indicated a good fit with the data (0.942), the fit was not acceptable according to the values achieved by the other indices (Table 3). The modification indices were reviewed to identify where linear constraints might be released to improve the model fit. The highest value suggested freeing the path associated with the variables: psychological exhaustion → psychosomatic problems (MI = 116.29). Freeing this path followed a theoretical basis, as the literature concluded that there is a significant and positive relationship between psychological exhaustion and psychosomatic problems [78,79]. Additionally, it did not invalidate this study's objective, as it continued to test the mediating role of feelings of guilt in the burnout process.

Table 3. Fit indices for the study models.

	χ^2	df	$RMSEA_{(90\%\ CI)}$	SRMR	GFI	AGFI	NNFI	CFI
Hypothesized model	168.645 *	9	$0.158_{(0.137–0.179)}$	0.093	0.942	0.820	0.688	0.866
Hypothesized rev. model	14.647	8	$0.034_{(0.000–0.061)}$	0.023	0.994	0.980	0.985	0.994
Alternative model	223.829 *	9	$0.183_{(0.163–0.204)}$	0.100	0.926	0.770	0.581	0.820
Alternative rev. model	154.856 *	8	$0.160_{(0.139–0.183)}$	0.062	0.945	0.806	0.678	0.877

* $p < 0.001$. Note 1. χ^2—Chi-square; df—degrees of freedom; $RMSEA_{(CI)}$—root mean square error of approximation (90% confidence intervals); SRMR—standardized root mean squared residual; GFI—goodness-of-fit index; AGFI—adjusted goodness of fit index; NNFI—non-normed fit index; and CFI—comparative fit index.

After this, the revised model—i.e., the "hypothesized model" revised—was estimated again, the final fit indices were as follows: $\chi^2_{(8)} = 14.647, p > 0.05$); GFI = 0.994; AGFI = 0.980; NNFI = 0.985; CFI = 0.994; RMSEA = 0.034 (90% CI = 0.000–0.061); and SRMR = 0.023 (Table 3). These values indicated a very good fit of the data to the overall revised hypothesized model.

All the paths were significant at $p \leq 0.001$ (Figure 2), and all hypotheses were confirmed. Specifically, self-efficacy was positively related to enthusiasm towards the job ($\gamma = 0.32$) and negatively related to psychological exhaustion ($\gamma = -0.22$). Social support presented a positive relationship with enthusiasm towards the job ($\gamma = 0.31$) and a negative relationship with psychological exhaustion ($\gamma = -0.18$). Regarding the hypotheses related to the burnout process, enthusiasm towards the job showed a negative relationship with indolence ($\beta = -0.21$), and psychological exhaustion showed a positive relationship with indolence ($\beta = 0.48$). In addition, enthusiasm towards the job presented a negative relationship with guilt ($\beta = -0.12$); psychological exhaustion obtained a positive relationship with guilt ($\beta = 0.17$); and a significant positive relationship was found between indolence and guilt (H7) ($\beta = 0.49$). Lastly, a significant positive relationship was found between guilt and psychosomatic problems (H8) ($\beta = 0.11$), and psychological exhaustion showed a positive relationship with psychosomatic problems ($\beta = 0.46$) (Figure 2). The revised model explained 32% of the variance in guilt and 27% of the variance in psychosomatic problems.

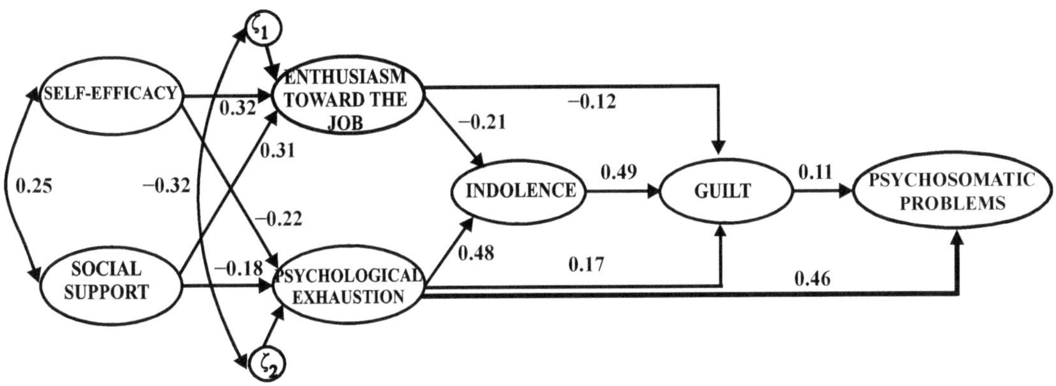

Figure 2. Standardized coefficients for the hypothesized model revised. Note. All relationships were significant at $p \leq 0.001$.

Using bootstrapping, the standardized indirect effect of indolence on psychosomatic problems was 0.09 ($p < 0.001$; bias corrected 95%, CI: 0.042 to 0.141), indicating that the relationship between indolence and psychosomatic problems was mediated by the variable of guilt (H7 and H8 were confirmed). However, the direct effect of indolence on psychosomatic problems remained significant ($\beta = 0.25, p < 0.001$; bias corrected 95%, CI: 0.161 to 0.332), indicating the partial mediation effect of the guilt variable.

The alternative model yielded a significant Chi2 value ($\chi^2_{(9)} = 223.829$, $p < 0.001$), which indicated an insufficient model fit according to this index. The fit to the data was adequate according to the GFI (0.926), but it was not acceptable according to the values achieved by other indices (Table 3). The modification indices were evaluated to improve the model fit. It appeared that releasing the constrained paths linking indolence with guilt (MI = 150.028, par change = 0.454), and psychological exhaustion with guilt (MI = 48.991, par change = 0.216) would improve the model fit. In addition, a review of the parameter estimations indicated that the relation between enthusiasm towards the job and psychosomatic problems was not significant ($\beta = 0.03, p = 0.390$).

With these results, we considered whether changing the model according to the modification indices would be a valid theoretical approach, because the highest modification index value suggested the freeing of the path associated with the variables indolence → guilt; however, there was no reason for considering this to be an adequate theoretical redesign for the alternative model.

In light of these results, an alternative revised model was evaluated, removing the non-significant relationship and adding the path psychological exhaustion → guilt (Figure 3). The fit indices were as follows: $\chi^2_{(8)}$ = 154.856, $p < 0.001$; GFI = 0.945; AGFI = 0.806; NNFI = 0.678; CFI = 0.877; and RMSEA = 0.160 (90% CI = 0.139–0.183) (Table 3). According to these results, the fit to the data of the alternative model redesign was not adequate.

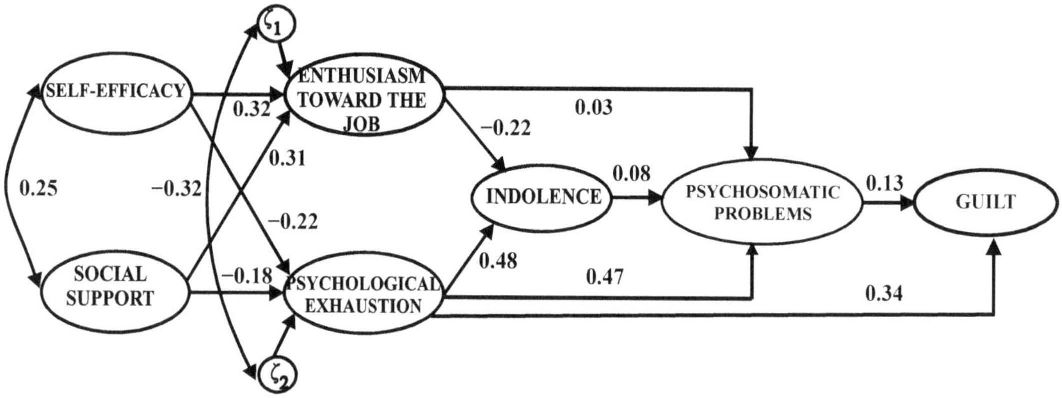

Figure 3. Standardized coefficients for the alternative model revised.

4. Discussion

This research sought to evaluate how guilt feelings mediate the burnout process and its relationship to psychosomatic problems, and to test the cross-national validation of the model of burnout developed by Gil-Monte [19]. The results supported that the relations represented in the hypothesized model, i.e., indolence → guilt → psychosomatic problems, are a good depiction of the burnout process and its relationship with psychosomatic problems. However, the relations depicted in the alternative model, i.e., indolence → psychosomatic problems → guilt, are not an adequate representation of the burnout process. The results provided support for the mediator role of feelings of guilt in the development of burnout and its consequences on the health of Brazilian teachers. This pattern suggests that higher levels of indolence lead to heightened feelings of guilt, which are, in turn, associated with the development of higher levels of psychosomatic problems, in line with the development of Profile 2 of burnout, hypothesized by the model of Gil-Monte.

Previous studies reached similar conclusions based on samples of teachers from Portugal and Spain [78]. In addition, the model has been supported for symptoms of depression in employees working with intellectually disabled people [4], and for alcohol intake and tobacco use as a consequence of troubles related to work in a sample of Chilean administration and customer service workers [80]. However, those previous studies did not test an alternative model, which is what makes this study original. It has also added new knowledge to the development of the burnout process, according to the model designed by Gil-Monte, by highlighting the relevance of developing feelings of guilt in explaining why job burnout leads to more serious psychosomatic problems.

The SBI theoretical model proposed two burnout development profiles. Both profiles feature indolence as a coping strategy that is employed in response to diminished enthusiasm towards the job and high psychological exhaustion. The feelings of guilt work as a "trigger variable" in the progress of burnout. Therefore, low or medium levels of guilt can be managed by personal coping strategies, i.e., Profile 1. However, when the feelings of guilt reach very high or critical levels, which cannot be managed by the individual without professional help, they accelerate the development of burnout into more serious health disorders, such as depression or psychosomatic problems, i.e., Profile 2 [24].

In addition, the results followed along the lines of other studies, which have pointed to self-efficacy [35,46] and social support [45,46] being relevant variables in preventing burnout in non-university teachers. When teachers show high self-efficacy and satisfaction with the perceived social support that they receive at work, their risk of burnout decreases.

It is necessary to highlight some limitations of this study. First, the cross-sectional data analysis presented limitations in determining the causal relationship between guilt and psychosomatic problems, making it challenging to establish whether guilt leads to psychosomatic problems or vice versa. Longitudinal studies are needed to draw conclusions on this issue. Second, the data derived from questionnaires increased the likelihood of common method variance effects. We employed various strategies to reduce the influence of these biases [81]: (a) participants' confidentiality was maintained; (b) participants did not know which items were associated with which scales; (c) back translation was carried out to minimize item ambiguity; and (d) an analysis using Harman's single factor test revealed that the total variance explained by one factor (32.81%) was less than 50% of the recommended threshold, indicating that common method bias is unlikely to significantly impact the study's findings. Third, participant selection was non-random.

5. Conclusions, Practical Implications, and Future Recommendations

The results of this study support the theoretical studies that have concluded that guilt is a significant variable in understanding the development of burnout [82–85]. This indicates that the feelings of guilt experienced by teachers play a significant role in explaining the different profiles of burnout progression [9] and its relationship with psychosomatic problems, which are closely associated with the development of guilt over time.

Feelings of guilt should be considered a symptom of burnout in order to achieve a more comprehensive diagnosis, distinguishing between individuals affected by the syndrome and recognizing its impact on health-related issues. While our research focused on a sample of teachers, burnout is also common among professionals in other helping professions (e.g., health, social services, and public servants). It may provide information for therapists to aid in the prevention, diagnosis, and treatment of different types of burnout syndrome—i.e., Profile 1 vs. Profile 2.

This study could also be useful in detecting the need for intervention programs to improve the social environment at educational centres and the need to train teachers in techniques for dealing with stress and burnout [86]. Principals and school administrators might help to promote collaborative relationships among teachers through programs for increasing social support, and by enhancing teachers' skills and capacities related to self-efficacy to prevent burnout and psychosomatic problems.

Future research should continue to investigate which situational (e.g., socialization in the professional role) [87,88] and individual factors (e.g., prosocial preferences and moral values) [89] cause guilt in the process of burnout and burnout Profile 2.

Author Contributions: Conceptualization, M.S.C. and P.R.G.-M.; methodology, M.S.C. and P.R.G.-M.; validation, M.S.C., P.G.-L. and P.R.G.-M.; formal analysis, M.S.C., P.G.-L. and P.R.G.-M.; investigation, M.S.C., P.G.-L. and P.R.G.-M.; resources, M.S.C., P.G.-L. and P.R.G.-M.; data curation, M.S.C.; writing—original draft preparation, M.S.C., P.G.-L. and P.R.G.-M.; writing—review and editing, M.S.C., P.G.-L. and P.R.G.-M.; visualization, M.S.C., P.G.-L. and P.R.G.-M.; supervision, M.S.C. and P.R.G.-M.; project administration, M.S.C. and P.R.G.-M.; funding acquisition, M.S.C. All authors have read and agreed to the published version of the manuscript.

Funding: This research received no external funding.

Institutional Review Board Statement: The study was conducted according to the guidelines of the Declaration of Helsinki, and approved by the Institutional Review Board of Pontifical Catholic University of Rio Grande do Sul (protocol code 02641012.5.0000.5336, 30 October 2012).

Informed Consent Statement: Informed consent was obtained from all subjects involved in the study.

Data Availability Statement: The raw data supporting the conclusions of this article will be made available by the authors upon request.

Conflicts of Interest: The authors declare no conflict of interest.

References

1. World Health Organization. *International Statistical Classification of Diseases and Related Health Problems*, 11th ed.; World Health Organization: Geneva, Switzerland, 2019. Available online: https://icd.who.int/ (accessed on 8 October 2024).
2. Maslach, C.; Jackson, S.E.; Leiter, M.P. *Maslach Burnout Inventory Manual*, 3rd ed.; Consulting Psychologists Press: Palo Alto, CA, USA, 1996.
3. Farber, B.A. Treatment strategies for different types of teacher burnout. *J. Clin. Psychol.* **2000**, *56*, 675–689. [CrossRef]
4. Gil-Monte, P.R. The influence of guilt on the relationship between burnout and depression. *Eur Psychol.* **2012**, *17*, 231–236. [CrossRef]
5. Paine, W.S. The burnout syndrome in context. In *The Burnout Syndrome: Current Research, Theory, Interventions*; Jones, J.W., Ed.; London House Press: Park Ridge, UK, 1982; pp. 1–29.
6. Tops, M.; Boksem, M.A.; Wijers, A.A.; van Duinen, H.; Den Boer, J.A.; Meijman, T.F.; Korf, J. The psychobiology of burnout: Are there two different syndromes? *Neuropsychobiology* **2007**, *55*, 143–150. [CrossRef] [PubMed]
7. Vanheule, S.; Declercq, F.; Meganck, R.; Desmet, M. Burnout, critical incidents and social support in security guards. *Stress Health* **2008**, *24*, 137–141. [CrossRef]
8. Gilmour, A.F.; Sandilos, L.E.; Pilny, W.V.; Schwartz, S.; Wehby, J.H. Teaching students with emotional/behavioral disorders: Teachers' burnout profiles and classroom management. *J. Emot. Behav. Disord.* **2022**, *30*, 16–28. [CrossRef]
9. Guidetti, G.; Viotti, S.; Gil-Monte, P.R.; Converso, D. Feeling guilty or not guilty. Identifying burnout profiles among Italian teachers. *Curr. Psychol.* **2018**, *37*, 769–780. [CrossRef]
10. Gillet, N.; Morin, A.J.S.; Colombat, P.; Ndiaye, A.; Fouquereau, E. Burnout profiles: Dimensionality, replicability, and associations with predictors and outcomes. *Curr. Psychol.* **2023**, *42*, 4504–4522. [CrossRef]
11. Leiter, M.P.; Maslach, C. Latent burnout profiles: A new approach to understanding the burnout experience. *Burn. Res.* **2016**, *3*, 89–100. [CrossRef]
12. Pyhältö, K.; Pietarinen, J.; Haverinen, K.; Tikkanen, L.; Soini, T. Teacher burnout profiles and proactive strategies. *Eur. J. Psychol. Educ.* **2020**, *36*, 219–242. [CrossRef]
13. Salmela-Aro, K.; Hietajärvi, L.; Lonka, K. Work burnout and engagement profiles among teachers. *Front. Psychol.* **2019**, *10*, 2254. [CrossRef]
14. Aguayo-Estremera, R.; Membrive-Jiménez, M.J.; Albendín-García, L.; Gómez-Urquiza, J.L.; Romero-Bejar, J.L.; De la Fuente-Solana, E.I.; Cañadas, G.R. Analyzing latent burnout profiles in a sample of Spanish nursing and psychology undergraduates. *Healthcare* **2024**, *12*, 438. [CrossRef] [PubMed]
15. Berjot, S.; Altintas, E.; Lesage, F.X.; Grebot, E. Burnout risk profiles among French psychologists. *Burn. Res.* **2017**, *7*, 10–20. [CrossRef]
16. Jones-Bitton, A.; Gillis, D.; Peterson, M.; McKee, H. Latent burnout profiles of veterinarians in Canada: Findings from a cross-sectional study. *Vet Rec.* **2023**, *192*, e2281. [CrossRef] [PubMed]
17. Angelini, G.; Mamprin, C.; Borrelli, I.; Santoro, P.E.; Gualano, M.R.; Moscato, U.; Fiorilli, C. Engaged teachers and well-being: The mediating role of burnout dimensions. *Health Psychol. Behav. Med.* **2024**, *12*, 2404507. [CrossRef]
18. Załuski, M.; Makara-Studzińska, M. Latent occupational burnout profiles of working women. *Int. J. Environ. Res. Public Health* **2022**, *19*, 6525. [CrossRef]
19. Gil-Monte, P.R. *CESQT: Cuestionario Para la Evaluación del Síndrome de Quemarse por el Trabajo [SBI: The Spanish Burnout Inventory]*; TEA: Madrid, Spain, 2011.
20. Maslach, C.; Leiter, M.P. Understanding burnout: New models. In *The Handbook of Stress and Health: A Guide to Research and Practice*; Cooper, C.L., Quick, J.C., Eds.; John Wiley & Sons: West Sussex, UK, 2017; pp. 36–56.
21. Eagly, A.H.; Chaiken, S. *The Psychology of Attitudes*; Harcourt Brace Jovanovich: Fort Worth, TX, USA, 1993.
22. Tangney, J.P.; Stuewig, J.; Mashek, D.J. Moral emotions and moral behavior. *Annu. Rev. Psych.* **2007**, *58*, 345–372. [CrossRef]
23. Vaish, A. The prosocial functions of early social emotions: The case of guilt. *Curr. Opin. Psychol.* **2018**, *20*, 25–29. [CrossRef]
24. Misiolek-Marín, A.; Soto-Rubio, A.; Misiolek, H.; Gil-Monte, P.R. Influence of burnout and feelings of guilt on depression and health in anesthesiologists. *Int. J. Environ. Res. Public Health* **2020**, *17*, 9267. [CrossRef]
25. Luck, T.; Luck-Sikorski, C. The wide variety of reasons for feeling guilty in adults: Findings from a large cross-sectional web-based survey. *BMC Psychol.* **2022**, *10*, 198. [CrossRef]
26. Motro, D.; Ordóñez, L.D.; Pittarello, A.; Welsh, D.T. Investigating the effects of anger and guilt on unethical behavior: A dual-process approach. *J. Bus. Ethics* **2018**, *152*, 133–148. [CrossRef]
27. Skatova, A.; Spence, A.; Leygue, C.; Ferguson, E. Guilty repair sustains cooperation, angry retaliation destroys it. *Sci. Rep.* **2017**, *7*, 46709. [CrossRef] [PubMed]
28. Le, T.T.; Jin, R. Vortex of regret: How positive and negative coping strategies correlate with feelings of guilt. *Acta Psycho.* **2024**, *247*, 104320. [CrossRef] [PubMed]

29. Muro, C.; Navarro-Prados, A.B.; Satorres, E.; Serra, E.; Meléndez, J.C. Coping and guilt in informal caregivers: A predictive model based on structural equations. *Psychol. Health Med.* **2023**, *28*, 819–830. [CrossRef] [PubMed]
30. Rose, S.; Palattiyil, G. Surviving or thriving? Enhancing the emotional resilience of social workers in their organisational settings. *J. Soc. Work* **2020**, *20*, 23–42. [CrossRef]
31. European Commission/EACEA/Eurydice. *Teachers in Europe: Careers, Development and Well-Being. Eurydice Report*; Publications Office of the European Union: Luxembourg, 2021. Available online: https://eurydice.eacea.ec.europa.eu/sites/default/files/teachers_in_europe_2020_chapter_1.pdf (accessed on 8 October 2024).
32. Bandura, A. *Self-Efficacy: The Exercise of Control*; Freeman: New York, NY, USA, 1997.
33. Barni, D.; Danioni, F.; Benevene, P. Teachers' self-efficacy: The role of personal values and motivations for teaching. *Front. Psychol.* **2019**, *10*, 1645. [CrossRef]
34. Lazarides, R.; Warner, L. Teacher self-efficacy. In *Oxford Research Encyclopedia of Education*; Oxford University Press: New York, NY, USA, 2020.
35. Daniilidou, A.; Platsidou, M.; Gonida, E. Primary school teacher's resilience: Association with teacher self-efficacy, burnout and stress. *Electron. J. Res. Educ. Psychol.* **2020**, *18*, 549–582. [CrossRef]
36. Mijakoski, D.; Cheptea, D.; Marca, S.C.; Shoman, Y.; Caglayan, C.; Bugge, M.D.; Gnesi, M.; Godderis, L.; Kiran, S.; McElvenny, D.M.; et al. Determinants of burnout among teachers: A systematic review of longitudinal studies. *Int. J. Environ. Res. Public Health* **2022**, *19*, 5776. [CrossRef]
37. Shakeel, S.; Khan, M.M.; Khan, R.A.A.; Mujtaba, B.G. Linking personality traits, self-efficacy and burnout of teachers in public schools: Does school climate play a moderating role? *Public Organ. Rev.* **2022**, *22*, 19–39. [CrossRef]
38. Friesen, D.C.; Shory, U.; Lamoureux, C. The role of self-efficacy beliefs and inclusive education beliefs on teacher burnout. *Soc. Sci. Humanit. Open* **2023**, *8*, 100599. [CrossRef]
39. Smetackova, I. Self-efficacy and burnout syndrome among teachers. *Eur. J. Soc. Behav. Sci.* **2017**, *20*, 228–241. [CrossRef]
40. Bayani, A.A.; Baghery, H. Exploring the influence of self-efficacy, school context and self-esteem on job burnout of Iranian muslim teachers: A path model approach. *J. Relig. Health* **2020**, *59*, 154–162. [CrossRef] [PubMed]
41. Mariani, A.M.; Piceci, L.; Melchiori, F.M. Protective factors for teachers' work stress: Psychoeducational programs based on self-efficacy and hope to reinforce personal resources. *Italian J. Educ. Res.* **2020**, *25*, 127–136.
42. Qiang, Y. A correlation study of self-efficacy and occupational burnout among university foreign language teachers. In Proceedings of the 2022 3rd International Conference on Modern Education and Information Management, Chengdu, China, 16–18 September 2022; Balakrishnan, V., Khan, I.A., Birkök, M.C., Eds.; Atlantis Press: Dordrecht, The Netherlands, 2022; pp. 234–240.
43. Schwarzer, R.; Hallum, S. Perceived teacher self-efficacy as a predictor of job stress and burnout: Mediation analyses. *Appl. Psychol.* **2008**, *57*, 152–171. [CrossRef]
44. Vidić, T.; Đuranović, M.; Klasnić, I. Student misbehaviour, teacher self-efficacy, burnout and job satisfaction: Evidence from Croatia. *Probl. Educ. 21st Cent.* **2021**, *79*, 657–673. [CrossRef]
45. Fiorilli, C.; Benevene, P.; De Stasio, S.; Buonomo, I.; Romano, L.; Pepe, A.; Addimando, L. Teachers' burnout: The role of trait emotional intelligence and social support. *Front. Psychol.* **2019**, *10*, 2743. [CrossRef]
46. Marcionetti, J.; Castelli, L. The job and life satisfaction of teachers: A social cognitive model integrating teachers' burnout, self-efficacy, dispositional optimism, and social support. *Int. J. Educ. Vocat. Guidance* **2023**, *23*, 441–463. [CrossRef]
47. Song, Y.; Zhao, W.; Wang, X.; Li, J. The impact of job stress on burnout in Chinese teachers: The mediating roles of social support and psychological empowerment. *Psychol. Sch.* **2024**, *61*, 253–271. [CrossRef]
48. Carlotto, M.S.; Câmara, S.G. Prevalence and predictors of Burnout Syndrome among public elementary school teachers. *Anal. Psicol.* **2019**, *2*, 135–146. [CrossRef]
49. Manzano, A.B.; León-Mejía, A.; Patino-Alonso, M.; Feu, S. Síndrome de burnout y apoyo social en maestros de educación primaria. [Burnout and social support in primary school teachers]. *Estud. Educ.* **2022**, *42*, 79–98.
50. Temam, S.; Billaudeau, N.; Vercambre, M.N. Burnout symptomatology and social support at work independent of the private sphere: A population-based study of French teachers. *Int. Arch. Occup. Environ. Health* **2019**, *92*, 891–900. [CrossRef]
51. Unterbrink, T.; Pfeifer, R.; Krippeit, L.; Zimmermann, L.; Rose, U.; Joos, A.; Hartmann, A.; Wirsching, M.; Bauer, J. Burnout and effort-reward imbalance improvement for teachers by a manual-based group program. *Int. Arch. Occup. Environ. Health* **2012**, *85*, 667–674. [CrossRef] [PubMed]
52. Capone, V.; Petrillo, G. Mental health in teachers: Relationships with job satisfaction, efficacy beliefs, burnout and depression. *Curr. Psychol.* **2020**, *39*, 1757–1766. [CrossRef]
53. Agyapong, B.; Obuobi-Donkor, G.; Burback, L.; Wei, Y. Stress, burnout, anxiety and depression among teachers: A scoping review. *Int. J. Environ. Res. Public Health* **2022**, *19*, 10706. [CrossRef]
54. Koutsimani, P.; Montgomery, A.; Georganta, K. The relationship between burnout, depression, and anxiety: A systematic review and meta-analysis. *Front. Psychol.* **2019**, *10*, 284. [CrossRef]
55. Sánchez-Narváez, F.; Velasco-Orozco, J.J.; Pérez-Archundia, E. Burnout syndrome and sleep quality in basic education teachers in Mexico. *Int. J. Environ. Res. Public Health* **2023**, *20*, 6276. [CrossRef]
56. Yang, Z.; Wang, D.; Fan, Y.; Ma, Z.; Chen, X.; Zhang, Y.; Fan, F. Relationship between sleep disturbance and burnout among Chinese urban teachers: Moderating roles of resilience. *Sleep Med.* **2023**, *108*, 29–37. [CrossRef]

57. Madigan, D.J.; Kim, L.E.; Glandorf, H.L.; Kavanagh, O. Teacher burnout and physical health: A systematic review. *Int. J. Educ. Res.* **2023**, *119*, 102173. [CrossRef]
58. Li, S.; Li, Y.; Lv, H.; Jiang, R.; Zhao, P.; Zheng, X.; Wang, L.; Li, J.; Mao, F. The prevalence and correlates of burnout among Chinese preschool teachers. *BMC Public Health* **2020**, *20*, 160. [CrossRef]
59. Marsollier, R.; Exposito, C.D.; Varela, J.J.; Miranda, R.; Guzman, P.; Lopez-Orellana, C. Burnout syndrome prevalence among Latin American teachers during the pandemic. *Ment. Health Prev.* **2024**, *34*, 200346. [CrossRef]
60. Ozamiz-Etxebarria, N.; Legorburu Fernández, I.; Lipnicki, D.M.; Idoiaga Mondragon, N.; Santabárbara, J. Prevalence of burnout among teachers during the COVID-19 pandemic: A meta-analysis. *Int. J. Environ. Res. Public Health* **2023**, *20*, 4866. [CrossRef]
61. Iriarte, C.; Erro-Garcés, A. Stress in teaching professionals across Europe. *Int. J. Educ. Res.* **2020**, *103*, 101623. [CrossRef]
62. Maratos, F.A.; Montague, J.; Ashra, H.; Welford, M.; Wood, W.; Barnes, C.; Sheffield, D.; Gilbert, P. Evaluation of a compassionate mind training intervention with school teachers and support staff. *Mindfulness* **2019**, *10*, 2245–2258. [CrossRef]
63. Nurdin, R.; Murni, A.W. Psychosomatic aspect of the COVID-19 pandemic. *Bioscientia Med. J. Biomed. Transl. Res.* **2022**, *6*, 2582–2590. [CrossRef]
64. Baessler, J.; Schwarzer, R. Evaluación de la autoeficacia: Adaptación española de la Escala de Autoeficacia general [Measuring optimistic self-beliefs: A Spanish adaptation of the General Self-Efficacy Scale]. *Ansiedad Estrés* **1996**, *2*, 1–8.
65. Gil-Monte, P.R. La Batería UNIPSICO: Propiedades psicométricas de las escalas que evalúan los factores psicosociales de demanda [The UNIPSICO questionnaire: Psychometric properties of the scales measuring psychosocial resource factors]. *Arch. Prev. Riesgos Labor.* **2016**, *19*, 86–94. [CrossRef]
66. Gil-Monte, P.R.; Carlotto, M.S.; Gonçalves, S. Validation of the Brazilian version of the "Spanish Burnout Inventory" in teachers. *Ver. Saude Publica* **2010**, *44*, 140–147. [CrossRef]
67. Gil-Monte, P.R.; Espejo, B.; Checa, I.; Gil-LaOrden, P.; Angeline, J.K.; Carlotto, M.S.; Converso, D.; Deroncele-Acosta, A.; Figueiredo-Ferraz, H.; Galarza, L.; et al. Factor structure and measurement invariance of the Spanish Burnout Inventory among professionals across 17 countries and regions. *Appl. Res. Qual. Life* **2023**, *18*, 869–892. [CrossRef]
68. World Medical Association. Declaration of Helsinki: Ethical principles for medical research involving human subjects. *JAMA* **2013**, *310*, 2191–2194. [CrossRef]
69. Kline, R.B. *Principles and Practice of Structural Equation Modeling*, 4th ed.; Guilford Publications: New York, NY, USA, 2016.
70. Hooper, D.; Coughlan, J.; Mullen, M.R. Structural equation modelling: Guidelines for determining model fit. *Electron. J. Bus. Res. Methods* **2008**, *6*, 53–60.
71. Kaplan, D. *Structural Equation Modeling: Foundations and Extensions*; Sage: Thousand Oaks, CA, USA, 2000.
72. Hu, L.-t.; Bentler, P.M. Cutoff criteria for fit indexes in covariance structure analysis: Conventional criteria versus new alternatives. *Struct. Equ. Model.* **1999**, *6*, 1–55. [CrossRef]
73. Lai, K. Fit difference between nonnested models given categorical data: Measures and estimation. *Struct. Equ. Model.* **2021**, *28*, 99–120. [CrossRef]
74. Hu, L.-t.; Bentler, P.M. Fit indices in covariance structure modeling: Sensitivity to underparameterized model misspecification. *Psychol. Methods* **1998**, *3*, 424–453. [CrossRef]
75. Browne, M.W.; Cudeck, R. Alternative ways of assessing model fit. In *Testing Structural Equation Models*; Bollen, K.A., Long, J.S., Eds.; Sage: Newbury Park, CA, USA, 1993; pp. 136–162.
76. Byrne, B.M. *Structural Equation Modeling with LISREL, PRELIS and SIMPLIS: Basic Concepts, Applications and Programming*; Lawrence Erlbaum Associates: Mahwah, NJ, USA, 1998.
77. Preacher, K.J.; Hayes, A.F. Asymptotic and resampling strategies for assessing and comparing indirect effects in multiple mediator models. *Behav. Res. Methods* **2008**, *40*, 879–891. [CrossRef]
78. Figueiredo-Ferraz, H.; Gil-Monte, P.R.; Grau-Alberola, E.; Ribeiro do Couto, B. The mediator role of feelings of guilt in the process of burnout and psychosomatic disorders: A cross-cultural study. *Front. Psychol.* **2021**, *12*, 751211. [CrossRef]
79. Łopatkiewicz, A.; Kwaśnicka, A.; Nowicki, P.; Furmańczyk, K.; Zieliński, W.; Woynarowska, M.; Krzych-Fałta, E. Occupational burnout and mental health. A study of psychiatric nurses from six European countries. *Adv. Cogn. Psychol.* **2023**, *19*, 80–91. [CrossRef]
80. Olivares-Faúndez, V.E.; Gil-Monte, P.R.; Figueiredo-Ferraz, H. The mediating role of feelings of guilt in the relationship between burnout and the consumption of tobacco and alcohol. *Jpn. Psychol. Res.* **2014**, *56*, 340–348. [CrossRef]
81. Podsakoff, P.M.; MacKenzie, S.B.; Lee, J.-Y.; Podsakoff, N.P. Common method biases in behavioral research: A critical review of the literature and recommended remedies. *J. Appl. Psychol.* **2003**, *88*, 879–903. [CrossRef]
82. Ekstedt, M.; Fagerberg, I. Lived experiences of the time preceding burnout. *J. Adv. Nurs.* **2005**, *49*, 59–67. [CrossRef]
83. Farber, B.A.; Miller, J. Teacher burnout: A psycho educational perspective. *Teach. Coll. Rec.* **1981**, *83*, 235–243. [CrossRef]
84. Maslach, C. *Burnout: The Cost of Caring*; Prentice Hall Press: New York, NY, USA, 1982.
85. Price, D.M.; Murphy, P.A. Staff burnout in the perspective of grief theory. *Death Educ.* **1984**, *8*, 47–58. [CrossRef]
86. Schoeps, K.; Tamarit, A.; de la Barrera, U.; González, R. Effects of emotional skills training to prevent burnout syndrome in schoolteachers. *Ansiedad Estrés* **2019**, *25*, 7–13. [CrossRef]
87. LaTronica-Herb, A.; Noel, T.K. Identity, agency, parenthood, and balance: Examining influential factors on former practitioners' decisions to leave P12 education. *Int. J. Educ. Res. Open* **2022**, *3*, 100172. [CrossRef]

88. Frögéli, E.; Eriksson, L.B. Obstacles experienced by socialization agents as they support new professionals' learning and adjustment: A systematic review of qualitative evidence. *Eur. J. Work Organ. Psychol.* 2023, *advance online publication*. [CrossRef]
89. Dar, N.; Usman, M.; Cheng, J.; Ghani, U. Social undermining at the workplace: How religious faith encourages employees who are aware of their social undermining behaviors to express more guilt and perform better. *J. Bus. Ethics* **2023**, *187*, 371–383. [CrossRef]

behavioral sciences

MDPI

Article

A Qualitative Exploration of the Process and Experience of Change in Moving on in My Recovery: An Acceptance and Commitment Therapy Based Recovery Group for Substance Use Disorder

Emma L. Shepley [1,2,*], Mike C. Jackson [1] and Lee M. Hogan [1,3,*]

[1] North Wales Clinical Psychology Programme, Bangor University, Bangor LL57 2DG, UK; mike.jackson@bangor.ac.uk
[2] Early Intervention in Psychosis, Betsi Cadwaladr University Health Board, Bangor LL57 2PW, UK
[3] Substance Misuse Services, Betsi Cadwaladr University Health Board, Rhyl LL18 3EY, UK
* Correspondence: emma.l.shepley@gmail.com (E.L.S.); lee.hogan@bangor.ac.uk (L.M.H.)

Abstract: Moving on in my recovery (MOIMR) is a new, acceptance and commitment therapy (ACT) based group intervention to support recovery from substance use disorder. It was co-developed by, and is co-facilitated with, people in recovery. This study used a grounded theory model to understand the process of change experienced by individuals who completed the group programme. Ten individuals who were abstinent from substances following their participation in MOIMR were interviewed. The model that emerged depicted a chronological series of processes that centred around a core category of gains derived from approaching their emotional vulnerability by leaning in to discomfort (e.g., difficult internal experiences like thoughts, emotions, and physical sensations) whilst pursuing activities that aligned to what mattered to them. Initial key processes indicated that participants experienced a degree of suffering from substance use prior to engagement. Group safety was a key element in fostering connection, normalisation, and cohesion, combined with psychological understanding being significantly derived from those with a lived experience of substance misuse and addiction. Later processes reflecting core ACT mechanisms such as letting go, value-guided action, and acceptance of difficult internal experiences took time to develop; many participants reported completing MOIMR more than once as a means of understanding these components. Limitations, along with implications for clinical practice and future research are discussed.

Keywords: substance use disorder; acceptance and commitment therapy; group therapy; recovery; behavioural change; qualitative; grounded theory

1. Introduction

Substance use disorder (SUD) is characterized as the habitual, compulsive, and continued use of alcohol and/or drugs despite problematic cognitive, behavioural, and/or physiological consequences [1]. SUD is a serious widespread concern; government statistics suggested that close to 300,000 people were in contact with substance misuse services in the UK between 2021 and 2022, a figure which had increased by over 13,000 from the previous year [2]. Common sequelae of SUD include significant distress, impaired functioning, financial crisis, and unemployment [3]. Importantly, SUD is a leading contributor of global disease [4]. The Office for National Statistics [5] showed that SUD-related deaths accounted for 10% of all preventable deaths in the UK in 2018. This was the fourth highest cause of preventable deaths after cancer (35%), diseases of the circulatory system (27%), and the respiratory system (14%).

1.1. Psychological Intervention in SUD

SUDs are often chronic in nature and frequently associated with comorbid mental health problems [6]. There is a long history of psychological intervention within SUD, with approaches drawn from a variety of traditions [7] such as contingency management, cognitive behavioural therapy, and motivational interviewing [8]. Reviews of these approaches have suggested that abstinence rates tend to be low and short-lived, with substantial dropout rates [9,10], although contingency management has shown superior outcomes [11]. Furthermore, there is a lack of empirical evidence for approaches that effectively address the comorbidity between SUD and mental health problems [12].

Group-based mutual aid interventions are recommended for promoting recovery from SUD [13]. What exactly constitutes recovery from SUD is hotly debated and agreement on a precise definition is not clear [14]. However, it is generally agreed that it is not sufficient for recovery to be achieved solely by abstinence and it requires improvements across a broad range of biopsychosocial domains [15]. International examples of recovery groups include the Twelve-Step Fellowships: Alcoholics Anonymous and Narcotic Anonymous [16] and SMART recovery [17]. Evidence has suggested that 12-step and non-12-step group outcomes are equivalent, whilst relapse following treatment remains high [18]. The UK government has recommended a wider choice of effective mutual aid groups for the treatment of SUD [19].

1.2. Contextual Behavioural Therapy in SUD

With the above points in mind, it is timely to investigate new group-based psychological interventions for SUD. Over the last decade, increasing attention has been given to the application of third-wave and contextual behaviour therapies in the treatment of SUD. These approaches focus on the use of mindfulness and acceptance strategies to reduce the likelihood that internal experiences (such as thoughts and emotions) will lead to substance use [20]. The main difference between contextual behavioural therapies and traditional cognitive behavioural therapies is the emphasis on the context and function of internal experiences, rather than on the content of them [21]. Contextual behaviour therapies, including acceptance and commitment therapy (ACT), have gathered interest over recent years as approaches for effectively addressing comorbidity between SUD and mental health problems; see [22].

ACT has been reviewed in multiple randomised controlled trials, and a recent review of meta-analytic evidence has found it to be an efficacious approach across a broad range of target conditions and has supported the transdiagnostic underpinnings of the approach [23]. Within the ACT framework, substance use is seen as a form of 'experiential avoidance' [24], whereby individuals use substances to avoid unwanted thoughts, feelings, and physiological experiences. ACT focusses on approaching these internal experiences with awareness and acceptance, rather than avoidance. Emphasis is also placed upon identifying personal values and supporting individuals to build a meaningful life aligned with these values [25]. The evidence base for the use of ACT in the treatment of SUD is growing: a meta-analysis by Gloster et al. [23] reported a significant small to medium effect favouring ACT over other treatments. Additionally, a systematic review by Byrne et al. [8] and a more recent systematic review and meta-analysis by Krotter et al. [26] found that ACT is useful in treating comorbid SUD and mental health problems.

1.3. Moving on in My Recovery

Coproduction has been found to be a vital component of psychological interventions within SUD [27]. Combining coproduction with evidence-based approaches, moving on in my recovery (MOIMR) [28] is a new group-based intervention for SUD. MOIMR draws on ACT to address SUD and mental health problems to support a transition out of substance misuse services. MOIMR was developed following consultation with people with lived experience of recovery and professionals working in the area to identify what was most helpful in the recovery process. It aims to bridge the gap between formal treatment provision and mutual aid. Sessions are co-facilitated by professionals and graduates of the programme. The programme is aimed at individuals who have achieved abstinence and are considering a transition out of treatment services.

MOIMR consists of twelve weekly, two-hour sessions. Topics considered include supporting wellbeing, dealing with anxiety and low mood, building/rebuilding relationships, planning for relapse, working with loss, self-identity, and stigma, all of which are delivered from an ACT-based perspective. Each session begins with a 'check-in', where group members discuss how they have applied MOIMR skills throughout the past week, and ends with a 'check-out' where group members agree on how they will apply learning throughout the next week by setting a challenge. The check-in and check-out also give group members the opportunity to share experiences and to offer support to others. The challenges that are set each week encourage commitment and action towards values. An initial pilot study demonstrated promising results including improved social functioning, reduced low mood and anxiety, and decreased experiential avoidance; improvements that were maintained at a three-month follow-up [28]. Plans are underway for a larger randomised control trial.

Research of psychological interventions in SUD (including ACT-based interventions) has largely focussed on quantitative measures [12,29]. However, it is recognized that this type of research does not uncover the deeper dimensions involved in the process of recovery and fails to explore mechanisms for change [14]. It has been proposed that future research should place a larger focus on understanding the change processes involved within recovery [30]. Thus, when evaluating therapeutic approaches it is important to investigate not only if an approach works, but also how it works for individuals.

A literature review found only one published study employing qualitative methodology to explore the application of ACT within an SUD population [12]. No studies were found which pertained to the processes of change during an ACT-based intervention for SUD. Grounded theory methodology [31] was selected for the present study due to the emphasis this approach places upon developing a model grounded in the experiences of participants. Grounded theory is appropriate when little is known about a phenomenon, and facilitates uncovering of the processes inherent to the area of inquiry [32], such as the process of change through engagement with a recovery group. Grounded theory has been applied to understanding the processes involved in therapeutic groups including mindfulness-based approaches for chronic pain [33] and distressing voice hearing [34]. The aim of the present study was to use grounded theory to develop a model of the change processes that occurred through engagement in MOIMR, derived from the experiences of participants who had made steps towards recovery.

2. Method

2.1. Design

Grounded theory methodology, following the procedures outlined by Strauss and Corbin [31], was used to generate and analyse data.

2.2. Participants

Participants were recruited via NHS substance misuse service staff within Betsi Cadwaladr University Health Board in Wales, UK. These staff members provided information about the study to all of those who met the recruitment inclusion criteria.

2.2.1. Inclusion and Exclusion Criteria

Participants met the inclusion criteria if they had completed MOIMR within the past 12 months and had attended a minimum of 9 out of the 12 group sessions. In order to take part, participants must have been in recovery and abstinent from substances for a minimum of three months after completing MOIMR.

2.2.2. Participant Characteristics

Ten participants took part in the research and none of these participants dropped out of the study. Within the pragmatic constraints of the project and sample, recruitment ceased at ten participants as by this point there were no further significant developments to the emerging theory. The sample comprised two female participants and eight male participants. All participants were originally from Britain and of white, Caucasian ethnicity. The mean age was 52.9 years ($SD = 7.0$), with ages ranging from 36 to 64 years. Participants were previously addicted to alcohol (n = 4), heroin (n = 2), crack cocaine (n = 1), amphetamines (n = 1) or multiple substances (n = 2). All participants reported long histories of addiction ranging from 15 to 35 years. The length of time in recovery at the point of interview ranged from 6 months to 2 years.

2.2.3. Ethical Considerations

Prior to agreeing to take part, all participants were provided with an information leaflet with details about the research. This leaflet clearly outlined how the data they provided would be confidentially treated. Informed consent was obtained from all participants. Participants were informed that participation was voluntary and they were free to withdraw at any point without their treatment within substance misuse services being impacted; no participants chose to withdraw. The capacity to give consent was assessed by asking participants to talk through their understanding of the benefits and potential risks of taking part in the research. The first author, who completed the interviews and analysis, was not involved in any aspect of the participants' care within substance misuse services.

2.3. Procedure

NHS substance misuse staff approached potential participants for the study and offered them an Information Sheet. Interested participants were asked to complete and return a form to state they were interested in taking part and were willing to be contacted by the researcher. The first author contacted participants over the telephone, answered questions about the research, and arranged to carry out face-to-face interviews.

A semi-structured interview schedule was used to gather data (see Supplementary Materials, S1: Interview Schedule). The schedule was drawn up by the research group; as the aims of the study were to examine change processes and turning points, the questions centred on these topics. Feedback was sought regarding the appropriateness of the questions from a MOIMR graduate and group facilitator prior to the commencement of the study. In line with grounded theory methodology, the interview schedule evolved throughout the data collection process. General topics included life before MOIMR, the experience of the group process, what learning was acquired from MOIMR, and what aspects were helpful and unhelpful. The interviews were conducted in a participant-centred manner, with open questions and follow-up questions and prompts where appropriate.

Ten interviews were conducted over four months between November 2019 and February 2020. All interviews took place within a clinical setting. Each interview was recorded using an encrypted dictaphone and transcribed by the first author with identifying information removed. The interviews were carried out in three stages. During the first stage, open questions were asked to allow initial ideas to emerge; examples included "How has MOIMR played a role in the recent changes you have made in your life?" and "Could I ask you to describe the most important things you learnt through MOIMR?". In keeping with theoretical sampling, ref. [31] the interview schedule was revised after each interview and evolved throughout the data collection process as categories and subcategories began to become clear; thus, during the second stage, questions were more focussed around the emerging categories (e.g., "Which skills or tools did you find most helpful?", which was focussed around the emerging category of 'action' and "Can you tell me about something difficult that has happened in your life recently, and how you applied MOIMR principles to cope with it?", which was focussed around the emerging subcategory of 'understanding the impact of maladaptive strategies'). The final stage was used to confirm hypotheses and strengthen the validity of the model. Participants were asked questions such as, "Were there some elements of MOIMR learning that longer took to understand and apply than others?"

The first author maintained a warm, engaged, and open approach when conducting the interviews. Only the author and the participant were present during all interviews. Plenty of time was given for participants to formulate their responses to questions and the author checked in with each participant at the end as to whether they felt the interview had been a true reflection of their experiences and if they had anything more to add. All participants were keen to share their stories and gave significant detail about their experiences. Therefore, the author did not feel it necessary to go back to participants for further clarification.

2.4. Data Analysis

All analysis was carried out by hand by the first author (see Supplementary Materials, S2: Worked example of analysis and model development process). In keeping with the grounded theory method, analysis was carried out throughout the study and was used to shape the data collection process. Open coding, using line-by-line analysis, was used initially to generate concepts. These concepts were transferred to cards, which were sorted and grouped into higher-order categories as the analysis took shape. Properties and dimensions of the categories were identified, and axial coding was used to clarify relationships between the categories. As the core category emerged, selective coding was employed, which involved revisiting the categories and delineating their relation to the core category. Constant comparison and memoing were used throughout to ask whether a concept had been seen before to note ideas and reflections and to use diagrams to support the development of the model.

2.4.1. Quality Assurance Methods

The first author made use of theoretical memoing to note preconceptions about the data and any emotional reactions to the data generated, with the intention of maintaining awareness of her perspective. Additionally, a coded transcript was audited by the second and third authors to ensure credibility within the coding and category generation.

2.4.2. Author Reflexive Statement

The author is a white, female trainee clinical psychologist with no personal experience of SUD or substance misuse services. Additionally, she had no professional experience in delivering groups to support recovery from SUD. That said, the author had professional experience in using ACT to support individuals presenting with various mental health problems. She holds the belief that ACT is an effective and helpful therapeutic approach.

The author was led by the data during the analysis. However, her lack of personal and professional experience with SUD could potentially have limited her ability to fully identify concepts related to this. In order to account for this, the third author, who is a clinical psychologist with extensive experience working with individuals with SUD, oversaw the analysis process. It is also worth noting that the third author was responsible for the development of MOIMR. Therefore, it is acknowledged that the emerging categories may have been influenced by the author's professional experience of and belief in the benefits of ACT and the third author's vested interest in MOIMR as an effective intervention. Efforts were made to account for this by intentionally searching for negative incidences, sorting codes according to those that were and were not in line with ACT, and actively encouraging participants to discuss any unhelpful aspects of MOIMR. The first author's independence from MOIMR made it easier for participants to discuss negative perspectives. Additionally, the second author was not involved with MOIMR and had less experience of using ACT. Therefore, the second author supported the first and third authors to recognise and look for biases during the analysis process.

3. Results

3.1. Interviews

The average length of interviews was M = 48 min (*SD* = 15.0), with interviews lasting between 20 and 80 min. The mean amount of data collected from the interviews was 7092 words (*SD* = 1883.5), with interview transcripts ranging from 3142 to 10,676 words.

3.2. Overview of the Model

Figure 1 is a model of the process of change made throughout MOIMR. Categories and subcategories are represented in Table 1 and highlighted in the text in bold. The model depicts the change processes that occurred through participants' engagement with MOIMR, grounded in the descriptions of participants' experiences. The model begins prior to MOIMR with an experience of suffering as a result of substance use, timing factors, and reaching a turning point of deciding to make changes. Positive preconceptions supported initial engagement with MOIMR. The first stages of the group experienced by participants were feeling safe in the group setting and then beginning to understand substance use from a psychological perspective, which were necessary for further changes to be made. Investment into MOIMR and recovery followed. A focus of MOIMR was to identify what is important in life (values) and support participants to take behavioural action that was consistent with this. Positive outcomes followed these stages, which had a bi-directional relationship with the processes, strengthening their continuation. Time was taken to reach the final stages of acceptance of emotions and making space for difficulty, which often involved completing MOIMR more than once.

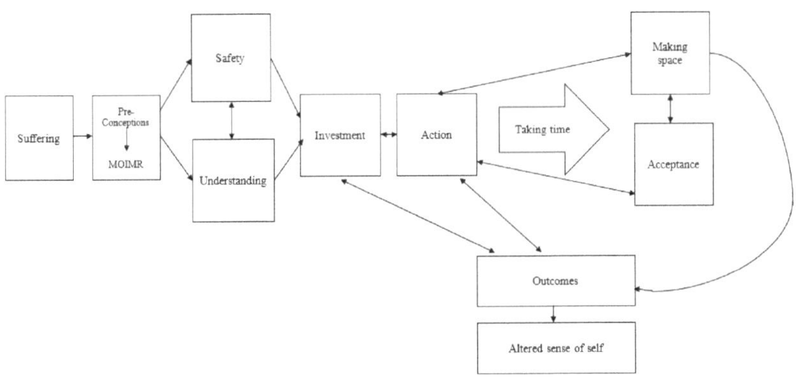

Figure 1. Model of the process of change through MOIMR.

Table 1. Categories and Subcategories.

Categories	Subcategories
A. Suffering	Detrimental impacts of addictive behaviours Feeling stuck Seeking help Timing factors Pre-conceptions
B. Safety	Scary at first "We were all in the same boat" Connection Shared journey Facilitation style

Table 1. *Cont.*

Categories	Subcategories
C. Understanding	Resonant "Puts in layman's terms" Balanced structure
D. Investment	Motivation Hearing the stories of others Seeing the benefits Snowballing effect Making changes in other areas
E. Action	Meaning Focus point Value-guided action Placing priority in recovery
F. Taking time	Completing MOIMR more than once
G. Making space for difficulty and discomfort	Understanding of maladaptive coping strategies "Leaning In" Making space for emotions Getting in touch with loss Mindfulness
H. Acceptance	"Letting Go" Gaining distance from thoughts
I. Outcomes	Integration De-stigmatised Achievement Confidence Improvements in relationships Enrichment Altruism
J. Altered sense of self	Opening to the possibility of a different life Reduced self-stigma New self

3.3. Core Category

The core category that emerged from the analysis and could be seen to some degree within all other categories, were the gains of engaging in MOIMR and recovery consistent behaviours. Given the group nature of MOIMR, these gains involved a strong social component.

For all participants, there was a great degree of suffering which had resulted from substance use prior to engaging with MOIMR. Thus, the reinforcement that was gained from engaging with recovery-consistent behaviours through MOIMR in terms of social connection and improvements in daily life was sufficient to support participants to overcome barriers including fear of being in a group setting, motivation, and the difficulty of getting in touch with some painful experiences. Engaging in recovery-consistent behaviours began to hold an increasingly greater degree of reward than engaging in substance use.

3.4. Category A: Suffering

This category represents the large degree of suffering that participants experienced prior to engaging with substance misuse services and prior to MOIMR. Participants explained that there had been several **detrimental impacts** resulting from their substance use, including within their families, relationships, and work, for example:

> P4: *"I wasn't seeing my daughter I was drinking more and more and more and then I lost me job as well… and it went downhill from there really…"*

Participants described **feeling stuck**, with a lack of meaning and a general dissatisfaction with life. This resulted in **seeking help** from substance misuse services; however, many participants described that they had been with these services for many years and had not made any significant changes in their substance use. Various **timing factors** were described by participants prior to MOIMR; physical and/or mental health problems were often mentioned. For example:

P5: *"I felt so low and got to such a low place... I was both physically and mentally drained... literally drained... and you know I felt there was only one way I could only go up here cos you know that was really how bad it was"*

Due to the culmination of these factors, all participants had a **turning point** story, which contained decisions made to take steps towards recovery. For all participants, this occurred prior to MOIMR:

P7: *"it was my time you know to turn it around... I just couldn't carry on like that... I'd had enough you know; it wasn't just the drugs it was all the crap that went with it. I couldn't do it anymore; mentally I felt like I was gonna have a nervous breakdown... I was on the edge"*

Many participants described **positive pre-conceptions** of MOIMR which they had developed through hearing of the benefits others had experienced. Others described positive experiences of other ACT-based recovery groups they had taken part in prior to MOIMR. These had led participants to want to take part in MOIMR.

P4: *"I'd seen the changes that some of the other lads made, and I thought yeah alright I'll give it a try"*

3.5. Category B: Safety

This category represents the first process that occurred when participants began MOIMR. Participants described that entering a social setting, after what had often been an extended period of isolation due to substance use, was **scary at first.**

P6: *"yeah anxiety ridden... I was really bad. I didn't live in the toilet but I spent a tiny bit longer than I should have done there... I'd been out of the world for so long and then coming back it was a real shock"*

This was alleviated through the creation of a non-judgemental environment; participants described the feeling that **"We were all in the same boat".** This process was enabled via warmth, genuineness, and openness on the part of the group facilitators. Group members began to feel safe to share experiences, of which they may have felt highly ashamed and kept hidden for many years. Hearing that others in the group had had similar experiences was de-stigmatising and normalising:

P3: *"it was good... open friendly people and it was very warm and welcoming... it was nice because people have been in your situation you know and you can tell that about the group... whereas you get a lot of judgemental people you know stigma and that... there's no feeling of that, no stigma or anything; it's just normal people who've had a bad time"*

P8: *"you speak about things and you think 'I was the only one who's been there', sort of thing and it sort of opens doors and you think 'Christ we're all in the same boat here'... it is good to hear I'm not the only one... I'm not a freak"*

Participants described a strong **connection** with other group members; many participants formed strong bonds and friendships. These positive relationships were important as participants often described having to separate themselves from existing friends and relationships which may have perpetuated substance use:

P8: *"at the start of the programme I was quite nervous thinking 'oh do I want to talk about that', 'should I mention this?' but eventually I'd open up... and being able to open up and offload that in front of people who understood that helped in a big way"*

P1: "*I made two very good friends out of it you know and that's been missing... that's been missing in my life... I hadn't made new friends for 20 years while I was on the drink*"

The connection evolved into a sense of a **shared journey towards recovery**:

P6: "*I think there's this thing with being in a group... even if it's not spoken it's an incentive purpose*"

The group employed a flattened hierarchy approach where the **facilitation style** involved a degree of self-disclosure and participation in weekly challenges etc. This contributed to the overall feeling of safety.

P5: "*there was no us and them... we were all in it together, helping each other out*"

3.6. Category C: Understanding

Participants described beginning to develop an understanding of their substance use; all explained that the content of the programme was extremely **resonant** with their own experiences:

P8: "*it was almost as though I wrote the bleeding thing... thinking oh he's [facilitator] got it all on paper what I've got in here [points to own head]*"

The material was described as accessible, using everyday language to explain ACT ideas and psychoeducation. Participants explained that having this understanding meant they felt able to begin to take steps to change their addictive behaviours:

P7: "*it* ***puts in layman's terms*** *what's going on mentally you know*"

P7: "*to understand what was going on and take it instead of getting all these emotions and not knowing, like I had done before... to be able to break it down and understand and how to deal with cravings as well...*"

Participants reported they appreciated the **balanced structure** which allowed opportunity for openness and sharing as well as covering structured topics each week. For example:

P3: "*there's like a topic in them [group sessions] and stuff; it was like keeping my mind awake and focussed... I've been to other groups and that's more like people just go there to have a chat really*"

3.7. Category D: Investment

Some participants described an initial lack of **motivation** to attend the group and a lack of or only partial investment in recovery. A sense of scepticism around the benefits of MOIMR was described, along with a reluctance to engage in group discussions and complete tasks set within the group:

P6: "*'should I go home?', 'should I not?' ...you know I just didn't really wanna engage*"

Participants described that motivation began to build through **hearing the stories of others** who had recovered through the group and through the peer facilitators.

P2: "*seeing the positivity of those people who'd done it, I'd say in my case, that gave me the will to do it*"

Participants described beginning to tentatively try things out and beginning to **see the benefits:**

P4: "*I sort of did start applying things and you know like more motivation came and I was, like, doing things more*"

Motivation continued to grow throughout the group, comparable to a **snowballing effect**:

P1: "*[we] set a challenge each week... for the first few weeks I never did one... but by the end of it I was doing every one*"

Participants described that they began to develop motivation to make **changes in other areas of their lives**, outside of their recovery:

> P7: "*it starts definitely with MOIMR like coming here volunteering...it led to all of this for me you know... I think if it weren't for that I'd probably have started using again*"

3.8. Category E: Action

This category refers to participants taking action to implement changes in their lives through changes in their behaviour. Participants described a lack of **meaning** prior to MOIMR:

> P1: "*empty I suppose is the word that strikes to mind... there was just nothing in my life no structure*"

Weekly attendance at MOIMR provided a **focus point** in the lives of participants. Engaging with the weekly challenges was described as giving participants a way of spending their time which felt productive, and supported participants to begin to implement structure into their lives.

> P2: "*it made me realise I had other things I wanted to do... I'd been through a phase of purposeless like I've got nothing to do, well there's no point doing that...*"

> P6: "*It's good cos in the chaos of the addiction I just lurched from one situation to another and everything was so up in the air*"

The idea of **considering one's values and using these to guide action** was emphasised in MOIMR with the metaphor of "anchor points"; for most participants, this meant using activities which were related to their values to guide them when difficulty arose. This gave participants a way of considering alternatives to their substance use which connected them with what was important to them.

> P1: "*If I start feeling down with the depression I don't think now 'right I'm gonna go and get a drink'... what I do now is use me anchor points which is music, fishing, decorating... I've got quite a few anchor points... reading books... the things I never, ever did before I went to the group*"

Participants described a process of placing **priority in recovery** and building a substance-free life. This was a difficult process; for many participants, it meant ending relationships and friendships that perpetuated addictive behaviours.

> P7: "*my partner did still use so I just always got dragged back in to it... so I had to get rid of him to stop, so that was a big thing you know... cos we were together 20 years*"

3.9. Category F: Taking Time

Several participants had **completed MOIMR more than once** and emphasised that without this they would have struggled to make considerable changes:

> P6: "*if anything, I'd say it doesn't all sink it at once... it took me doing it twice to really absorb it*"

Those who had only completed the group once discussed wanting to do it again, suggested they felt the group should be longer or that there should be a follow-on group. Some participants explained that some of the processes (see Categories H & I) took a long time to grasp and explained that without completing the group more than once they would have struggled to apply them.

3.10. Category G: Moving from a Place of Avoidance to Making Space for Difficulty and Discomfort

Participants described a long history of substance use as a means of avoiding uncomfortable emotions and a lifestyle which involved avoidance of numerous situations:

> P1: "*I just hid behind the bottle*"

MOIMR supported participants to **understand the consequences of maladaptive coping styles** (typically using substances to manage uncomfortable thoughts or emotions):

> P7: *"I'd of just wanted a hit I wouldn't have even... even just simple things like paying bills... learning if there's a problem dealing with it straight away cos if you bury your head in the sand they just get worse"*

The term **"lean in"** is used within MOIMR which refers to moving towards, rather than avoiding difficulties that arise. This was typically used to refer to internal experiences including thoughts and memories, and situations that arose in life. Although all participants described some aspect of this, this idea was more apparent in the descriptions of participants who had completed MOIMR more than once. For example, this quote is from a participant who had completed MOIMR three times:

> P4: *"you sort of turn to that fear and just like do it... it's been really hard but now I see the benefits are brilliant"*

Participants were able to describe how they had applied this to their day-to-day lives, for example, one participant described a recent experience of losing a loved one:

> P8: *"I think the whole family was expecting me to crash you know, to go back down the bad line but what I did instead of that I sort of threw myself in to everything. I organised the burial, the funeral, everything... I knew through the programme like dwelling on things and just thinking 'well one bag will switch it off for today', it's not gonna stop it's gonna carry on; I knew that"*

Participants also described learning to **make space for emotions**, both pleasant and unpleasant, and the idea of a valued life being one that involves the experience of some unpleasant emotions. This was also apparent to a greater degree within the descriptions of participants who had completed MOIMR more than once.

> P9: *"I'm gonna get peaks and troughs as you do that's life not an excuse to use... that's how it was before you know"*

Participants described beginning to acknowledge thoughts rather than pushing them away:

> P10: *"I think I'd learned to lock them away [thoughts] and, yeah, by doing that they're just gonna keep coming back and you'll have to deal with it"*

MOIMR supported participants to **get in touch with losses**. Loss was very evident in the lives of participants, for whom their addictive behaviours may have been a means of blocking out the pain associated with loss. Loss was also a common consequence of substance use. For others, loss was relevant to the drugs themselves. All participants explained that through MOIMR they got in touch with their losses, and all explained that this was the most difficult part of the group and their overall experience of recovery.

> P7: *"facing that loss without drugs, learning that cos you're sedated for so long all your emotions are sedated as well... so facing that, having to think about that instead of just pushing it to the back of my mind... that was the hardest thing"*

Mindfulness strategies were described by some participants as a means of allowing space for and coping with the intensity of emotions:

> P7: *"If I have a craving, it's ok don't panic...I breathe do my mindfulness... it helped me not to react to my emotions mindfulness did"*

Although mindfulness concepts are relevant to many of the processes (e.g., the mindfulness concept of observing thoughts), using mindfulness as an explicit strategy was not discussed at all by some participants, suggesting that it was not something that everyone took on board.

3.11. Category H: Acceptance

This category reflects another process which was more apparent within the descriptions of participants who had completed MOIMR more than once. The idea of **"letting go"** is emphasised within MOIMR. For all participants, this referred to trying to let go of regrets about their past behaviour and their past selves, such as years spent with little focus in life other than seeking substances, or the impact of substance use on relationships. Some participants described fully applying this idea, whereas some were clear that there were some things they did not feel they could let go of.

> P8: *"I've carried a rucksack full of problems my whole life... I try to let it go now, what's done is done"*

> P10: *"I've let go of feelings about my addiction... there's still a few things that I have a lot of problems about letting go, mainly with family"*

These contrasting responses indicate for some, there was an element of remaining struggle with their past selves and past behaviour towards others.

Some participants described the process of learning to gain **distance from thoughts.** This involved the application of mindfulness principles and learning to take an *"observer"* perspective on one's thoughts in relation to addiction. For example:

> P7: *"before I was like no, no, no don't, don't, don't... and you're mentally at war with yourself... but understanding, ok, I'm just craving... accepting that I'm craving and then saying 'no thank you... I'm not doing it today'"*

This captures the process of moving from a place of being "at war" with one's mind to being "at peace".

3.12. Category I: Outcomes

Integration of MOIMR into the lives of participants was facilitated via the check-in process at the start of each group. Participants explained that hearing from others about how they had applied the group principles helped them to think about how they could apply it to their own lives:

> P2: *"I picked up on it so much more because other people had brought it up in their check in... so it's reiterating an important point of the course, so that checking in process is great"*

All participants described a gradual process of integrating learning from MOIMR, which led to positive outcomes. These positive outcomes supported participants to continue to apply MOIMR principles

Participants described feeling **de-stigmatised** and having an increased sense of self-worth

> P8: *"I don't feel as little anymore... as much of a waste of space... more of an equal, you know"*

A sense of **achievement** from the acknowledgement of their success in recovery by self and others was described:

> P7: *"it's little steps and every time I feel proud and a little rewarded"*

A number of participants found that by engaging with others in the group, by carrying out weekly challenges, and by moving towards difficulty gave an increased sense of **confidence:**

> P5: *"I've been very much more confident; I can take things in my stride without panicking, 'oh what am I going to do?' 'I must have a drink'"*

Through mentalising, being able to see others' perspectives, and without the strain that substance use placed on relationships, several participants spoke about **improvements in their relationships with others.**

Participants described an overall **enrichment** of their lives:

> P9: *"I've learnt to go and appreciate the outdoor walks and mountains... go swimming with my son. I enjoy things like that now they're not a chore I love doing them... I'm in touch with that side of me now"*

All participants spoke about wanting to **altruistically** use their own experience of recovery to help others. Most participants described wanting to stay involved with MOIMR groups as facilitators and many also described aspirations towards careers in recovery work:

> P3: *"That's what I'm perusing now... going into you know helping people... caring and stuff, maybe... becoming like a keyworker myself or helping people"*

This final subcategory reflected an investment in the identity as someone in recovery.

3.13. Category J: Altered Sense of Self

This category refers to the process of altered perspectives participants held about themselves and their lives, which was apparent as a later process in all participants' experiences of MOIMR and recovery in general.

Participants spoke about beginning to **open to the possibility of a different life** outside of one dominated by substance use:

> P1: *"It just made you realise that alcohol wasn't your life whereas before it was; I was always thinking 'right where's the next drink coming from?'... before the group I didn't like me, I didn't like the world... and now, I'm slowly but surely getting to like myself again"*

MOIMR addresses the ideas of both stigma and **self-stigma**. Participants described realising that a lot of the perceived stigma they felt was internally generated and that their assumptions of how they were viewed by others were not necessarily accurate:

> P7: *"you don't know what other people are thinking, you know, you're just presuming cos you're judging people by your own standards; so you just put yourself down mentally so you think everyone else is thinking the same, but they don't..."*

> P8: *"I've always had this fear that it's written all over me you know, druggie, and all this sort of thing but it wasn't so"*

Finally, a sense of **new self** was reflected in the way participants spoke about their past selves and their past addictive behaviour:

> P9: *"I've reinvented myself in a way... regrown... cos I never got chance, did I, 'cause I was always consumed by drugs"*

4. Discussion

This study is the first attempt to build a qualitative model of the process of change from an ACT-based therapy group to support recovery from SUD. The study's findings are considered in the context of the existing literature and established theory. Clinical implications, suggestions for future research, and the limitations of the study are also outlined.

Principally, MOIMR can be conceptualised as a group programme that is underpinned by an ACT-based model that increases participants' willingness to experience their emotional vulnerability. Unlike, traditional cognitive therapy, which seeks to modify the content of thoughts and beliefs [35], MOIMR encourages participants to move towards their difficult thoughts, emotions, and physical sensations, to make space for them, and to open up to these internal experiences without seeking to change them, using skills such as leaning in. It also encourages diffusion from internal experiences, such as thoughts and memories, using skills such as letting go. What is clear from the experiences of the group participants is that prior to attending MOIMR they had worked hard to avoid leaning in: in fact, they had used substances and employed other behaviours to move away from discomfort for many years and the consequences resulted in a high degree of suffering, self-blame, and shame.

Participants were able to identify two mechanisms and benefits of leaning in towards difficult experiences. First, in moving away (i.e., through excessive substance use) despite the short-term benefit of experiential avoidance, they experienced a high degree of suffering in the long term. The detrimental long-term impact of substance use had increased to the point where this form of experiential avoidance was no longer effective. This is consistent with reinforcement theories of addiction (for a recent review see Wise & Koob [36]) and with the ACT-based explanation of addiction [24]. Leaning in naturally reduced the negative consequences of damaging maladaptive coping strategies.

A second benefit of leaning in was that it enabled participants to connect to those things that really mattered to them (e.g., organising a funeral despite the discomfort of experiencing a loss). Of note, leaning in to emotional vulnerability is not an attempt to eradicate discomfort, as one moves towards those things that matter then feelings of discomfort increase rather than decrease (e.g., thoughts of failing and feelings of doubt can become more prominent). In choosing to lean in and in making space for discomfort, participants were able to derive reinforcement from many other areas of their lives (e.g., in helping others), which resulted in feelings of pride, reward, and confidence.

Participants learned the MOIMR skills through their own direct experience and vicariously by observing the change and positive outcomes shared by their peers. In fact, listening to the experiences of change from others in recovery (often those with more recovery time or from those who had completed the programme previously) was deemed highly beneficial. The importance of peer role models such as these has been recognised in the literature and identified in other qualitative accounts of recovery [37].

The safety within the group facilitated skill attainment, although many only felt ready to embark on the MOIMR style of recovery after experiencing the group for the second time. The practical steps delivered in *"layman's terms"*—of what was a new/novel concept—described by those with lived experience supported the process of change. There was a recognition that change occurred through the doing: it required investment and action; again, the experience of a shared journey, modelling by facilitators, and the commitment to challenges were crucial to the change process. A process of change from initial scepticism and ambivalence, followed by increased commitment, and then taking action towards change is consistent with the contemplation—preparation—action process depicted by Prochaska and DiClemente's Stages of Change Model [38].

The social support, connection, and identification that resulted from engaging with MOIMR was highly positively reinforcing, and thus supported the continuation of recovery-consistent behaviours and was sufficient to support participants to overcome barriers. Entering a group setting after often long periods of social isolation was an intimidating experience for participants. The non-judgemental and warm atmosphere of the group setting was essential in alleviating this initial discomfort. Participants began to feel safe to share experiences and described that hearing similar experiences from others in the group was extremely normalising and de-stigmatising. This supported an ongoing sense of connection and identification with the group and led to the development of a shared purpose within the group in terms of a movement towards recovery. Elements of this category are related to social support, which is a well-established component of successful recovery groups [39].

Participants' descriptions of a sense of belonging and shared purpose were consistent with the components of a psychological sense of community [40]. These findings were in line with previous qualitative studies, such as DeLucia, Bergman, Formoso, and Weinberg [41] who investigated the successful components of recovery groups from a 12-step perspective. The altered sense of self-described by participants (e.g., *"I've reinvented myself in a way"*) was a position that offered new insights and opportunities. The MOIMR facilitated insights that were transformative (see Miller & C'de Baca, [42]).

4.1. Clinical Recommendations

Together with the findings of the pilot study [28], the current study supports the benefits of MOIMR as an intervention to promote recovery from SUD. Participants suggested that the group should have a follow-on group.

The structure of MOIMR, particularly the check-in was especially helpful and appeared to be key to several of the categories, including group cohesion, increased the sense of safety, understanding, and application of group learning into daily life. Weekly challenges were also important to support the application of group learning and strengthen commitment. The coproduced element of MOIMR was reflected in participants' accounts. Consulting with those with experience of recovery from SUD in the development of MOIMR meant that the group closely resonated with the participants' own experiences. Additionally, hearing from peer facilitators who had graduated from MOIMR, and who had made considerable changes as a result, was extremely helpful. These points hold implications for the development and delivery of psychological group therapy in general, both within substance misuse services and across mental health services more widely.

4.2. Limitations and Suggestions for Future Research

An important limitation of the current study was the focus on participants who had benefited from MOIMR. Although this allowed a greater focus on change processes towards recovery, it limited the model's ability to account for those who did not achieve change. This focus was pragmatic given the time and resource constraints of the research. It is acknowledged that this meant only partial saturation was met and the constant comparison method could not be fully applied. It would be beneficial for future research to test the validity of and develop the current model by recruiting participants who did not benefit from, or who dropped out of MOIMR. It would be helpful to examine whether variation in the categories of the current model can account for both change and lack of change. Additionally, it would be helpful for future research to consider including substance misuse service staff with experience in delivering MOIMR to examine whether the model is consistent with their observations of change processes within service users. Further sampling in this way would allow the research to reach full saturation.

Input was sought from a graduate of MOIMR in the design of the study and development of the interview schedule. However, it may have been helpful to draw further on this input during the coding process, given the author's lack of personal experience of addiction. Lastly, the current study recruited a relatively small, entirely Caucasian and majority male sample of low to middle socioeconomic status. This is fairly representative of the population who typically access substance misuse services in North Wales, UK, where the majority of MOIMR groups are offered; however, this sample limits the explanatory power of the model. If MOIMR were to become available more widely, it would be beneficial to test the model within more diverse samples.

5. Conclusions

Overall, this study adds to our understanding of recovery from SUD and how ACT can support this process. Using grounded theory methodology, a model was developed to explain the process of change through an ACT-based recovery group. The model depicts the core processes involved in this change, which follow a chronological order, centred around a core category of approaching one's emotional vulnerability.

Supplementary Materials: The following supporting information can be downloaded at: https://www.mdpi.com/article/10.3390/bs14121237/s1, S1: Interview Schedule; S2: Worked example of analysis and model development process.

Author Contributions: Conceptualization, E.L.S., M.C.J. and L.M.H.; Formal analysis, E.L.S.; Investigation, E.L.S.; Methodology, E.L.S.; Resources, L.M.H.; Supervision, M.C.J. and L.M.H.; Visualization, L.M.H.; Writing—original draft, E.L.S.; Writing—review & editing, E.L.S., M.C.J. and L.M.H. All authors have read and agreed to the published version of the manuscript.

Funding: This research received no external funding.

Institutional Review Board Statement: This study was conducted in accordance with the Declaration of Helsinki. The study was approved by the University of Bangor on 4 July 2019 (reference: 2019-16553) and the NHS Wales Research Ethics Committee on 19 September 2019 (reference: 19/WA/0220).

Informed Consent Statement: Informed consent was obtained from all subjects involved in this study.

Data Availability Statement: The data presented in this study are available on request from the corresponding author due to participant privacy restrictions.

Conflicts of Interest: Author L.M.H. was responsible for the development of the recovery groups to which this research pertains.

References

1. American Psychiatric Association. *Diagnostic and Statistical Manual of Mental Disorders*, 5th ed.; American Psychiatric Publishing: Arlington, VA, USA, 2013.
2. Office of National Statistics (GOV.UK). Adult Substance Misuse Treatment Statistics 2021 to 2022: Report. 2023. Available online: https://www.gov.uk/government/statistics/substance-misuse-treatment-for-adults-statistics-2021-to-2022/adult-substance-misuse-treatment-statistics-2021-to-2022-report (accessed on 3 October 2024).
3. Franco, S.; Olfson, M.; Wall, M.M.; Wang, S.; Hoertel, N.; Blanco, C. Shared and specific associations of substance use disorders on adverse outcomes: A national prospective study. *Drug Alcohol Depend.* **2019**, *201*, 212–219. [CrossRef] [PubMed]
4. Degenhardt, L.; Charlson, F.J.; Ferrari, A.J.; Santomauro, A.; Erskine, H.; Mantilla-Herrara, A.; Whiteford, H.; Leung, J.; Naghavi, M.; Griswold, M.; et al. The global burden of disease attributable to attributable to drug and alcohol use in 195 countries and territories, 1990–2016: A systematic analysis for the Global Burden of Disease Study 2016. *Lancet* **2018**, *382*, 1564–1574. [CrossRef]
5. Office for National Statistics. Avoidable Mortality in the UK: 2018. 2020. Available online: https://www.ons.gov.uk/peoplepopulationandcommunity/healthandsocialcare/causesofdeath/bulletins/avoidablemortalityinenglandandwales/2018#avoidable-mortality-by-cause (accessed on 23 March 2020).
6. Kessler, R.C.; Chiu, W.T.; Demler, O.; Walters, E. Prevalence, Severity, and Comorbidity of 12-Month DSM-IV Disorders in the National Comorbidity Survey Replication. *Arch. Gen. Psychiatry* **2005**, *62*, 617–627. [CrossRef] [PubMed]
7. Byrne, S.P.; Haber, P.; Baillie, A.; Costa, D.S.J.; Fogliati, V.; Morley, K. Systematic reviews of mindfulness and acceptance and commitment therapy for alcohol use disorder: Should we be using Third Wave Therapies? *Alcohol Alcohol.* **2019**, *54*, 159–166. [CrossRef] [PubMed]
8. Volkow, N.D.; Blanco, C. Substance use disorders: A comprehensive update of classification, epidemiology, neurobiology, clinical aspects, treatment and prevention. *World Psychiatry* **2023**, *22*, 203–229. [CrossRef]
9. Prendergast, M.L.; Podus, D.; Chang, E.; Urada, D. The effectiveness of drug abuse treatment: A meta-analysis of comparison group studies. *Drug Alcohol Depend.* **2002**, *67*, 53–72. [CrossRef] [PubMed]
10. Lappan, S.N.; Brown, A.W.; Hendricks, P.S. Dropout rates of in-person psychosocial substance use disorder treatments: A systematic review and meta-analysis. *Addiction* **2020**, *115*, 201–217. [CrossRef]
11. Ginley, M.K.; Pfund, R.A.; Rash, C.J.; Zajac, K. Long-term efficacy of contingency management treatment based on objective indicators of abstinence from illicit substance use up to 1 year following treatment: A meta-analysis. *J. Consult. Clin. Psychol.* **2021**, *89*, 58–71. [CrossRef]
12. Johnson, L.; Elsegood, K.; Lennox, C. A qualitative evaluation of an ACT-based substance misuse treatment programme for service users within a secure mental health setting. *Adv. Dual Diagn.* **2019**, *12*, 117–131. [CrossRef]
13. Department of Health. *Alcohol-Use Disorders: Diagnosis Assessment and Management of Harmful Drinking and Alcohol Dependence CG115. NICE Clinical Guidelines*; Department of Health: London, UK, 2011.
14. Witkiewitz, K.; Pfund, R.A.; Tucker, J.A. Mechanisms of Behavior Change in Substance Use Disorder with and Without Formal Treatment. *Annu. Rev. Clin. Psychol.* **2022**, *18*, 497–525. [CrossRef] [PubMed]
15. Witkiewitz, K.; Montes, K.S.; Schwebel, F.J.; Tucker, J.A. What Is Recovery? *Alcohol Res. Curr. Rev.* **2020**, *40*, 1. [CrossRef] [PubMed] [PubMed Central]
16. Wilson, B. *Alcoholics Anonymous*; Alcoholics Anonymous World Services Inc.: New York, NY, USA, 1955.
17. Horvath, T.; Velten, E. SMART Recovery: Addition Recovery from a Cognitive-Behavioral Perspective. *J. Ration. Emot. Cogn. Behav. Ther.* **2000**, *18*, 181–191. [CrossRef]
18. Dennis, M.L.; Foss, M.A.; Scott, C. An eight-year perspective on the relationship between the duration of abstinence and other aspects of recovery. *Eval. Rev.* **2007**, *31*, 585–612. [CrossRef]
19. HM Government. From Harm to Hope: A 10-Year Drugs Plan to Cut Crime and Save Lives. December 2021. Available online: https://assets.publishing.service.gov.uk/media/629078bad3bf7f036fc492d1/From_harm_to_hope_PDF.pdf (accessed on 3 December 2024).

20. Balandeh, E.; Omidi, A.; Ghaderi, A. A Narrative Review of Third-Wave Cognitive-Behavioral Therapies in Addiction. *Addict. Health* **2021**, *13*, 52–65. [CrossRef]
21. Fang, S.; Ding, D. The differences between acceptance and commitment therapy (ACT) and cognitive behavioral therapy: A three-level meta-analysis. *J. Context. Behav. Sci.* **2023**, *28*, 149–168. [CrossRef]
22. Lebeaut, A.; McGrew, S.J.; Slotts, A.L.; Vujanovic, A.A. Third Wave Behavioral Treatment for Comorbid SUD and Emotional Disorders. In *Treating Comorbid Substance Use and Emotional Disorders. CBT: Science into Practice*; Wolitzky-Taylor, K., Ed.; Springer: Cham, Switzerland, 2024. [CrossRef]
23. Gloster, A.T.; Walder, N.; Levin, M.; Twohig, M.; Karekla, M. The empirical status of acceptance and commitment therapy: A review of meta-analyses. *J. Context. Behav. Sci.* **2020**, *18*, 181–192. [CrossRef]
24. Hayes, S.C.; Wilson, K.G.; Gifford, E.V.; Follette, V.M.; Strosahl, K. Experiential avoidance and behavioral disorders: A functional dimensional approach to diagnosis and treatment. *J. Consult. Clin. Psychol.* **1996**, *64*, 1152–1168. [CrossRef]
25. Hayes, S.C.; Stosahl, K.D.; Wilson, K. *Acceptance and Commitment Therapy: The Process and Practice of Mindful Change*, 2nd ed.; The Guilford Press: New York, NY, USA, 2012.
26. Krotter, A.; Aonso-Diego, G.; González-Menéndez, A.; González-Roz, A.; Secades-Villa, R.; García-Pérez, A. Effectiveness of acceptance and commitment therapy for addictive behaviors: A systematic review and meta-analysis. *J. Context. Behav. Sci.* **2023**, *32*, 100773. [CrossRef]
27. Park, S. Beyond patient-centred care: A conceptual framework of co-production mechanisms with vulnerable groups in health and social service settings. *Public Manag. Rev.* **2020**, *22*, 452–474. [CrossRef]
28. Hogan, L.M.; Bagheri, M.; Cox, W.M.; Morgan, D.B.; Rettie, H.C. A pilot study of the Moving on in My Recovery program for people in recovery from substance use. *J. Addict. Dis.* **2024**, 1–9. [CrossRef]
29. Neale, J.; Allen, D.; Coombes, L. Qualitative research methods within the addictions. *Addiction* **2005**, *100*, 1584–1593. [CrossRef]
30. Orford, J. Asking the right questions in the right way: The need for a shift in research on psychological treatments for addiction. *Addiction* **2008**, *103*, 875–885. [CrossRef] [PubMed]
31. Strauss, A.; Corbin, J. *Basics of Qualitative Research: Techniques and Procedures for Developing Grounded Theory*, 4th ed.; Sage Publications: Thousand Oaks, CA, USA, 2015.
32. Birks, M.; Mills, J. *Grounded Theory: A Practical Guide*, 2nd ed.; Sage Publications: London, UK, 2015.
33. Guiffrida, D.A.; McGuinness, S.; Carter, R.; Miller, D.; Farah, J. A qualitative study of clients with chronic pain who participated in an integrative mind/body psychotherapy intervention. *J. Psychother. Integr.* 2023; *advance online publication*. [CrossRef]
34. McHale, C.; Hayward, M.; Jones, F.W. Building a Grounded Theory of Engagement in Mindfulness-Based Group Therapy for Distressing Voices. *Qual. Health Res.* **2018**, *28*, 2169–2182. [CrossRef]
35. Beck, A.T. Cognitive therapy: Past, present, and future. *J. Consult. Clin. Psychol.* **1993**, *61*, 194. [CrossRef] [PubMed]
36. Wise, R.A.; Koob, G.F. The development and maintenance of drug addiction. *Neuropsychopharmacology* **2014**, *39*, 254–262. [CrossRef] [PubMed]
37. Scannell, C. Voices of hope: Substance use peer support in a system of care. *Subst. Abuse Res. Treat.* **2021**, *15*, 11782218211050360. [CrossRef] [PubMed]
38. Prochaska, J.O.; DiClemente, C.C. Transtheoretical therapy: Toward a more integrative model of change. *Psychother. Theory Res. Pract.* **1982**, *19*, 276–288. [CrossRef]
39. Vigdal, M.I.; Moltu, C.; Bjornestad, J.; Selseng, L.B. Social recovery in substance use disorder: A metasynthesis of qualitative studies. *Drug Alcohol Rev.* **2022**, *41*, 974–987. [CrossRef]
40. Ashford, R.D.; Brown, A.; Canode, B.; Sledd, A.; Potter, J.S.; Bergman, B.G. Peer-based recovery support services delivered at recovery community organizations: Predictors of improvements in individual recovery capital. *Addict. Behav.* **2021**, *119*, 106945. [CrossRef] [PubMed]
41. DeLucia, C.; Bergman, B.G.; Formoso, D.; Weinberg, L.B. Recovery in Narcotics Anonymous from the Perspectives of Long-Term Members: A Qualitative Study. *J. Groups Addict. Recovery* **2015**, *10*, 3–22. [CrossRef]
42. Miller, W.R.; C'de Baca, J. *Quantum Change: When Epiphanies and Sudden Insights Transform Ordinary Lives*; Guilford Press: New York, NY, USA, 2001.

behavioral sciences

MDPI

Article

Behavioural Systems Mapping of Solid Waste Management in Kisumu, Kenya, to Understand the Role of Behaviour in a Health and Sustainability Problem

Joanna Davan Wetton [1,*], Micaela Santilli [1], Hellen Gitau [2], Kanyiva Muindi [2], Nici Zimmermann [3], Susan Michie [1] and Michael Davies [3]

1 Centre for Behaviour Change, Department of Clinical, Educational and Health Psychology, University College London, London WC1E 7HB, UK; micaela.santilli.21@ucl.ac.uk (M.S.); s.michie@ucl.ac.uk (S.M.)
2 African Population and Health Research Center, P.O. Box 10787, Nairobi 00100, Kenya; hgitau@aphrc.org (H.G.); kmuindi@aphrc.org (K.M.)
3 Institute for Environmental Design and Engineering, The Bartlett Faculty of the Built Environment, University College London, London WC1H 0NN, UK; n.zimmermann@ucl.ac.uk (N.Z.); michael.davies@ucl.ac.uk (M.D.)
* Correspondence: jo.davanwetton@ucl.ac.uk

Abstract: Poor solid waste management in Kisumu, Kenya, contributes to adverse health, social, and environmental outcomes as a result of open burning, illegal dumping, and reliance on landfills. Taking Kisumu as a case study, we use behavioural systems mapping (BSM) for the purpose of understanding the role of behaviour in this complex problem. We qualitatively analysed transcripts from focus groups and interviews with 45 stakeholders in Kisumu to construct a BSM of the perceived actors, behaviours, and behavioural influences affecting waste management, as well as causal links. Influences were analysed using the capability, opportunity, and motivation model of behaviour (COM-B). The resulting BSM connects 24 behaviours by 12 different actors and 49 unique influences (30 related to opportunity, 16 to motivation, and 3 to capability). It reflects three sub-systems: policy-making, public waste management, and the policy–public interface. Six key feedback loops are described, which suggest that cycles of underfunding are interlinked with problematic practices around the build-up, handling, and segregation of waste and conflicting public and political views around responsibility. We demonstrate how the BSM method can be used with transcript data and provide steps that others can follow to inform the design of systemic behaviour change interventions. Further research to validate and adapt this approach may extend the learnings to other countries and health and sustainability challenges.

Keywords: behaviour change; COM-B model; behaviour change wheel; systems thinking; behavioural systems mapping; waste management; Kenya

1. Introduction

Global sustainability and health crises mean that governments urgently need to change a multitude of interconnected actions of citizens and organisations. In environmental policy contexts, behaviour change has often been equated with individual-level approaches and seen in contrast to systemic approaches. However, there is increasing recognition that effective environmental policies will need to be informed by an understanding of the causes and consequences of human behaviours in complex socio-technical systems. Although systems mapping and modelling approaches are widely used in the development of national and local environmental policies, few approaches are designed to represent the role of people's behaviours, and few are linked to frameworks for designing behaviour change interventions. Behavioural systems mapping is a recent approach developed in connection with the Behaviour Change Wheel framework (Michie et al., 2011) for the purposes of understanding and changing human behaviour in complex systems and for informing policy decisions (Allison et al., 2024; Hale et al., 2022; West et al., 2020). In this paper, we apply behavioural systems mapping to the major challenge of municipal solid waste management (MSWM) in Kisumu County, Kenya.

1.1. The Problem of Municipal Solid Waste Management

Globally, growing quantities of municipal solid waste contribute to adverse environmental, social and health outcomes (Chen et al., 2020; Kaza et al., 2018; Vergara & Tchobanoglous, 2012; Wilson & Velis, 2015). In low- and middle-income countries, the problem is exacerbated by the prevalence of open dumping and burning (Ferronato & Torretta, 2019; Kaza et al., 2018; United Nations Environment Programme, 2016), low standards of formal waste management and reliance on informal waste picking (Aparcana, 2017; Ferronato & Torretta, 2019; Wilson & Velis, 2015). In sub-Saharan Africa, MSWM remains a major challenge despite past and ongoing strategies at local, national, regional and continental levels (Ayeleru et al., 2020; Friedrich & Trois, 2011; Güneralp et al., 2017; United Nations Environment Programme, 2018). The majority of waste ends up in controlled or uncontrolled landfill sites, where its decomposition leads to greenhouse gas emissions, contamination of soil and water, and associated diseases (Friedrich & Trois, 2011; United Nations Environment Programme, 2018), which have the greatest impacts on vulnerable groups such as those living in poverty and in proximity to dumpsites (Awuor et al., 2019; Ma & Hipel, 2016; Sibanda et al., 2017).

This long-standing challenge is driven by a complex set of factors, including population growth, increasing urbanisation and economic development, in conjunction with a lack of municipal financial resources, infrastructure, technical expertise and management planning (Henry et al., 2006; Sibanda et al., 2017; Srivastava et al., 2015). It is also characterised by complex interactions between local government, private and informal waste sectors, and the public (Ma & Hipel, 2016). Because of these complexities and its resistance to change, MSWM in LMICs has been described as a 'wicked problem' (Chan, 2016; Ferrans et al., 2019; Salvia et al., 2021; Shah et al., 2019). This refers to problems that are 'ill-defined, ambiguous, and contested, and feature multi-layered interdependencies and complex social dynamics' (Termeer et al., 2015, p. 680) and that imply a need for systems thinking (Gray, 2018; Kreuter et al., 2004; Lönngren & Svanström, 2016).

Despite understanding that urban waste management involves a complex interplay of human behaviours, existing systems research in low- and middle-income countries has mainly focused on modelling flows of waste itself (Sudhir et al., 1997; Sufian & Bala, 2006, 2007; Talyan et al., 2007). An exception is research by Gutberlet et al. (2017), who used a systems thinking approach to map the interconnected actions and actors involved in waste management in Kisumu, Kenya. Drawing on transcripts from participatory modelling activities, their analysis aimed to represent key actions and actors involved in the flow of waste materials to identify weak links that could be potential points for intervention. These included a mix of changes to citizen behaviours, such as reducing waste, sorting at source, and improving disposal practices; changes to actors' roles, namely entrepreneurs and local governors; and changes to financial and market systems. This study demonstrates the feasibility and benefits of mapping actors and their actions within the waste system, although the authors noted that their simplified map may benefit from further analysis. One aspect that their analysis did not aim to capture is the range of influences on people's behaviours within the system. Understanding influences on behaviour (including and in addition to the role of other people's behaviours) is a key starting point in developing effective interventions to change behaviour (Craig et al., 2008; Hale et al., 2020; Michie et al., 2011, 2014; Michie & Johnston, 2012).

1.2. Behavioural Systems Mapping

Behavioural systems mapping (BSM) is a recent approach developed in the field of behavioural science for the purpose of helping to understand and change human behaviour in complex systems (Allison et al., 2024; Hale et al., 2020; West et al., 2020). It involves making explicit the actors, behaviours, and influences on behaviour within a system, as well as the nature of the relationships connecting these. The method may vary depending on the type of systems map being produced. For example, types of systems mapping that depict causal relationships may include (but are not limited to) connection circles (Mildeová, 2013), fuzzy cognitive mapping (Groumpos, 2010; Kosko, 1986), and causal loop diagrams (Bala et al., 2017; Coletta et al., 2020). Behavioural systems mapping is not intended to replace other systems mapping methods but aims to guide and specify what type of information should be usefully represented in the systems for understanding and changing behaviour. For example, it is slightly different from behavioural system dynamics, in which psychological and behavioural explanations of phenomena are incorporated into quantitative systems models (Barnabè & Davidsen, 2019; Lane, 2017), in that behavioural systems mapping is a qualitative approach that focuses on framing and analysing issues primarily in terms of the human behaviours involved.

A behavioural systems map is a tool to help understand what is causing people's current behaviours and what needs to be altered to change behaviours and the system as a whole (Hale et al., 2022; West et al., 2020). This may be improved by linking influences in the map to existing theories and models of behaviour (Allison et al., 2024; Department for Environment, Food & Rural Affairs, 2023a, 2023b; Hale et al., 2022). A useful model in this context is the capability, opportunity, and motivation model of behaviour (COM-B) (Michie et al., 2011), which proposes that these three conditions are necessary for any behaviour to occur (Figure 1). Capability, opportunity, and motivation form an interacting system with behaviour, making COM-B particularly compatible with systems mapping (Michie et al., 2011; West & Michie, 2020). The COM-B model forms the basis of the Behaviour Change Wheel framework, which can be used for designing interventions that address these behavioural influences (Michie et al., 2011).

In the initial development of the approach, BSM was used in a participatory process to address the decarbonisation of homes in Wales (Hale et al., 2022). While stakeholder participation is widely recognised as beneficial to the process and outcomes of systems mapping by increasing the validity and utility of maps (Antunes et al., 2015; Barbrook-Johnson & Penn, 2021), there are situations where this is impractical or inefficient. In such contexts, previous research demonstrates that it is feasible and valuable to derive systems maps from textual data, particularly transcripts of open or semi-structured interviews with stakeholders (Eker & Zimmermann, 2016; Kim & Andersen, 2012; Turner et al., 2013a, 2013b). Several methods have been developed for deriving causal maps from transcripts (Eker & Zimmermann, 2016; Kim & Andersen, 2012; Turner et al., 2013b; Yearworth & White, 2013). Key features of these approaches include identifying causal relationships in the initial steps of coding and maintaining an audit trail from the original transcripts to the final systems map, often facilitated by computer-aided qualitative data analysis software (CAQDAS).

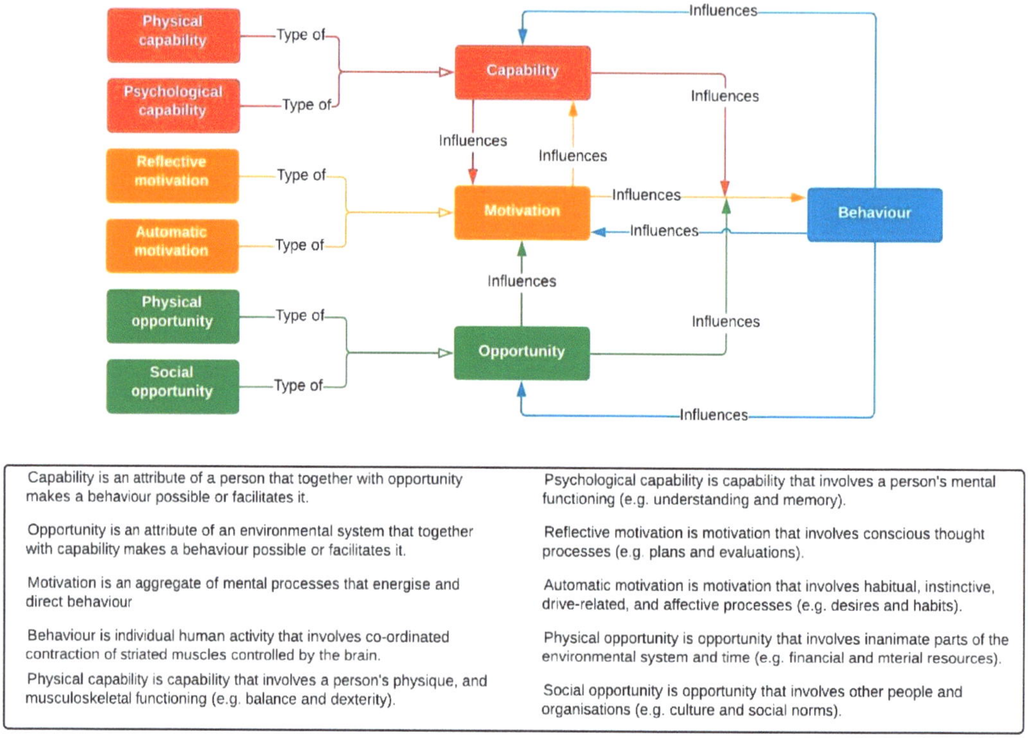

Figure 1. The COM-B model of behaviour. Reproduced with permission from West and Michie (2020).

1.3. The Present Study

In this study, we aimed to draw upon transcripts to build a BSM without the direct participation of stakeholders in the construction of the map and to detail our methodology so that others may benefit from this extension of the method. To do this, we focus on municipal waste management in Kisumu, Kenya, as a case study. Data were gathered through participatory focus groups, interviews, and workshops involving stakeholders from local government, industry, academia, community-based organisations, and residents' associations, all aimed at exploring health and sustainability issues in Kisumu County. The data were collected as part of the Complex Urban Systems for Sustainability and Health (CUSSH) project (Davies et al., 2021; Moore et al., 2021), which led to two related studies focusing on waste management in Kisumu through the lenses of system dynamics and attention theory (Dianati et al., 2021; Salvia et al., 2021). This study complements the previous two by focusing on the systemic role of people's behaviour in driving waste management challenges and linking this to a behavioural science framework.

Our research questions are as follows: (1) Which actors, behaviours, and influences on behaviour contribute to the current system of solid waste management in Kisumu? (2) What are the causal pathways and feedback loops connecting these behaviours and influences? We anticipate the outcomes of this study may help to advance the application of BSM using transcripts as a primary data source, as well as generating behavioural findings that can help to inform policy design and implementation through close collaboration between the CUSSH project and the Kisumu County Government.

2. Materials and Methods

2.1. Case Study: Solid Waste Management in Kisumu, Kenya

Kisumu County in Kenya can be seen as a case study for the waste management crisis in sub-Saharan Africa. Kisumu City, the county's capital, is Kenya's third largest city. Located in the West of the country on the edge of Lake Victoria, Kisumu forms an important national and international hub for transport and commerce. Nevertheless, at the time of our data collection in 2019, more than half of the county's population was categorised as poor, and around half were estimated to live in informal settlements (Simiyu et al., 2019). The county's population of around 1.1 million (Kenya National Bureau of Statistics, 2019) was estimated to generate between 200 and 500 tonnes of solid waste per day (Dianati et al., 2021; Oyake-Ombis, 2017; Sibanda et al., 2017). Up to 40% of waste is collected and, until 2022, was taken to the city's main landfill, Kachok dumpsite, where it had accumulated since 1975 and was periodically burned to free up capacity (Awuor et al., 2019; Dianati et al., 2021). The majority of the county's waste is openly burned or illegally dumped on vacant land, on roadsides, and in drainage channels, where it contributes to poor sanitation, disease and air pollution (Dianati et al., 2021; Gutberlet et al., 2017; Sibanda et al., 2017). This unsustainable situation will be further strained as the Kenyan population is expected to grow over the next few decades, accompanied by continued urbanisation and changing patterns of consumption (Dianati et al., 2021; Munala & Moirongo, 2011; Sibanda et al., 2017).

Previous attempts to improve waste management in Kisumu have faced difficulties. Plans to establish a new landfill at a distance from the overflowing Kachok dumpsite were delayed for years, mainly because of resident resistance in the proposed locations (Awuor et al., 2019; Dianati et al., 2021). The Kisumu Integrated Solid Waste Management Plan, developed and revised by the county government, outlined a 10-year strategy from 2015 to 2025 that aimed to reduce waste at source, improve waste collection and recycling rates, and establish more environmentally sustainable methods of waste disposal (County Government of Kisumu, 2017). These outcomes were to be achieved through planning, investment in infrastructure, legal reforms, and public–private partnerships, as well as grassroots-level initiatives such as community clean-ups designed to build public capacity and willingness to participate in waste management. However, the strategy did not follow the original implementation schedule, and in 2019, it failed to bring about substantial changes (Awuor et al., 2019; Dianati et al., 2021; Sibanda et al., 2017).

2.2. Participants

Our data were transcripts from in-depth interviews and focus groups with 45 participants representing seven stakeholder groups, listed in Table 1. Participants were invited by the study researchers or a research partner in the Kisumu County Government with a purposive, snow balling approach to recruitment based on their expertise and familiarity with the waste management sector. We also included transcript data from a workshop of mixed stakeholders who were partners in a funding application for waste management in Kisumu. Workshop participants comprised partners from the CUSSH project, the Kisumu County Government and local universities (including some participants who also took part in the focus groups).

Table 1. Stakeholder groups interviewed.

Stakeholder Group	Number of Participants
Kisumu County climate change directorate	10
Kisumu County officials	8
Community-based organisations (CBOs) providing waste management and waste-to-energy services	9
Industrial associations of commerce and manufacturing	2
Academic researchers in sustainability, health, and waste management from local universities	8
Residents' associations	7
Local factory-based industry	1

2.3. Data Collection

Focus groups and interviews were facilitated using a 3 h discussion guide written in English (Table S1, Supplementary File S1). This was developed for the wider programme of CUSSH research in Kisumu and therefore did not specifically address the present research questions. The discussion guide aimed to elicit a wide range of insights related to the CUSSH project's aims around city health and sustainability goals (which were shared with participants), local decision-making, and the development and implementation of city interventions.

Focus groups and interviews were conducted over two days in July 2019 in a hotel venue near Milimani, Kisumu. Interviews were in English, with some clarifications and prompts in Kiswahili. The research team (J.D.W., H.G., K.M., and N.Z.) facilitated each discussion in pairs. All are women social scientists with postgraduate training and experience in conducting qualitative interviews for research. For focus groups, at least one Kenyan researcher facilitated each discussion and provided any necessary translation between English and Kiswahili. Because stakeholder group sizes varied between 1 and 10 (Table 1), discussions varied in length. Participants were offered regular breaks with refreshments. All discussions were audio recorded and transcribed in English.

A separate workshop for partners from the CUSSH project, the Kisumu County Government, and local universities was held at the same hotel venue prior to the interviews. The same researchers (J.D.W., H.G., K.M., and N.Z.) were present and contributed to the discussion. The meeting was held in English and focused on discussing a joint programme of research and interventions around solid waste management. The workshop was audio recorded and transcribed in English.

3. Analyses

The analysis followed nine steps, each outlined in more detail below:

1. Familiarisation with transcripts;
2. Qualitative coding of transcripts to identify actors, behaviours, influences on behaviour, and perceived causal relationships between these;
3. Construction of an initial behavioural systems map;
4. Expert review (round 1);
5. Revision and simplification (round 1);
6. Expert review (round 2);
7. Revision and simplification (round 2);
8. Selection of illustrative quotes and linking to the COM-B model of behaviour;
9. Identification of causal pathways and feedback loops.

3.1. Step 1: Familiarisation with Transcripts

J.D.W. read each transcript and associated coding generated in another analysis (Salvia et al., 2021) and produced researcher memos to capture reflections from reading the transcripts.

3.2. Step 2: Qualitative Coding of Transcripts

J.D.W. coded the transcripts inductively in NVivo 12 Pro software by adding new codes under pre-determined categories of 'actor', 'behaviour', 'influence on behaviour', or 'relationship' (Table 2). These are the component parts that build up a behavioural systems map. Descriptions were developed by two researchers (J.D.W. and S.M.) prior to coding.

Table 2. Coding categories.

Coding Category	Description
Actor	An individual, group, organisation, or sector that enacts a behaviour seen as relevant to the issue.
Behaviour	An action that is directly or indirectly observable.
Influence on behaviour	A variable that directly or indirectly affects the likelihood, frequency, or characteristics of a behaviour and is not itself a behaviour.
Relationship	An observed, perceived or expected causal relationship between behaviours and/or influences on behaviours, expressed explicitly or implicitly.

Behaviour and influence codes were named in such a way that they could form variables in the behavioural systems map (i.e., could be said to increase or decrease). Relationships between variables were coded using the 'relationship' feature in NVivo. Each relationship was coded as 'positive' (same direction of change; as A goes up, B goes up and vice versa) or 'negative' (opposite direction of change; as A goes up, B goes down and vice versa). The NVivo relationships feature was also used to record which actors performed each behaviour.

3.3. Step 3: Construction of Initial Behavioural Systems Map

To select variables that were likely to be relevant and important to the system of waste management, three sets of criteria were examined for inclusion of variables in the behavioural systems map:

(a) Code mentioned at least three times and in at least three transcripts;
(b) Code mentioned at least three times and in at least two transcripts;
(c) Code mentioned at least two times and in at least two transcripts.

Criterion A is the most conservative, while Criterion C is the least conservative. Criterion B was selected and applied as the best compromise. All relationships between the selected variables were included, as were the actors associated with each behaviour.

J.D.W. constructed the initial behavioural systems map as a diagram in Vensim PLE version 8.0 (https://vensim.com/), a system dynamics open-source software (Supplementary File S2). Colours were used to distinguish behaviour and influence variables. Arrows were used to represent causal relationships, with '+' and '−' denoting positive and negative relationships.

3.4. Step 4: Expert Review (Round 1)

The initial behavioural systems map was separately reviewed by three pairs of researchers: those who collected the data (K.M. and G.H.); system dynamics experts from the CUSSH project, not involved in the data collection; and behaviour change experts who were not involved with the CUSSH project. Each pair of reviewers was sent a copy of the initial behavioural systems map, background information, and written instructions. Reviewers were asked to inspect the map and consider the following questions:

- To what extent does the diagram capture the most relevant and important information?
- Are there parts of the diagram that are too complex or too simple?
- Are there any variables or links missing?
- Are there any variables or links that are not needed?
- Are there any variables or links that seem incorrect?
- Do you have any other feedback points?

J.D.W. met with each pair of researchers and facilitated a semi-structured discussion based on the questions above. Each meeting was audio recorded and transcribed. Suggested changes to the map were categorised according to whether they related to the map in general or a specific part and whether the suggestion was to add, remove, or change variables or relationships.

3.5. Step 5: Revision and Simplification (Round 1)

J.D.W. re-read all transcripts and researcher memos and suggested changes to the map before making revisions and simplifications. The revised version of the map (round 1) was constructed in Vensim PLE version 8.0. Any variables that did not pertain to the existing system of solid waste management (i.e., pertained to an imagined ideal or future system) were removed. Some variables were re-named or combined. Then, the researcher made and recorded changes to the map suggested by the reviewers and the reasons for them. At this stage, based on the feedback received and re-reading of transcripts and memos, the map was organised into two sub-systems to aid readability, named *policy* and *waste 'on the ground'* (Figure S2, Supplementary File S2).

3.6. Step 6: Expert Review (Round 2)

The revised behavioural systems map was separately reviewed by two of the authors (S.M. and N.Z.) and an additional researcher from the CUSSH project. They were asked to provide feedback from the perspective of behaviour change (S.M.), system dynamics (N.Z.), or in-depth familiarity with the transcript data (additional researcher). Each was sent a copy of the revised map background information and asked to consider the questions above. J.D.W. met with each reviewer to discuss their feedback. Each meeting was audio recorded and transcribed, and suggested changes were recorded and categorised as before (see step 4).

3.7. Step 7: Revision and Simplification (Round 2)

The revised version of the map (round 2) was made using Kumu software (version 2). Kumu was chosen for its interactive features, which could increase the usability of the final map. As before, J.D.W. made and recorded changes to the map suggested by the reviewers. At this stage, based on the additional feedback received and to further aid readability, the two sub-systems in the map (see step 5) were re-organised into three sub-systems, named *policy-making*, *public waste management*, and *policy–public interface*.

3.8. Step 8: Selection of Illustrative Quotes and Linking to the COM-B Model of Behaviour

J.D.W. selected illustrative quotes from the transcript data that described each variable and provided context (Tables S1 and S2, Supplementary File S3). These were included as an interactive feature in Kumu so that viewers can click on a variable to view the quotes. To link the map to the COM-B model of behaviour, influence variables were categorised into capability, opportunity, or motivation factors, and these were colour-coded in the map.

3.9. Step 9: Identification of Causal Pathways and Feedback Loops

J.D.W. identified the balancing and reinforcing feedback loops present in the map. This is a typical step in the analysis and interpretation of causal systems maps, particularly causal loop diagrams because feedback loops can underlie important dynamics of a system. In a reinforcing feedback loop, there is a 'snowball effect' whereby a change in one variable ultimately leads to more change in that variable in the same direction, reinforcing the change. In a balancing feedback loop, change in a variable instead leads to a self-correcting effect, which limits runaway increase or decrease. In the Results section, we do not exhaustively describe every feedback loop in the map; short loops of two or three variables can be spotted relatively easily, but we focus on more complex loops, which may be harder to identify in the map and less obvious as potential drivers of the issue.

4. Results

Figure 2 shows the behavioural systems map of solid waste management in Kisumu. We recommend viewing this map interactively at https://kumu.io/JoHale/waste-in-kisumu (accessed 1 October 2024), where it is possible to zoom in and out and click on variables for illustrative quotes.

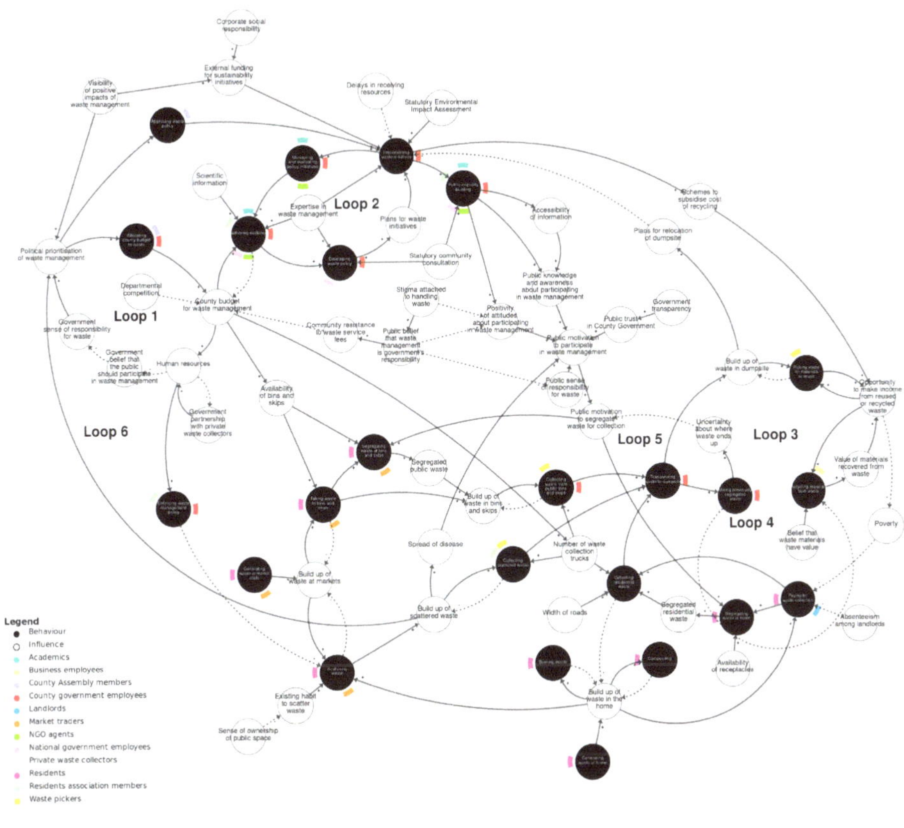

Figure 2. Behavioural systems map of solid waste management in Kisumu. Behaviours are shown as black circles. Actors (the people doing the behaviours) are shown as colour-coded flags around the edge of each behaviour. Influences on behaviour are shown as grey circles. Causal relationships are shown as arrows. Solid arrows are used for positive relationships (+). Dashed arrows are used for negative relationships (−). We recommend viewing this figure interactively online at https://kumu.io/JoHale/waste-in-kisumu (accessed on 1 October 2024).

The overall map is organised into three sub-systems, which were identified through expert review and serve to help navigate the map by grouping the variables into related domains. The three sub-systems are *policy-making, public waste management*, and the *policy–public interface*. The *policy-making* sub-system describes processes of developing and implementing waste policy involving the county government, county assembly, national government, NGOs, and others. The *public waste management* sub-system describes practices happening 'on the ground', such as generating, segregating, mixing, collecting, transporting, picking, and burning waste. The *policy–public interface* sub-system connects these two sub-systems and describes the interplay between policy consultation and transparency and public attitudes and motivations.

4.1. Which Actors, Behaviours, and Influences on Behaviour Contribute to the Current System of Solid Waste Management in Kisumu?

In Table 3, we list the behaviours within each sub-system of the behavioural systems map and the actor(s) connected to them. Illustrative quotes describing each behaviour are provided in Table S1 (Supplementary File S3), or they can be viewed by clicking on each behaviour in the interactive online map.

Table 3. Behaviours and actors within three sub-systems of waste management in Kisumu.

Sub-System	Behaviour	Actor(s) Connected to the Behaviour
Policy-making	Allocating county budget to waste	County assembly members, county government employees
	Approving waste policy	County assembly members
	Developing waste policy	National government employees, county government employees
	Enforcing waste management policy	County government employees, residents association members
	Gathering evidence	Residents association members, academics, NGO agents, national government employees, county government employees
	Implementing waste initiatives	County government employees
	Monitoring and evaluating policy initiatives	Academics, NGO agents, county government employees
Public waste management	Burning waste	Residents
	Collecting residential waste	Private waste collectors
	Collecting scattered waste	Residents' association members, waste pickers
	Collecting waste from public bins and skips	County government employees, waste pickers
	Composting	Residents
	Generating waste at home	Residents
	Generating waste at market stalls	Residents, market traders
	Mixing previously segregated waste	Private waste collectors, county government employees
	Paying for waste collection	Residents, landlords
	Picking waste for materials to reuse	Waste pickers
	Recycling materials from waste	Business employees
	Scattering waste	Residents, market traders
	Segregating waste at bins and skips	Residents, market traders
	Segregating waste at home	Residents
	Taking waste to bins and skips	Residents, market traders
	Transporting waste to dumpsite	Private waste collectors, county government employees
Policy–public interface	Public capacity building	Residents association members, academics, NGO agents, national government employees, county government employees

Table 4 lists the influences on behaviour, categorised according to the COM-B model into capability, opportunity, and motivation variables. These can be viewed in the interactive online map by clicking 'show COM-B'. Illustrative quotes describing each influence are provided in Table S2 (Supplementary File S3), or they can be viewed by clicking on each influence in the interactive online map.

Table 4. Influences on behaviour categorised according to COM-B.

Sub-System	COM-B Domain (*N* Influences)	Influence on Behaviour
Policy-making	Capability (1)	Expertise in waste management
	Motivation (6)	Corporate social responsibility
		Government belief that the public should participate in waste management
		Government sense of responsibility for waste
		Plans for relocation of dumpsite
		Plans for waste initiatives
		Political prioritisation of waste management
	Opportunity (10)	County budget for waste management
		Delays in receiving resources
		Departmental competition
		External funding for sustainability initiatives
		Government partnership with private waste collectors
		Human resources
		Schemes to subsidise cost of recycling
		Scientific information
		Statutory Environmental Impact Assessment
		Visibility of positive impacts of waste management
Public waste management	Capability (1)	Uncertainty about where waste ends up
	Motivation (5)	Belief that waste materials have value
		Existing habit to scatter waste
		Opportunity to make income from reused or recycled waste
		Public motivation to segregate waste for collection
		Sense of ownership of public space
	Opportunity (15)	Absenteeism among landlords
		Availability of bins and skips
		Availability of receptacles
		Build-up of scattered waste
		Build-up of waste at markets
		Build-up of waste in bins and skips
		Build-up of waste in dumpsite
		Build-up of waste in the home
		Number of waste collection trucks
		Poverty
		Segregated public waste
		Segregated residential waste
		Spread of disease
		Value of materials recovered from waste
		Width of roads

Table 4. *Cont.*

Sub-System	COM-B Domain (*N* Influences)	Influence on Behaviour
Policy–public interface	Capability (1)	Public knowledge and awareness about participating in waste management
	Motivation (5)	Positivity of attitudes about participating in waste management
		Public belief that waste management is government's responsibility
		Public motivation to participate in waste management
		Public sense of responsibility for waste
		Public trust in county government
	Opportunity (5)	Accessibility of information
		Community resistance to waste service fees
		Government transparency
		Statutory community consultation
		Stigma attached to handling waste

Only three variables related to people's capability (knowledge and skills). In other words, stakeholders did not often point to people's abilities as the main influences shaping people's current actions. The majority of influences described in the transcripts are related to opportunity (features of people's physical and social environments), followed by motivational influences (automatic or reflective mental processes that drive behaviour). This is consistent with the nature of Kisumu's waste management situation as a highly systemic problem made up of many interactions between different actors and local sites and infrastructure.

4.2. What Are the Causal Pathways and Feedback Loops Connecting These Behaviours and Influences?

We next describe the main causal pathways and feedback loops within each sub-system of the map and the connections between sub-systems. Not all possible pathways and loops are described exhaustively; we focus on those that appear to explain important patterns within and between the sub-systems and be relevant to add to stakeholders' knowledge (as expressed in the transcript data) of the waste management challenges in Kisumu.

4.2.1. Policy-Making Sub-System

Figure 3 shows the policy-making sub-system. Within this sub-system, there are two main reinforcing loops. The first reinforcing loop ('Loop 1') involves the behaviour *allocating county budget to waste* by county government employees and county assembly members. It represents that the less county budget allocated to waste, the less *county budget for waste management* and the fewer *human resources*. Human resources also depend on *government partnership with private waste collectors* (forming a balancing loop) and influence *enforcing waste management policy*. With fewer human resources, the greater the *government belief that the public should participate in waste management*, and the less *government sense of responsibility for waste*. The less sense of responsibility, the less *political prioritisation of waste management* and the less allocating of budget, completing the loop. *Departmental competition* was also described as an influence on county budget for waste management.

The second main reinforcing loop ('Loop 2') connects behaviours by county government employees and others of *gathering evidence, developing waste policy, implementing waste initiatives, and monitoring and evaluating policy initiatives*. There are several external influences on these behaviours, including scientific information, expertise in waste management, statutory environmental impact assessments, and delays in receiving resources.

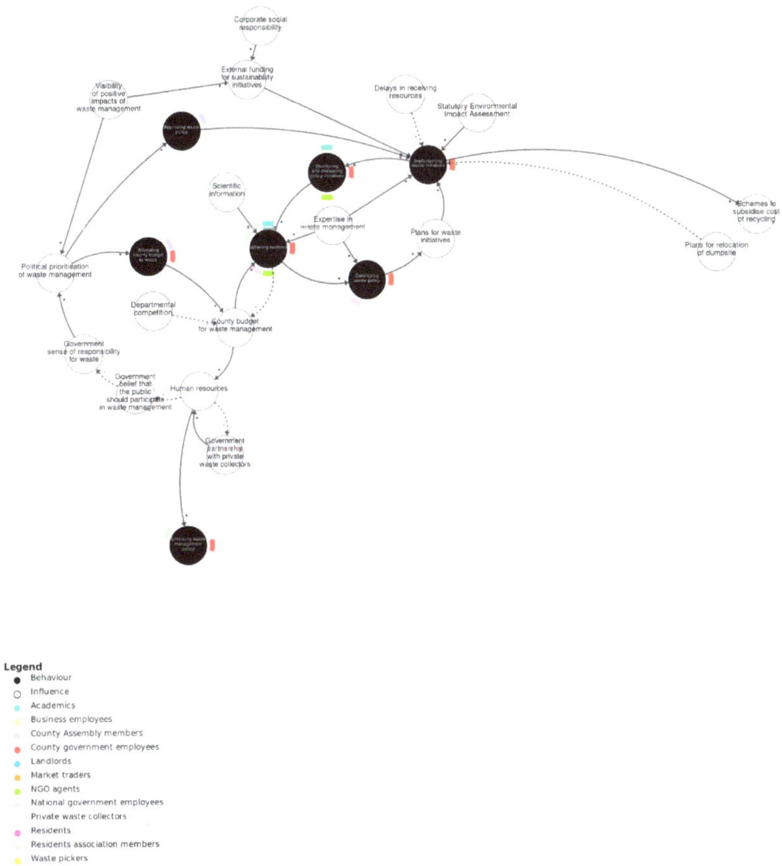

Figure 3. Policy-making sub-system. Loop 1 and Loop 2 are labelled with pale grey text. We recommend viewing this figure interactively online at https://kumu.io/JoHale/waste-in-kisumu (accessed on 1 October 2024).

The two feedback loops are connected in several ways. First, county budget for waste management and gathering evidence forms a balancing loop, whereby (for instance) more budget allows more gathering of evidence, which depletes the budget. Secondly, implementing waste initiatives depends on county assembly members *approving waste policy*, which is influenced by the political prioritisation of waste management. Thirdly, *visibility of positive impacts of waste management* influences both political prioritisation and also *external funding for sustainability initiatives*, which then influences implementation.

4.2.2. Public Waste Management Sub-System

Figure 4 shows the public waste management sub-system. Two main sources of waste are represented in this sub-system. The first is *generating waste at market stalls*. As a consequence, a *build-up of waste at markets* influences market traders and residents *taking waste to bins and skips*. The *availability of bins and skips* influences taking waste to bins and skips and segregating waste there. The second source of waste is residents *generating waste at home*. A build-up of waste in the home leads to *burning waste*, *composting*, and *paying for waste collection*. Build-up of waste in the home and at markets both lead to *scattering waste*, which is influenced by an *existing habit to scatter waste*, affected by *sense of ownership of public space*.

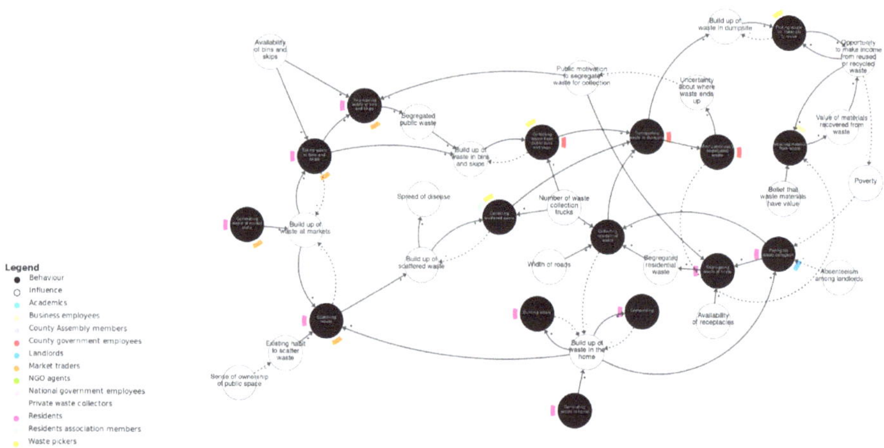

Figure 4. Public waste management sub-system. Loops 3–5 are labelled with pale grey text. We recommend viewing this figure interactively online at https://kumu.io/JoHale/waste-in-kisumu (accessed on 1 October 2024).

As waste builds up in bins and skips, in homes, and scattered in public, this leads to collecting waste and transporting it to the dumpsite. Collecting waste is influenced by the *number of waste collection trucks*. This is reflected in the actors depicted as involved in waste collection (which are not necessarily exhaustive): *collecting waste from bins and skips* is performed by county government employees and waste pickers; *collecting residential waste* is performed by private waste collectors; and *collecting scattered waste* is performed by waste pickers and residents' association members.

Transporting waste to the dumpsite is part of several feedback loops that we will describe here. In Loop 3, *transporting waste to the dumpsite* influences a build-up of waste there. This leads to *picking waste materials to reuse*, which influences *opportunity to make income from reused or recycled waste*, in turn influencing *poverty*, which influences *paying for waste collection*, and this feeds back to *collecting residential waste* and *transporting waste to dumpsite*. However, the opportunity to make income also depends on the *value of materials recovered from waste* for recycling. This is part of Loop 4: transporting waste to the dumpsite leads to *mixing previously segregated waste* (within the same truck or upon entering the dumpsite), and with more mixing, the less recycling can be carried out. In Loop 5, mixing previously segregated waste also leads to *uncertainty about where waste ends up*, which influences *public motivation to segregate waste for collection*, which in turn influences the segregating of waste at bins and skips and at home.

4.2.3. Policy–Public Interface Sub-System

Figure 5 shows the policy–public interface sub-system. This sub-system includes one behaviour, *public capacity building*, by national and county government employees, NGOs, academics, and residents' association members. This includes activities such as community education and clean-up days, which were described as having the purpose of increasing aspects of public capability, opportunity, and/or motivation to engage in waste management.

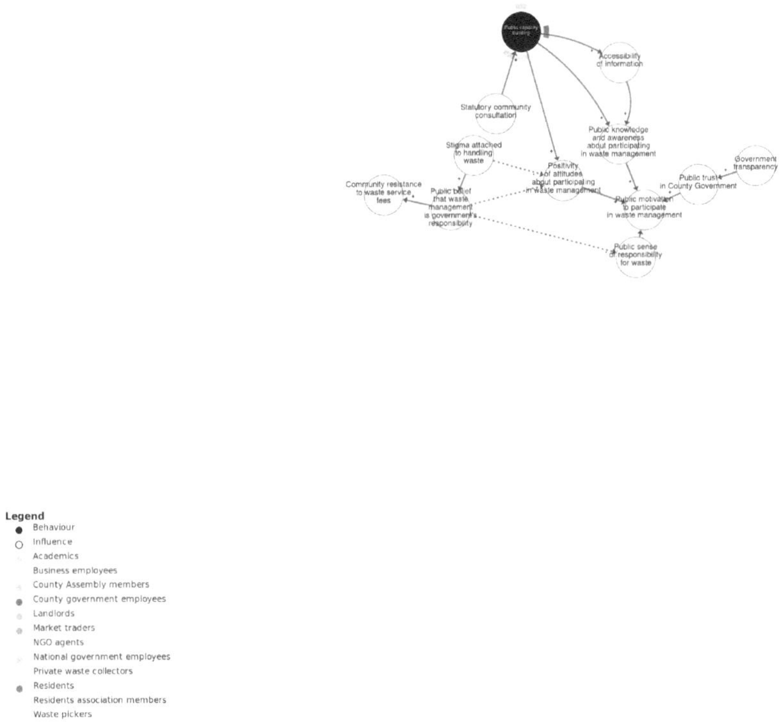

Figure 5. Public–policy interface sub-system. We recommend viewing this figure interactively online at https://kumu.io/JoHale/waste-in-kisumu (accessed on 1 October 2024).

Public capacity building is part of a causal pathway that connects the policy-making sub-system to the public waste management sub-system. Capacity building follows from implementing waste management initiatives and is influenced by the requirement for the government to undertake *statutory community consultation*. Public capacity building positively influences *public knowledge, awareness, and attitudes about participating in waste management*, which in turn positively influence *public motivation to participate in waste management* and to segregate waste for collection.

The policy–public interface sub-system contains several other direct and indirect influences on public motivation to participate in waste management. These include *public trust in county government*, which is influenced by *government transparency*, and *public sense of responsibility for waste*, influenced by the *belief that waste management is the government's responsibility*. This belief is influenced by *stigma attached to handling waste*, which also influences the positivity of attitudes about participating in waste management.

4.2.4. Connections Between the Sub-Systems

We have already described how public capacity building is part of a causal pathway that connects from the policy-making sub-system to the public waste management sub-system. Here, we describe other relationships and feedback loops that connect behaviours within different sub-systems.

In the policy-making sub-system, allocating county budget for waste management influences the *availability of bins and skips* and the *number of waste collection trucks*, which affect behaviours in the public waste management sub-system. The number of trucks influences *collecting scattered waste* and in turn the *build-up of scattered waste*. With more build-up of scattered waste comes greater political prioritisation of waste management (or vice versa), which influences allocating county budget and thus forms a feedback loop (Loop 6). Other influences from the policy-making sub-system to the public waste management sub-system include *enforcing waste policy*, which negatively influences *scattering waste* and *schemes to subsidise the cost of recycling*, which positively influence the *opportunity to make income from reused or recycled waste*.

From the public waste management sub-system, a build-up of waste in the dumpsite was identified to positively influence *plans for relocating the dumpsite*. As waste built up in the past, this led to more intense plans for relocation. Relocation of the dumpsite could ease pressure on the need to implement (other) waste management initiatives, which is part of the policy-making sub-system.

5. Discussion

This study aimed to use the case study of municipal waste management in Kisumu, Kenya, to develop a behavioural systems map (BSM) representing the actors, behaviours, and influences on behaviour that contribute to the county's waste challenges and to analyse the behavioural influences using the COM-B model of behaviour. We also aimed to demonstrate the usability of transcript data to build a BSM and document our methodology so that others may build on it. Our step-by-step analysis involved qualitatively coding transcripts to thoroughly identify the behavioural components that stakeholders described as contributing to Kisumu's waste management issues, as well as relationships among these, and transferring this information into a BSM that was refined through two documented rounds of expert review. The resulting BSM allowed us to identify causal pathways and feedback loops connecting the behaviours of multiple actors in the public and policy spheres. Similar to Gutberlet et al.'s previous systems mapping study of household waste management in Kisumu (Gutberlet et al., 2017), we depict a complex system involving many of the same actors at county, city, business, and household levels. However, whereas Gutberlet et al. focus predominantly on actions that happen to waste (or products before they become waste), our data led us to also map a range of policy-making behaviours.

The overall behavioural system of MSWM in Kisumu can be viewed in three sections, or 'sub-systems'. The first relates to local policy-making. It encompasses the roles of government employees, assembly members, non-governmental organisations (NGOs), and academics in evidence-gathering, policy development and approval, implementation, and monitoring. Feedback loops in this part of the BSM suggest that the government's lack of human resources reinforces, and is reinforced by, a lack of political prioritisation for waste management in budgets (in agreement with Sibanda et al., 2017), which is motivated by the view that the public should participate to meet the shortfall. This problematic cycle also hampers a more virtuous policy cycle of developing, implementing, monitoring, and evaluating waste policy. The more money diverted to gathering evidence, the less is available for human resources. While previous studies have found that budgetary and human resource constraints are barriers to effective MSWM in Kenyan and other sub-Saharan African cities (Gatura & Mberu, 2019; Kaza et al., 2018; Sibanda et al., 2017; UNEP, 2024; Zhang et al., 2024), our study illustrates how these factors can be tied up in cycles of behaviours that perpetuate a lack of resources for implementing evidence-based policies.

The second section of the BSM pertains to the actions of residents, businesses, traders, and civil groups in the processes of generating waste—particularly at homes and markets—and then dealing with it through more or less desirable routes. This section includes considerable overlap with Gutberlet et al.'s map (Gutberlet et al., 2017), specifically actions such as generating, composting, burning, sorting, collecting, transporting, dumping, and picking/scavenging waste, although our BSM goes into less granular detail and includes influences on the beahviours. Feedback loops in this part of the BSM suggest that public motivation to segregate waste (which would be desirable for recycling and recovering value) is undermined (Salvia et al., 2021) by the practice of mixing any waste that was segregated at bins or skips when these are emptied into trucks to take the waste to the dumpsite. This occurs because there are too few bins, skips, and trucks (due to the lack of waste budget) to operate a preferable system of keeping waste streams segregated. Consequentially, there are fewer opportunities for government, businesses, or residents to recycle materials or recover income from waste. This is important for the promotion of a more circular economy, which has not only environmental but also socio-economic benefits through the creation of livelihoods (Boon & Anuga, 2020; Debrah et al., 2022). Lack of political will, funding, and public awareness have been previously identified as barriers to circular waste management in sub-Saharan Africa (Debrah et al., 2022; Muheirwe et al., 2022); our findings add that undermining public motivation may play a role.

The third section of the BSM describes some of the interface between policy-makers and the public, which is characterised by capacity-building efforts, such as community education and clean-up events. While these efforts are designed to increase the capability, opportunity, and motivation of residents to engage with waste management, two critical factors could influence their success: first, public trust in the county government (linked to government transparency around budgets and accountability), and second, the public's belief that waste management is the government's responsibility. Disagreement over government and public responsibility for waste management in Kisumu was prominent in our transcript data (Salvia et al., 2021). This aligns with Gutberlet et al.'s finding that the responsibilities of the city/county are a point of confusion that needs to be addressed (Gutberlet et al., 2017). Our findings add that the public's viewpoint may partly stem from the undesirability of handling waste, while the government's viewpoint relates to their lack of budget to deal with it.

A key contribution of this study is the use of the COM-B model to analyse the influences on behaviour represented in the BSM (Hale et al., 2022). This takes us further than previous studies in understanding the *types* of factors that drive behaviour in the waste management system. Capability factors (knowledge and skill) were only seen to play a small role. Most influences on behaviour in our map related to opportunities afforded by the physical environment, such as waste infrastructure and financial resources, and (to a lesser extent) social influences, such as the social stigma around waste handling. A range of motivational factors were also seen to play a role, particularly actors' (often opposing) beliefs and attitudes surrounding waste management and sense of responsibility, as well as plans and existing habits.

5.1. Practical and Scientific Implications

Our findings have practical implications for MSWM intervention in Kisumu and places facing similar waste issues. Where there is a mismatch between government and public attitudes about who should take responsibility for waste management, it may be important to facilitate dialogues between government officials and community representatives to address the disagreement and develop a collaborative approach. The CUSSH project has subsequently helped facilitate such dialogues through a programme of public engagement between residents, local policy-makers, journalists, and other stakeholders (Kisumu, n.d.). Increasing the visibility of positive impacts of waste management, e.g., through campaigns highlighting health and sustainability benefits, could also help to increase both political prioritisation and external investment of funding (Johnson et al., 2017). In addition to this, increasing the transparency of government decision-making and expenditure could help to build public trust (Alessandro et al., 2021) and avoid undermining public capacity-building efforts that are already in place (although previous research suggests this may not be guaranteed (Grimmelikhuijsen et al., 2013)). Efforts could be improved by shifting the emphasis away from informing, educating, and persuading residents to designing behaviour change interventions that address the physical opportunity barriers they are also facing (Bortoleto, 2014; Dioba et al., 2024; Nordlund et al., 2011), such as limited availability of waste receptacles, unaffordable home waste collections (Sibanda et al., 2017), and landlord absenteeism. This is not only relevant for Kisumu and locations in the global south but applies just as much to global north cities where there is also over-reliance on informational approaches to reduce littering (Chaudhary et al., 2021).

Scientifically, this study contributes to the new and growing literature on behavioural systems mapping (Allison et al., 2024; Chadwick et al., 2021; Craven, 2017; Craven & Healy, 2021; Department for Environment, Food & Rural Affairs, 2023a, 2023b; Hale et al., 2022; Lunetto et al., 2022; West et al., 2020; Zhu et al., 2023). The main feature of behavioural systems mapping (relative to other systems mapping approaches) is that it makes explicit the role of specific actors, behaviours, and influences on behaviour and how these are connected in a system (Hale et al., 2022). This approach offers much more nuance than traditional qualitative studies of barriers and enablers to behaviour change (which usually list factors in relation to one 'target' behaviour), while still enabling the use of frameworks such as the Behaviour Change Wheel (BCW) to aid in identifying suitable types of intervention. Previously published BSM studies have involved participatory stakeholder workshops and interviews (Allison et al., 2024; Chadwick et al., 2021; Hale et al., 2022; Zhu et al., 2023), although two projects have drawn upon wider data sources, including literature reviews (Allison et al., 2024; Zhu et al., 2023). Training in BSM led by the UCL Centre for Behaviour Change and other institutions has also focused primarily on group model-building approaches. Our study demonstrates the feasibility of constructing BSMs from transcript data when access to stakeholders is no longer possible and provides a detailed step-by-step approach that others can follow and adapt.

5.2. Strengths, Limitations, and Future Research

A strength of this study is the application of behavioural theory in building and interpreting the BSM. Many systems science studies of waste management (Termeer et al., 2015; Gray, 2018; Lönngren & Svanström, 2016; Dianati et al., 2021) and other environmental and health issues model material stocks and flows and treat policies or behaviours as extraneous variables. Studies that do incorporate human behaviour in systems models rarely link to theories about the determinants of behaviour. This makes it hard to connect insights from the systems map/model to interventions that could change behaviour. In our study, the use of the COM-B model bridges that gap by linking the components of the map to a coherent intervention design framework, the BCW. Additional research could build on the present study by using the BCW to explore potential intervention options in detail with local stakeholders (West et al., 2019).

Another strength of this study is that it draws from a wide range of stakeholder perspectives (Salvia et al., 2021), providing different views of MSWM issues 'on the ground'. Forty-five people from varied roles in local government, industry, academia, and community organisations took part in the discussions that formed our dataset, providing rich insight into waste issues and how these connected with the wider context of climate and health policy-making in Kisumu. Most of the stakeholders (with the exception of industry) took part in group discussions, which can reduce reliance on individual views. Combining such a range of perspectives is a key tenet of systems thinking approaches, and it can lend fairness, accuracy, and legitimacy to resulting systems maps (Antunes et al., 2015; Hale et al., 2022).

These benefits are more fully realised when stakeholders take part in the mapping process itself (Antunes et al., 2015), and a limitation of the study is that we could not give participants that opportunity due to project constraints during the COVID-19 pandemic. We mitigated this partly through two rounds of expert review by behavioural scientists, systems scientists, and local researchers to improve the quality of the BSM. However, a valuable next step would be to engage local stakeholders in interpreting, challenging, and using the BSM as a tool for building joint understandings. This could also present an opportunity to include any additional perspectives that could have been missing among those interviewed. Our inclusion of interactive features in the online version of the BSM (e.g., to view sub-systems, toggle COM-B colour-coding, and click on elements to read illustrative quotes from the transcripts) could help stakeholders engage with the map.

The successful use of transcript data to create a BSM is also a strength of the study. We were able to reuse data collected for other purposes within the CUSSH project to carry out a rich behavioural analysis that complements two other studies on the same issue (Dianati et al., 2021; Salvia et al., 2021). Re-analysis of data is not only good for scientific efficiency (Pronk, 2019) but can offer benefits through the opportunity to triangulate insights gained through different methods.

However, compared with group model-building workshops, our qualitative coding of transcripts was a very time-intensive method. This limitation has been acknowledged in previous studies (Eker & Zimmermann, 2016; Kim & Andersen, 2012; Yearworth & White, 2013) and could present a barrier to following our steps. Part of the reason was that our transcripts were very long and not specifically directed by the research questions. The analysis could be quicker by collecting or editing transcript data to be more focused. By increasing access to and knowledge of AI-assisted qualitative analysis (Carvalho et al., 2024; Christou, 2023; Hamilton et al., 2023; Lee et al., 2020), made possible by recent large language models and generative AI, future research could potentially make use of these tools to increase the efficiency of coding and systems modelling (Liu & Keith, 2024).

Finally, it is important to note that the data analysed in the present study were collected in 2019, and in the time elapsed, there will have been changes to MSWM in Kisumu. One of the most significant changes has been the relocation of the Kachok dumpsite (Sibanda et al., 2017). Work began in 2021 to establish a new dumpsite in the Muhoroni sub-county and decommission the old site (Breath of fresh air in Kisumu as Kachok dumpsite is finally levelled, 2022; Nyabundi, n.d.), with plans to convert the Kachok site into a recreational garden, although this has not yet been realised (Kachok: Locals lose hope as promise of converting Kisumu dumpsite to garden wastes away, 2023). This and other developments could alter the picture of MSWM in our BSM, underscoring the relevance of further work to engage local stakeholders in interpreting, challenging, and using the map. Nevertheless, the issues discussed reflected long-term patterns of behaviour that have persisted for decades and continue to hinder solid waste management in sub-Saharan African contexts (Adedara et al., 2023; Ayeleru et al., 2020; Debrah et al., 2022). Thus, recent and future developments in Kisumu are unlikely to alter all the lessons learned from this case study and do not detract from the wider value of the project in advancing BSM.

This map was specifically developed to understand the MSWM in Kisumu. We recognise that the behaviours, influences, and actors identified in this map may vary in other nations or different cities within Kenya. While some general trends may be applicable to other sub-Saharan African cities, we recommend that this map be validated and adapted for use in different contexts to ensure its relevance and accuracy in other case scenarios.

6. Conclusions

This study developed a behavioural systems map (BSM) to represent the actors, behaviours, and influences contributing to municipal solid waste management challenges in Kisumu, Kenya. Applying the COM-B model revealed that physical opportunity and motivational factors predominantly influence behaviour in this context. Through qualitative analysis of transcript data, we identified interconnected processes in local policy-making, public waste handling, and interactions between policy-makers and the public. The BSM revealed critical feedback loops that suggest that cycles of underfunding are interlinked with problematic practices around the build-up, handling, and segregation of waste and conflicting public and political views around responsibility.

Our findings suggest the need for collaborative dialogues between government and community representatives, increased transparency in decision-making, and interventions addressing physical opportunity and motivation barriers. Overcoming these barriers could help to promote more circular waste management practices, which can have additional benefits, such as generating income. This study contributes to behavioural systems mapping methodology by demonstrating the feasibility of constructing BSMs from transcript data. Future research and collaborative dialogues to improve MSWM could involve local stakeholders in interpreting and using BSMs, potentially employing AI-assisted analysis to enhance efficiency in BSM construction.

Supplementary Materials: The following supporting information can be downloaded at https://www.mdpi.com/article/10.3390/bs15020133/s1, Supplementary File S1: Interview discussion guide. Supplementary File S2, Figure S1: Draft behavioural systems map for review (round 1). Figure S2: Draft behavioural systems map for review (round 2). Supplementary File S3, Table S1: Illustrative quotes for behaviours and actors within three sub-systems of waste management in Kisumu. Table S2: Illustrative quotes for influences on behaviour categorised according to COM-B.

Author Contributions: Conceptualisation, J.D.W., N.Z., and S.M.; methodology, J.D.W., H.G., K.M., N.Z., and S.M.; formal analysis, J.D.W.; investigation, J.D.W., H.G., K.M., N.Z., and M.D.; writing—original draft preparation, J.D.W., M.S., and K.M.; writing—review and editing, J.D.W., M.S., H.G., K.M., N.Z., and S.M.; visualisation, J.D.W.; supervision, N.Z., S.M., and M.D.; project administration, H.G. and K.M.; funding acquisition, N.Z., S.M., and M.D. All authors have read and agreed to the published version of the manuscript.

Funding: This research was funded in whole or in part by the Wellcome Trust [grant number 209387/Z/17/Z]. For the purpose of open access, the author has applied a CC BY public copyright licence to any author-accepted manuscript version arising from this submission.

Institutional Review Board Statement: The study was conducted in accordance with the Declaration of Helsinki and approved by the UCL Bartlett School of Environment, Energy and Resources (protocol code 20180103_IEDE_STA_ETH, date of approval 23 January 2018). Work in Kenya received ethical approval from the Amref Health Africa's Ethics and Scientific Research Committee (Ref: ESRC-P506-2018, date of approval 2018) and a research permit from the National Commission for Science, Technology and Innovation (NACOSTI) (Ref: NACOSTI/P/19/99937/31473, date of approval 2019).

Informed Consent Statement: Informed consent was obtained from all subjects involved in the study.

Data Availability Statement: Data collected and generated by this research are considered confidential.

Acknowledgments: The authors would like to thank the participants for the precious time and information provided. We thank Evans Gichana for assistance with collection of the data analysed in this study. We thank Kaveh Dianati, Irene Pluchinotta, and Giuseppe Salvia for providing expert review of draft behavioural systems maps and comments on draft versions of this paper.

Conflicts of Interest: The authors declare no conflicts of interest. The funders had no role in the design of the study; in the collection, analyses, or interpretation of data; in the writing of the manuscript; or in the decision to publish the results.

References

Adedara, M. L., Taiwo, R., & Bork, H.-R. (2023). Municipal solid waste collection and coverage rates in sub-saharan african countries: A comprehensive systematic review and meta-analysis. *Waste, 1*(2), 24. [CrossRef]

Alessandro, M., Cardinale Lagomarsino, B., Scartascini, C., Streb, J., & Torrealday, J. (2021). Transparency and trust in government. evidence from a survey experiment. *World Development, 138*, 105223. [CrossRef]

Allison, A. L., Frost, R., & Murtagh, N. (2024). Promoting planting in front gardens: A systematic approach to intervention development. *UCL Open Environment, 6*(1), e3147. [CrossRef]

Antunes, P., Stave, K., Videira, N., & Santos, R. (2015). Using participatory system dynamics in environmental and sustainability dialogues. In M. Ruth (Ed.), *Handbook of research methods and applications in environmental studies* (pp. 346–374). Edward Elgar Publishing. [CrossRef]

Aparcana, S. (2017). Approaches to formalization of the informal waste sector into municipal solid waste management systems in low- and middle-income countries: Review of barriers and success factors. *Waste Management, 61*, 593–607. [CrossRef]

Awuor, F. O., Nyakinya, B., Oloo, J., Oloko, M., & Agong', S. G. (2019). How Did kachok dumpsite in kisumu city develop into a crisis? *Urban Forum, 30*(1), 115–131. [CrossRef]

Ayeleru, O. O., Dlova, S., Akinribide, O. J., Ntuli, F., Kupolati, W. K., Marina, P. F., Blencowe, A., & Olubambi, P. A. (2020). Challenges of plastic waste generation and management in sub-Saharan Africa: A review. *Waste Management, 110*, 24–42. [CrossRef]

Bala, B. K., Arshad, F. M., & Noh, K. M. (2017). Modelling of solid waste management systems of Dhaka city in Bangladesh. In B. K. Bala, F. M. Arshad, & K. M. Noh (Eds.), *System dynamics: Modelling and simulation* (pp. 249–274). Springer. [CrossRef]

Barbrook-Johnson, P., & Penn, A. (2021). Participatory systems mapping for complex energy policy evaluation. *Evaluation, 27*(1), 57–79. [CrossRef]

Barnabè, F., & Davidsen, P. I. (2019). Exploring the potentials of behavioral system dynamics: Insights from the field. *Journal of Modelling in Management, 15*(1), 339–364. [CrossRef]

Boon, E. K., & Anuga, S. W. (2020). Circular economy and its relevance for improving food and nutrition security in sub-saharan africa: The case of ghana. *Materials Circular Economy, 2*(1), 5. [CrossRef]

Bortoleto, A. P. (2014). Driving forces and barriers for waste prevention behaviour. In *Waste prevention policy and behaviour*. Routledge.

(2022, June 20). *Breath of fresh air in Kisumu as Kachok dumpsite is finally levelled.* Nation. Available online: https://nation.africa/kenya/counties/kisumu/breath-of-fresh-air-in-kisumu-as-kachok-dumpsite-is-finally-levelled-3853778 (accessed on 1 October 2024).

Carvalho, T., Negm, H., & El-Geneidy, A. (2024). A Comparison of the Results from Artificial Intelligence-based and Human-based Transport-related Thematic Analysis. *Findings*. [CrossRef]

Chadwick, P., Paske, K., & Baars, V. (2021, January 12). *Applying behavioural science to reduce bullying, harassment and sexual misconduct within academia.* Centre for Behaviour Change. Available online: https://www.ucl.ac.uk/behaviour-change/news/2021/jan/applying-behavioural-science-reduce-bullying-harassment-and-sexual-misconduct-within (accessed on 1 October 2024).

Chan, J. K. H. (2016). The ethics of working with wicked urban waste problems: The case of Singapore's semakau landfill. *Landscape and Urban Planning, 154*, 123–131. [CrossRef]

Chaudhary, A. H., Polonsky, M. J., & McClaren, N. (2021). Littering behaviour: A systematic review. *International Journal of Consumer Studies*, *45*(4), 478–510. [CrossRef]

Chen, T., Gozgor, G., Koo, C. K., & Lau, C. K. M. (2020). Does international cooperation affect CO2 emissions? Evidence from OECD countries. *Environmental Science and Pollution Research*, *27*(8), 8548–8556. [CrossRef] [PubMed]

Christou, P. A. (2023). The use of artificial intelligence (ai) in qualitative research for theory development (1st edition). *The Qualitative Report*, *28*(9), 2739–2755.

Coletta, V. R., Pagano, A., Pluchinotta, I., Fratino, U., Scrieciu, A., Nanu, F., & Giordano, R. (2020). Causal loop diagrams for supporting nature based solutions participatory design and performance assessment. *Journal of Environmental Management*, *6*, 111668. [CrossRef] [PubMed]

County Government of Kisumu. (2017). *Kisumu integrated solid waste management plan (KISWaMP) by horizon 2030*; County Government of Kisumu.

Craig, P., Dieppe, P., Macintyre, S., Michie, S., Nazareth, I., & Petticrew, M. (2008). Developing and evaluating complex interventions: The new medical research council guidance. *BMJ*, *337*, a1655. [CrossRef]

Craven, L. K. (2017). System effects: A hybrid methodology for exploring the determinants of food in/security. *Annals of the American Association of Geographers*, *107*(5), 1011–1027. [CrossRef]

Craven, L. K., & Healy, M. (2021). *Barriers and enablers to the repair of electrical equipment: Application of the system effects methodology (EV0285)*; Department for Environment, Food and Rural Affairs.

Davies, M., Belesova, K., Crane, M., Hale, J., Haines, A., Hutchinson, E., Kiesewetter, G., Mberu, B., Mohajeri, N., Michie, S., Milner, J., Moore, G., Osrin, D., Pineo, H., Pluchinotta, I., Prasad, A., Salvia, G., Symonds, P., Taylor, J., . . . Wilkinson, P. (2021). The CUSSH programme: Learning how to support cities' transformational change towards health and sustainability. *Wellcome Open Research*, *6*, 100. [CrossRef]

Debrah, J. K., Teye, G. K., & Dinis, M. A. P. (2022). Barriers and Challenges to waste management hindering the circular economy in sub-saharan africa. *Urban Science*, *6*(3), 57. [CrossRef]

Department for Environment, Food & Rural Affairs. (2023a). *Barriers and enablers to reducing plate waste in hospitality settings A behavioural systems mapping project using the system effects method (PB1158)*. Available online: https://sciencesearch.defra.gov.uk/ProjectDetails?ProjectId=21323 (accessed on 1 October 2024).

Department for Environment, Food & Rural Affairs. (2023b). *Barriers to the use of timber in construction: A behavioural systems mapping project using the system effects method (PB1195)*. Available online: https://sciencesearch.defra.gov.uk/ProjectDetails?ProjectId=21391 (accessed on 1 October 2024).

Dianati, K., Schäfer, L., Milner, J., Gómez-Sanabria, A., Gitau, H., Hale, J., Langmaack, H., Kiesewetter, G., Muindi, K., Mberu, B., Zimmermann, N., Michie, S., Wilkinson, P., & Davies, M. (2021). A system dynamics-based scenario analysis of residential solid waste management in Kisumu, Kenya. *Science of The Total Environment*, *777*, 146200. [CrossRef]

Dioba, A., Kroker, V., Dewitte, S., & Lange, F. (2024). Barriers to pro-environmental behavior change: A review of qualitative research. *Sustainability*, *16*(20), 8776. [CrossRef]

Eker, S., & Zimmermann, N. (2016). Using textual data in system dynamics model conceptualization. *Systems*, *4*(3), 28. [CrossRef]

Ferrans, L., Avellán, T., Müller, A., Hettiarachchi, H., Dornack, C., & Caucci, S. (2019). Selecting sustainable sewage sludge reuse options through a systematic assessment framework: Methodology and case study in Latin America. *Journal of Cleaner Production*, *242*, 118389. [CrossRef]

Ferronato, N., & Torretta, V. (2019). Waste mismanagement in developing countries: A review of global issues. *International Journal of Environmental Research and Public Health*, *16*(6), 1060. [CrossRef] [PubMed]

Friedrich, E., & Trois, C. (2011). Quantification of greenhouse gas emissions from waste management processes for municipalities—A comparative review focusing on Africa. *Waste Management*, *31*(7), 1585–1596. [CrossRef]

Gatura, C., & Mberu, B. (2019). Chapter 12: Assessing solid waste management policies in Kenya. In *Breaking cycles of risk accumulation in african cities*. UN Habitat. Available online: https://unhabitat.org/sites/default/files/2020/03/un_report_2019_ebook_high_res.pdf (accessed on 1 October 2024).

Gray, S. (2018). Measuring systems thinking. *Nature Sustainability*, *1*(8), 388–389. [CrossRef]

Grimmelikhuijsen, S., Porumbescu, G., Hong, B., & Im, T. (2013). The effect of transparency on trust in government: A cross-national comparative experiment. *Public Administration Review*, *73*(4), 575–586. [CrossRef]

Groumpos, P. P. (2010). Fuzzy cognitive maps: Basic theories and their application to complex systems. In M. Glykas (Ed.), *Fuzzy cognitive maps: Advances in theory, methodologies, tools and applications* (pp. 1–22). Springer. [CrossRef]

Güneralp, B., Lwasa, S., Masundire, H., Parnell, S., & Seto, K. C. (2017). Urbanization in Africa: Challenges and opportunities for conservation. *Environmental Research Letters*, *13*(1), 015002. [CrossRef]

Gutberlet, J., Kain, J.-H., Nyakinya, B., Oloko, M., Zapata, P., & Zapata Campos, M. J. (2017). Bridging weak links of solid waste management in informal settlements. *The Journal of Environment & Development*, *26*(1), 106–131. [CrossRef]

Hale, J., Hastings, J., West, R., Lefevre, C. E., Direito, A., Bohlen, L. C., Godinho, C., Anderson, N., Zink, S., Groarke, H., & Michie, S. (2020). An ontology-based modelling system (OBMS) for representing behaviour change theories applied to 76 theories. *Wellcome Open Research*, *5*, 177. [CrossRef] [PubMed]

Hale, J., Jofeh, C., & Chadwick, P. (2022). Decarbonising existing homes in wales: A participatory behavioural systems mapping approach. *UCL Open: Environment*, *4*. [CrossRef]

Hamilton, L., Elliott, D., Quick, A., Smith, S., & Choplin, V. (2023). Exploring the use of AI in qualitative analysis: A comparative study of guaranteed income data. *International Journal of Qualitative Methods*, *22*, 16094069231201504. [CrossRef]

Henry, R. K., Yongsheng, Z., & Jun, D. (2006). Municipal solid waste management challenges in developing countries—Kenyan case study. *Waste Management*, *26*(1), 92–100. [CrossRef] [PubMed]

Johnson, O., Muhoza, C., Osano, P., Senyagwa, J., & Kartha, S. (2017). *Catalysing investment in sustainable energy infrastructure in Africa: Overcoming financial and non-financial constraints*. Stockholm Environment Institute. Available online: https://www.jstor.org/stable/resrep02834 (accessed on 1 October 2024).

(2023, April 13). *Kachok: Locals lose hope as promise of converting Kisumu dumpsite to garden wastes away*. Nation. Available online: https://nation.africa/kenya/counties/kisumu/kachok-locals-lose-hope-as-promise-of-converting-kisumu-dumpsite-to-garden-wastes-away-4197834 (accessed on 1 October 2024).

Kaza, S., Yao, L. C., Bhada-Tata, P., & Van Woerden, F. (2018). *What a waste 2.0: A global snapshot of solid waste management to 2050*. World Bank. Available online: https://www.worldbank.org/en/news/infographic/2018/09/20/what-a-waste-20-a-global-snapshot-of-solid-waste-management-to-2050 (accessed on 1 October 2024).

Kenya National Bureau of Statistics. (2019). *2019 Kenya population and housing census volume I: Population by county and sub-county*. Kenya National Bureau of Statistics. Available online: https://www.knbs.or.ke/?wpdmpro=2019-kenya-population-and-housing-census-volume-i-population-by-county-and-sub-county (accessed on 1 October 2024).

Kim, H., & Andersen, D. F. (2012). Building confidence in causal maps generated from purposive text data: Mapping transcripts of the Federal Reserve. *System Dynamics Review*, *28*(4), 311–328. [CrossRef]

(n.d.). *Kisumu*. CUSSH. Available online: https://projectcussh.org/cities/kisumu/ (accessed on 18 December 2024).

Kosko, B. (1986). Fuzzy cognitive maps. *International Journal of Man-Machine Studies*, *24*(1), 65–75. [CrossRef]

Kreuter, M. W., De Rosa, C., Howze, E. H., & Baldwin, G. T. (2004). Understanding wicked problems: A key to advancing environmental health promotion. *Health Education & Behavior*, *31*(4), 441–454. [CrossRef]

Lane, D. C. (2017). 'Behavioural system dynamics': A very tentative and slightly sceptical map of the territory. *Systems Research and Behavioral Science*, *34*(4), 414–423. [CrossRef]

Lee, L. W., Dabirian, A., McCarthy, I. P., & Kietzmann, J. (2020). Making sense of text: Artificial intelligence-enabled content analysis. *European Journal of Marketing*, *54*(3), 615–644. [CrossRef]

Liu, N. Y., & Keith, D. (2024, August 4–8). *The transformative potential of large language models for system dynamics modeling* [Paper presentation]. The 2024 International System Dynamics Conference, Bergen, Norway. Available online: https://proceedings.systemdynamics.org/2024/ (accessed on 1 October 2024).

Lönngren, J., & Svanström, M. (2016). Systems thinking for dealing with wicked sustainability problems: Beyond functionalist approaches. In W. Leal Filho, & S. Nesbit (Eds.), *New developments in engineering education for sustainable development* (pp. 151–160). Springer International Publishing. [CrossRef]

Lunetto, M., Hale, J., & Michie, S. (2022). Achieving effective climate action in cities by understanding behavioral systems. *One Earth*, *5*(7), 745–748. [CrossRef]

Ma, J., & Hipel, K. W. (2016). Exploring social dimensions of municipal solid waste management around the globe—A systematic literature review. *Waste Management*, *56*, 3–12. [CrossRef]

Michie, S., Atkins, L., & West, R. (2014). *The behaviour change wheel: A guide to designing interventions*. Silverback Publishing.

Michie, S., & Johnston, M. (2012). Theories and techniques of behaviour change: Developing a cumulative science of behaviour change. *Health Psychology Review*, *6*(1), 1–6. [CrossRef]

Michie, S., van Stralen, M. M., & West, R. (2011). The behaviour change wheel: A new method for characterising and designing behaviour change interventions. *Implementation Science*, *6*, 42. [CrossRef] [PubMed]

Mildeová, S. (2013). Research problem description and definition: From mental map to connection circle. *Journal on Efficiency and Responsibility in Education and Science*, *6*(4), 328–335. [CrossRef]

Moore, G., Michie, S., Anderson, J., Belesova, K., Crane, M., Deloly, C., Dimitroulopoulou, S., Gitau, H., Hale, J., Lloyd, S. J., Mberu, B., Muindi, K., Niu, Y., Pineo, H., Pluchinotta, I., Prasad, A., Roue-Le Gall, A., Shrubsole, C., Turcu, C., . . . Osrin, D. (2021). Developing a programme theory for a transdisciplinary research collaboration: Complex Urban Systems for Sustainability and Health. *Wellcome Open Research*, *6*, 35. [CrossRef]

Muheirwe, F., Kombe, W., & Kihila, J. M. (2022). The paradox of solid waste management: A regulatory discourse from Sub-Saharan Africa. *Habitat International*, *119*, 102491. [CrossRef]

Munala, G., & Moirongo, B. O. (2011). The need for an integrated solid waste management in kisumu, kenya. *Journal of Agriculture, Science and Technology, 13*(1). Available online: http://journals.jkuat.ac.ke/index.php/jagst/article/view/138 (accessed on 1 October 2024).

Nordlund, A., Eriksson, L., & Garvill, J. (2011). Barriers and facilitators for pro-environmental behaviour. In *Environmental policy and household behaviour*. Routledge.

Nyabundi, D. (n.d.). *Kisumu county gets land in Chiga to relocate Kachok dumpsite*. The Standard. Available online: http://www.standardmedia.co.ke/counties/article/2001339750/kisumu-county-gets-land-in-chiga-to-relocate-kachok-dumpsite (accessed on 12 October 2024).

Oyake-Ombis, L. (2017). *Awareness of environmentally sound solid waste management by communities and municipalities in Kenya*. UNDP. Available online: https://www.ke.undp.org/content/kenya/en/home/library/environment_energy/Sound-waste-management-bycommunities.html (accessed on 1 October 2024).

Pronk, T. E. (2019). The time efficiency gain in sharing and reuse of research data. *Data Science Journal, 18*, 10. [CrossRef]

Salvia, G., Zimmermann, N., Willan, C., Hale, J., Gitau, H., Muindi, K., Gichana, E., & Davies, M. (2021). The wicked problem of waste management: An attention-based analysis of stakeholder behaviours. *Journal of Cleaner Production, 326*, 129200. [CrossRef]

Shah, K. U., Niles, K., Ali, S. H., Surroop, D., & Jaggeshar, D. (2019). Plastics waste metabolism in a Petro-Island state: Towards solving a "wicked problem" in Trinidad and Tobago. *Sustainability, 11*(23), 6580. [CrossRef]

Sibanda, L. K., Obange, N., & Awuor, F. O. (2017). Challenges of solid waste management in Kisumu, Kenya. *Urban Forum, 28*(4), 387–402. [CrossRef]

Simiyu, S., Cairncross, S., & Swilling, M. (2019). Understanding Living Conditions and Deprivation in Informal Settlements of Kisumu, Kenya. *Urban Forum, 30*(2), 223–241. [CrossRef]

Srivastava, V., Ismail, S. A., Singh, P., & Singh, R. P. (2015). Urban solid waste management in the developing world with emphasis on India: Challenges and opportunities. *Reviews in Environmental Science and Bio/Technology, 14*(2), 317–337. [CrossRef]

Sudhir, V., Srinivasan, G., & Muraleedharan, V. R. (1997). Planning for sustainable solid waste management in urban India. *System Dynamics Review, 13*(3), 223–246. [CrossRef]

Sufian, M. A., & Bala, B. K. (2006). Modelling of electrical energy recovery from urban solid waste system: The case of Dhaka city. *Renewable Energy, 31*(10), 1573–1580. [CrossRef]

Sufian, M. A., & Bala, B. K. (2007). Modeling of urban solid waste management system: The case of Dhaka city. *Waste Management, 27*(7), 858–868. [CrossRef] [PubMed]

Talyan, V., Dahiya, R. P., Anand, S., & Sreekrishnan, T. R. (2007). Quantification of methane emission from municipal solid waste disposal in Delhi. *Resources, Conservation and Recycling, 50*(3), 240–259. [CrossRef]

Termeer, C. J. A. M., Dewulf, A., Breeman, G., & Stiller, S. J. (2015). Governance capabilities for dealing wisely with wicked problems. *Administration & Society, 47*(6), 680–710. [CrossRef]

Turner, B. L., Gates, R., Wuellner, M., Dunn, B., & Tedeschi, L. (2013a, July 21–25). *An investigation into land use changes and consequences in the northern great plains using systems thinking and dynamics* [Paper presentation]. The 31st International Conference of the System Dynamics Society, Cambridge, MA, USA. Available online: https://openprairie.sdstate.edu/nrm_pubs/104 (accessed on 1 October 2024).

Turner, B. L., Kim, H., & Andersen, D. F. (2013b). Improving coding procedures for purposive text data: Researchable questions for qualitative system dynamics modeling. *System Dynamics Review, 29*(4), 253–263. [CrossRef]

UNEP. (2024). *Global waste management outlook 2024*. Available online: https://wedocs.unep.org/bitstream/handle/20.500.11822/44939/global_waste_management_outlook_2024.pdf?sequence=3 (accessed on 1 October 2024).

United Nations Environment Programme. (2016). *Waste management: Global status*. United Nations. [CrossRef]

United Nations Environment Programme. (2018). *Africa waste management outlook | international environmental technology centre*. Available online: https://www.unep.org/ietc/resources/publication/africa-waste-management-outlook (accessed on 1 October 2024).

Vergara, S. E., & Tchobanoglous, G. (2012). Municipal solid waste and the environment: A global perspective. *Annual Review of Environment and Resources, 37*(1), 277–309. [CrossRef]

West, R., & Michie, S. (2020). A brief introduction to the COM-B Model of behaviour and the PRIME theory of motivation. *Qeios*. [CrossRef]

West, R., Michie, S., Atkins, L., Chadwick, P., & Lorencatto, F. (2019). *Achieving behaviour change: A guide for local government and partners*; Public Health England. Available online: https://assets.publishing.service.gov.uk/government/uploads/system/uploads/attachment_data/file/875385/PHEBI_Achieving_Behaviour_Change_Local_Government.pdf (accessed on 1 October 2024).

West, R., Michie, S., Chadwick, P., Atkins, L., & Lorencatto, F. (2020). *Achieving behaviour change: A guide for national government and partners*; Public Health England. Available online: https://assets.publishing.service.gov.uk/government/uploads/system/uploads/attachment_data/file/933328/UFG_National_Guide_v04.00__1___1_.pdf (accessed on 1 October 2024).

Wilson, D. C., & Velis, C. A. (2015). Waste management--still a global challenge in the 21st century: An evidence-based call for action. *Waste Management & Research: The Journal of the International Solid Wastes and Public Cleansing Association, ISWA, 33*(12), 1049–1051. [CrossRef]

Yearworth, M., & White, L. (2013). The uses of qualitative data in multimethodology: Developing causal loop diagrams during the coding process. *European Journal of Operational Research, 231*(1), 151–161. [CrossRef]

Zhang, Z., Chen, Z., Zhang, J., Liu, Y., Chen, L., Yang, M., Osman, A. I., Farghali, M., Liu, E., Hassan, D., Ihara, I., Lu, K., Rooney, D. W., & Yap, P.-S. (2024). Municipal solid waste management challenges in developing regions: A comprehensive review and future perspectives for Asia and Africa. *Science of The Total Environment, 930*, 172794. [CrossRef] [PubMed]

Zhu, H., de Bont, C., Gruber, T., & Dong, H. (2023, October). *Mapping Health-Seeking Behaviours and Influences in Rural China: A behavioural systems approach.* Relating Systems Thinking and Design (SD12) Symposium. Available online: https://rsdsymposium.org/wp-content/uploads/2024/06/Mapping-Health-Seeking-Behaviours-and-Influences-in-Rural-China_-A-behavioural-systems-approach.pdf (accessed on 1 October 2024).

behavioral sciences

MDPI

Article

Physical Exercise and Sleep Quality Among Chinese College Students: The Mediating Role of Self-Control and the Moderating Role of Mindfulness

Xiaopeng Li [1], Chengli Xu [1], Wanyi Chen [2,*] and Jing Tian [1]

[1] School of Physical Education and Sports, Central China Normal University, Wuhan 430079, China; xiaoepngli@mails.ccnu.edu.cn (X.L.); xuchengli007@163.com (C.X.); taratianjing@ccnu.edu.cn (J.T.)

[2] School of Psychology, South China Normal University, Guangzhou 510631, China

* Correspondence: psychenwy@m.scnu.edu.cn

Abstract: Although a few studies have examined the relationship between physical exercise and sleep quality, the underlying mechanisms of this association remain unclear. This study aims to investigate how and under what conditions physical exercise can promote the sleep quality among Chinese college students, with a focus on how self-control mediates and mindfulness moderates this relationship. Data were collected through convenient sampling from five universities in China, with a total of 1028 college students aged 16 to 29 participating in the study. Participants were recruited to complete the self-report questionnaires measuring their physical exercise, self-control, sleep quality and mindfulness. Results showed that physical exercise significantly and positively predicts sleep quality among Chinese college students. Further moderated mediation analyses indicated that self-control plays a significant mediating role, while mindfulness plays a moderating role in this relationship. Additionally, simple slopes analyses found that the moderating effect of mindfulness is more pronounced among individuals with lower levels of mindfulness compared to those with higher levels. The findings suggest that physical exercise can enhance sleep quality by improving self-control. Furthermore, physical exercise has a beneficial impact on self-control and sleep quality among college students with low mindfulness, while mindfulness itself exerts a distinct positive influence among those with high mindfulness.

Keywords: physical exercise; sleep quality; self-control; mindfulness

1. Introduction

According to a survey conducted by the World Health Organization, a quarter of adolescents have been reported feeling nervous, irritable or experiencing sleep difficulties each week (World Health Organization, 2021), and sleep disorders have emerged as a significant threat to public health worldwide (Hale et al., 2020). Notably, insomnia is particularly prevalent among college students, with an incidence rate as high as 18.5%, which is much higher than that of other age groups (Koyanagi & Stickley, 2015). Currently, poor sleep quality is a particularly serious problem among Chinese college students (Wu et al., 2021). A survey conducted in China indicates that 25.7% of Chinese college students experience sleep problems, a figure far exceeding the 7.4–15.0% reported in the general population (Q. Q. Liu et al., 2018). Therefore, numerous initiatives aimed at enhancing the sleep quality of Chinese college students have been proposed. In this context, researchers have been widely concerned with how physical exercise affects the sleep quality of college students.

In addition, as research in positive psychology has been progressively deepened, certain positive protective factors, including self-control (J. Liu et al., 2020) and mindfulness (Lentz & Brown, 2019), have garnered increasing attention. Previous studies have found that self-control plays a significant mediating role between physical exercise and health problems such as sedentary behavior (Boat et al., 2024), and a strong link exists between sedentary behavior and sleep quality among Chinese college students (X. Zhang et al., 2022), meaning that self-control likely serves as a mediator in the relationship between physical exercise and sleep quality among college students. Therefore, we introduced self-control to further examine whether it mediates the relationship between physical exercise and sleep quality. In addition, previous studies have proven that mindfulness is a strong enhancer that can enhance the positive impact of physical exercise on a healthy lifestyle (Ruffault et al., 2016), and mindfulness can play a moderating role between healthy lifestyle and sleep quality in college students (L. Zhang et al., 2022). This suggests, from an alternative theoretical perspective, that mindfulness might serve as a regulatory factor in the process by which physical exercise influences the sleep quality of college students. Therefore, the present study introduces mindfulness to explore its moderating role in the above mediating model. Although the positive relationship between physical exercise and sleep quality has been proved (Mahfouz et al., 2020), research on the potential mediating and moderating mechanisms of this relationship is still limited. It is necessary to explore the influencing factors and potential influence mechanisms of physical exercise on the sleep quality of college students. Therefore, this study constructed a moderated mediation model to explore the underlying mechanisms between physical exercise and sleep quality.

1.1. Physical Exercise and Sleep Quality

Physical exercise is a physical activity with a certain intensity, frequency, and du-ration to improve health (Jiang et al., 2009). On the one hand, studies have shown that regular physical exercise is a positive and non-drug treatment for those with poor sleep quality. Specifically, physical exercise can improve the negative psychological emotions of college students, such as depression (Slykerman et al., 2020), anxiety (Patterson et al., 2021), and stress (Herawati & Gayatri, 2019), which could further improve their sleep quality. On the other hand, experimental studies have also shown that regular physical exercise in individuals can increase melatonin secretion levels in individuals, which can enhance their sleep quality (Chennaoui et al., 2015). All these benefits of physical exercise mentioned above can help to improve college students' sleep quality. In consideration of the above, we proposed the following hypothesis:

Hypothesis 1. *Physical exercise may have a positive impact on sleep quality among Chinese college students.*

1.2. The Mediating Role of Self-Control

Self-control is the ability of an individual to regulate reactions to overcome impulses, which requires individuals to independently adjust their behavior and conform to social expectations and their own values by changing their own behavior, way of thinking, and level of consciousness (MacLean et al., 2014). It has been verified that an individual's self-control is consistently and closely related to health behaviors. Specifically, an individual's self-control is positively related to health-promoting behaviors and negatively related to health-damaging behaviors (Hagger et al., 2019a). Poor sleep quality among college students due to sleep latency is an unhealthy behavior that implies a failure of individual self-control (Kroese et al., 2016). This means that college students succumb to other temptations before going to sleep, resulting in delayed sleep and poor sleep quality. Based on the fact that self-control is a limited resource, relevant studies further show that college students expend a lot of self-control resources during the day, resulting in the least self-control resources at night. This means there is a greater tendency for sleep procrastination in individuals with relatively depleted self-control resources, which can lead to poorer sleep quality (Bernecker & Job, 2020).

Physical exercise has been shown to be an effective way to improve individual self-control. Specifically, individuals who participate in regular physical exercise tend to have higher levels of self-control, which in turn affects the management of individuals' resources to implement goal-directed behaviors to achieve long-term goals, such as developing healthy sleep habits (Eysenck et al., 2007). Interestingly, it has been reported that self-control can play a mediating role between physical exercise and healthy lifestyle habits in college students (Hagger et al., 2019b), and an experimental study has been also observed that aerobic exercise may be a potentially effective intervention to enhance self-control in female college students, which could be beneficial in helping college students to develop their healthy habits (Chen et al., 2019). Sleep quality is an important organizing component of healthy lifestyle habits. Although there is no direct evidence that self-control can directly mediate the relationship between physical exercise and sleep quality, considering the similarities between sleep quality and healthy lifestyle habits, we hypothesized that self-control may play a mediating role in the relationship between physical exercise and sleep quality among college students. Thus, we proposed the following hypothesis:

Hypothesis 2. *Self-control may act as a mediator in the link between physical exercise and sleep quality among college students.*

1.3. The Moderating Role of Mindfulness

Mindfulness refers to being aware of the present reality or current experience in an accepting or non-judgmental way (Brown & Ryan, 2003). Previous research has shown that high mindfulness could promote physical and mental health such as sleep quality, positive effects, and self-control (Bajaj et al., 2016; Lyddy et al., 2021). In recent years, a growing number of studies have confirmed that high levels of mindfulness can play an enhancing or buffering role in self-control and sleep quality in college students, such as a study by Lentz and Brown (Lentz & Brown, 2019), who suggested that the relationship between physical exercise and sleep quality was intensified for college students with high mindfulness.

According to the re-perceiving model of mindfulness, mindfulness can help people re-perceive the moment-by-moment experience with greater objectivity, get rid of automatic behavioral and emotional patterns, and facilitate adaptive responses to negative stimulation (Shapiro et al., 2006), which means that mindfulness can buffer the adverse effects of negative factors on an individual. Indeed, it is also true that previous studies have confirmed that mindfulness can buffer the adverse effects of negativity, such as in Davis et al. (2016), who showed that mindfulness can relieve college students' anxiety, depression, and other negative psychological emotions, which has been proven to be one of the important factors for promoting the ability of college students to improve their sleep quality. In other words, mindfulness acts as a buffer with respect to psychological distress for individuals, which can help people avoid sleep disorders and improve sleep quality on a psychological level. Furthermore, according to the protection–protection model, two different protective factors will interact with each other, increasing or decreasing the outcome (Boksem et al., 2006). Specifically, the enhancing interaction hypothesis suggests that the effect of one protective factor (e.g., physical exercise) on its outcome (e.g., self-control) may be enhanced by another protective factor (e.g., mindfulness). Namely, individuals with high levels of mindfulness showed stronger associations between physical exercise and self-control than individuals with low levels of mindfulness. For example, a study indicated that the relationships between physical exercise and self-control were moderated by mindfulness, in that they were stronger for adolescents with higher levels of mindfulness (Stocker et al., 2019). Another study indicated that the direct effect of deprivation on sleep quality and its indirect effect through social anxiety were both moderated by mindfulness, in that those two effects were weaker in individuals with high levels of mindfulness (Xiong et al., 2023). Thus, mindfulness serves as an important protective factor that can reinforce the positive effects of physical exercise. In other words, the link between physical exercise and sleep quality, as well as the link between physical exercise and self-control, may be moderated by mindfulness. Above all, we propose the hypothesis as follows:

Hypothesis 3. *Mindfulness would moderate the relationship between physical exercise and sleep quality as well as physical exercise and self-control.*

1.4. Research Objective

Although the precise mechanisms remain not fully elucidated, substantial evidence suggests significant associations between physical exercise, sleep quality, self-control, and mindfulness. We posit that integrating these factors into a comprehensive model could effectively broaden the research perspective on sleep quality among college students. Taken together, we constructed a moderated mediation model in this study (Figure 1).

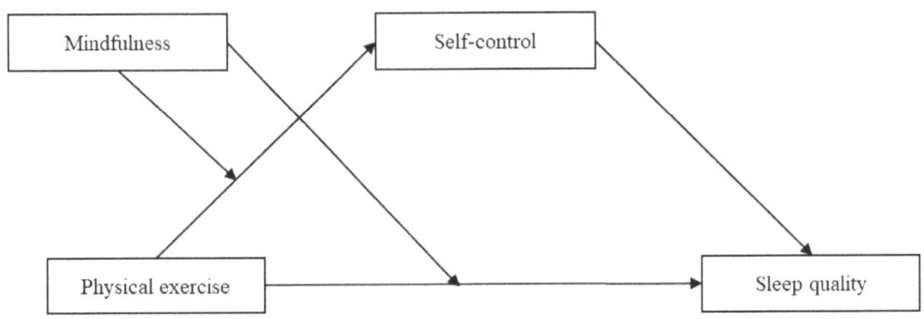

Figure 1. The proposed moderated mediation model.

The objective of our study was to investigate the impact of physical exercise on sleep quality among college students, while examining the mediating role of self-control and the moderating role of mindfulness in this relationship. Our findings aim to uncover the underlying mechanisms contributing to poor sleep quality among college students and to offer solutions to enhance sleep quality among Chinese college students.

2. Methods

2.1. Participants

A total of 1141 students participated in our study. After excluding participants who provided incomplete information and those who completed the survey in an unrealistically short time, the final sample consisted of 1028 participants. Among them, there were 487 (47.37%) males and 541 (52.63%) females. Their average age was 19.14 years old (SD = 1.85), ranging from 16 to 29 years old. Among the participants, 399 were freshmen (38.79%), 395 were sophomores (38.45%), 105 were juniors (10.17%), and 129 were seniors (12.76%). Additionally, there were 19 first-year graduate students (1.90%), 32 second-year graduate students (3.10%), and 50 third-year graduate students (4.83%).

2.2. Procedure

This study was conducted in accordance with the principles of the Declaration of Helsinki (World Medical Association, 2013) and approved by the Ethics Committee for Scientific Research at the authors' institution. Data were collected through convenience sampling from 5 comprehensive universities in Hubei Province, a major province in central China. The survey was conducted through an online platform called Wen Juan Xing (https://www.wjx.cn/) from 24 May to 21 June 2024. Prior to the study, all participants received an electronic informed consent, which provided detailed information about the survey and its procedure. Participants were also informed that they could terminate their participation at any time without any repercussions. Students who agreed to participate then completed the surveys by scanning the Quick Response (QR) code of the questionnaire at their school using their mobile phones or computers. It took approximately 10 min for all participants to complete the anonymous self-reported questionnaires.

3. Measures

3.1. Physical Exercise

Physical exercise was assessed using the Physical Activity Rating Scale (PARS-3), developed by Liang (1994). This scale consists of three items measuring the exercise intensity, exercise time, and exercise frequency of the participants to assess their physical activity level. Exercise frequency, exercise time, and exercise intensity were scored from 1–5. The physical activity level of the test subjects was calculated according to the formula of physical activity amount = exercise intensity $\times$ (exercise time $-$ 1) $\times$ exercise frequency. The higher the score measured by the scale, the higher the level of physical activity of the participants. Cronbach's alpha coefficient for the PARS-3 was 0.79.

3.2. Sleep Quality

This study used the Chinese version of the Pittsburgh Sleep Quality Index (PSQI, Liu, 1996), which was adapted from the original scale developed by Buysse et al. (1989). Previous studies have shown that the Chinese version of the PSQI has demonstrated good reliability and validity (Zheng et al., 2016). The PSQI consists of seven dimensions, including 19 items measuring individuals' subjective sleep quality, sleep latency, sleep duration, habitual sleep efficiency, sleep disturbance, sleep medication used, and daytime dysfunction. All items were scored from 0–3 and the total score ranged from 0–21. In the original scale, higher scores indicate poorer sleep quality. For better understanding, we have reversed all the items in this study. The higher the score, the better the individual's sleep quality. In this study, Cronbach's alpha for the PSQI was 0.82.

3.3. Self-Control

The Chinese version of the Self-Control Scale was used in our study (Tan & Guo, 2008). This scale comprises five dimensions, including 19 items that measure individuals' self-control through resisting temptation, impulse control, healthy habits, task performance, and entertainment temperance. Participants responded to the 19 items on a five-point Likert-type scale ranging from 1 (not at all) to 5 (very much), with a higher total score indicating better self-control. In the current study, the items demonstrated acceptable reliability (Cronbach's $\alpha = 0.82$).

3.4. Mindfulness

In this study, we used the Child and Adolescent Mindfulness Measure (CAMM, Greco et al., 2011) to measure the participants' level of mindfulness. The CAMM consists of 10 items. Participants rated their agreement with these items on a five-point Likert scale, ranging from 0 (never) to 4 (always). All responses were averaged after reversing the reverse-scored item. The higher the score, the higher the level of mindfulness in daily life. In this study, Cronbach's alpha of the CAMM was 0.81.

3.5. Control Variables

Gender and age were included as control variables in our study because previous studies found that they were closely associated with the main variables in this study (Lueke & Assar, 2024; Li et al., 2016).

3.6. Data Analysis

Data management and analysis were performed using SPSS 29.0 and the PROCESS macro developed by Hayes in 2013 (Version 3.5; https://www.processmacro.org/download.html, accessed on 1 November 2024). First, missing data accounted for less than 5% and were handled using the expectation maximization (EM) approach before conducting subsequent analyses (Schlomer et al., 2010). Next, a Harman single factor test was conducted to address potential common method biases (Podsakoff et al., 2003). Third, descriptive analysis of the main variables and Pearson correlation analysis were performed. Considering that data standardization in moderated mediation analysis helps to eliminate scale differences, reduce multicollinearity, and enhance model interpretability and stability (Hayes & Rockwood, 2016), we standardized the data.

Fourth, we conducted a Bootstrap analysis using the SPSS PROCESS macro (model 8) suggested by Hayes to test the proposed moderated mediation model. In addition, simple slopes analyses were performed to test all the potential significant interaction effects. Bootstrap confidence intervals (95% CIs) based on 5000 random samples of the data were utilized to determine the significance of the regression coefficients in Model 8. The effects were considered significant if the 95% CI did not include a zero value (Preacher et al., 2007). In addition, simple slopes analyses were conducted to examine all potential significant interaction effects. The simple slope test, also known as the pick-a-point approach or spotlight analysis (Hayes, 2017), is a conditional hypothesis test that assesses whether the relationship between an independent variable and a dependent variable is significant at specific values of the moderator (Hayes, 2015; Memon et al., 2019). In our analysis, we used the ± 1 standard deviation method to probe the effects of mindfulness at different levels. This approach allows us to evaluate the moderating effects of mindfulness without altering its continuous nature, thereby providing a detailed understanding of how mindfulness influences the relationships between physical exercise and sleep quality, as well as physical exercise and self-control.

4. Results

4.1. Analysis of Common Method Bias

Considering that this study adopts the method of the questionnaire survey, there may be the risk of common method bias (Tehseen et al., 2017). Although this study took some measures to reduce the common method bias in the process of data distribution, such as selecting a measurement instrument with high reliability and validity, anonymous responding, and using reverse scoring for scale items, the common method bias may still exist. Thus, we tested it by using the Harman single-factor method (Podsakoff et al., 2003). The results showed that there were 10 factors with eigenvalues greater than 1, among which the variation explained by the first factor was 14.79%, which was less than the critical criterion of 40%. Therefore, it could be concluded that there was no significant common method bias in the data of this study.

4.2. Preliminary Analyses

The means (M), standard deviations (SD), and correlations for all of the observed variables are presented in Table 1. As hypothesized, physical exercise was positively correlated with both self-control ($r = 0.32$, $p < 0.001$) and sleep quality ($r = 0.26$, $p < 0.001$).

Self-control was positively correlated with both sleep quality (r = 0.40, p < 0.001) and mindfulness (r = 0.29, p < 0.001). Mindfulness was positively correlated with sleep quality (r = 0.51, p < 0.001).

Table 1. Descriptive statistics and interrelations among all of the observed variables.

Variables	*M*	*SD*	1	2	3	4	5	6
1. Gender [a]	1.53	0.50	1					
2. Age	19.14	1.85	−0.03	1				
3. Physical exercise	2.48	1.03	−0.34 ***	0.22 ***	1			
4. Self-control	3.30	0.63	−0.07 *	0.23	0.32 ***	1		
5. Sleep quality	−4.93	2.9	−0.11 ***	0.02	0.26 ***	0.40 ***	1	
6. Mindfulness	2.47	0.72	−0.10 **	0.06	0.13 ***	0.29 ***	0.51 ***	1

Note. N = 1028. *** p < 0.001, ** p < 0.01, * p < 0.05. [a] 0 = male, 1 = female.

4.3. Testing for the Proposed Moderated Mediation Model

In this study, we adopted Hayes's (2013) PROCESS macro (Model 8) to examine the proposed moderated mediation model. The main results of the moderated mediation analysis were shown in Figure 2 and Table 2.

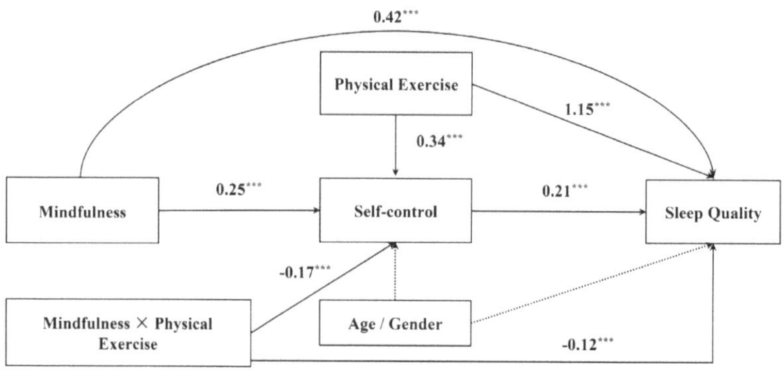

Figure 2. Results for the hypothesized moderated mediation model. Note: N = 1028. *** p < 0.001.

Table 2. Regression results for the conditional indirect effect (moderated mediation).

Model									
Model 1: Total effect model (outcome variable: sleep quality)									
R	R^2	*F*	df_1	df_2	*p*	β	*SE*	*t*	*p*
0.26	0.07	24.97	3	1024	<0.001				
Constant						5.41 ***	0.97	5.59	<0.001
Gender						−0.03	0.03	−0.84	0.40
Age						−0.04	0.03	−1.15	0.25
Physical exercise						0.26 ***	0.03	7.80	<0.001
Model 2: Mediator variable model (outcome variable: self-control)									
R	R^2	*F*	df_1	df_2	*p*	β	*SE*	*t*	*p*
0.45	0.21	53.25	5	1022	<0.001				
Constant						1.61 **	0.24	6.60	<0.001
Gender						0.07	0.04	1.84	0.06
Age						−0.02	0.01	−1.81	0.07
Physical exercise						0.34 ***	0.03	11.03	<0.001
Mindfulness						0.25 ***	0.03	8.69	<0.001
Physical exercise × Mindfulness						−0.17 ***	0.03	−6.48	<0.001

Table 2. *Cont.*

Model									
Model 3: Dependent variable model (outcome variable: sleep quality)									
R	R^2	F	df_1	df_2	p	β	SE	t	p
0.6	0.36	97.18	6	1021	<0.001				
Constant						0.01	0.03	0.60	0.55
Gender						−0.12	0.27	−0.68	0.50
Age						−0.04	0.03	−1.42	0.16
Physical exercise						1.15 ***	0.03	5.19	<0.001
Self-control						0.21 ***	0.03	7.47	<0.001
Mindfulness						0.42 ***	0.03	16.26	<0.001
Physical exercise × Mindfulness						−0.12 ***	0.02	−4.96	<0.001
Conditional direct effect analysis at values of mindfulness ($M \pm SD$)									
						β	Boot SE	LLCI	ULCI
$M - 1SD$ (1.75)						0.27 ***	0.04	0.19	0.35
M (2.47)						0.15 ***	0.03	0.09	0.21
$M + 1SD$ (3.22)						0.03	0.04	−0.04	0.10
Conditional indirect effect analysis at values of mindfulness ($M \pm SD$)									
						β	Boot SE	LLCI	ULCI
$M - 1SD$ (1.75)						0.51 ***	0.04	0.42	0.59
M (2.47)						0.34 ***	0.03	0.28	0.40
$M + 1SD$ (3.22)						0.17 ***	0.04	0.09	0.24

Note. *** $p < 0.001$, ** $p < 0.01$.

After controlling for gender and age, moderated mediation analyses were conducted. As expected, physical exercise showed a positive and significant total effect on sleep quality, with a regression coefficient being 0.26 (95% CI [0.19, 0.32], $p < 0.001$). When self-control was included as a mediator in the regression equation, physical exercise could still significantly predict sleep quality (β = 0.13, 95% CI [0.07, 0.19], $p < 0.001$). Moreover, self-control showed a positive and significant effect on sleep quality (β = 0.36, 95% CI [0.30, 0.42], $p < 0.001$). Physical exercise also significantly predicted self-control (β = 0.35, 95% CI [0.28, 0.41], $p < 0.001$). Furthermore, a Sobel test was employed to examine the significance of the indirect effect of self-control. Results showed that self-control significantly mediated the relationship between physical exercise and sleep quality ($Z = -8.08$, $p < 0.001$). These results provided compelling evidence that physical exercise can improve the sleep quality of college students, and this relationship is mediated by self-control. Thus, Hypotheses 1 and 2 were supported.

The solid line represents a significant effect and the dashed line represents a non-significant effect.

To test Hypothesis 3, mindfulness was included as a moderator in the regression equation. These results showed that mindfulness could positively and significantly predict self-control (β = 0.25, 95% CI [0.19, 0.30], $p < 0.001$) and sleep quality (β = 0.42, 95% CI [0.37, 0.48], $p < 0.001$). Furthermore, two interaction effects were further analyzed. The results showed that there was a significant physical exercise × mindfulness effect on self-control (β = −0.17, 95% CI [−0.22, −0.12], $p < 0.001$) in the mediator variable model. Furthermore, the effect of physical exercise × mindfulness on sleep quality (β = −0.12, 95% CI [−0.17, −0.07], $p < 0.001$) was also significant in the dependent variable model. These results suggest that both the relationship between exercise and sleep quality and the relationship between exercise and self-control were moderated by mindfulness. Hypothesis 3 was supported.

Additionally, simple slope analyses were conducted to further explain the moderating effect. Specifically, these analyses investigated whether the slopes for individuals with high mindfulness capacity (one standard deviation above the mean) differed from those of individuals with low mindfulness capacity (one standard deviation below the mean) in both mediator and dependent variable models. For visual inspection of the direction and strength of the moderating effect, we report the simple slope plots (see Figures 3 and 4). As shown in Figure 3, physical exercise could positively and significantly predict self-control for college students with both high and low mindfulness. Interestingly, the effect of physical exercise on self-control was stronger for those with lower mindfulness ($\beta = 0.51$, $t = 12.23$, 95% CI [0.42, 0.58], $p < 0.001$) than for those with higher mindfulness ($\beta = 0.17$, $t = 4.28$, 95% CI [0.06, 0.24], $p < 0.001$). Furthermore, as shown in Figure 4, the effect of physical exercise on sleep quality was positive and significant for college students with low mindfulness ($\beta = 0.27$, $t = 6.77$, 95% CI [0.19, 0.35], $p < 0.001$), whereas it was not significant for those with high mindfulness ($\beta = 0.03$, $t = 0.88$, 95% CI [−0.04, 0.10], $p > 0.05$). These findings indicate that physical exercise has a beneficial impact on self-control and sleep quality among individuals with low mindfulness, while mindfulness itself exerts a distinct influence among those with high mindfulness. Specifically, for individuals with low mindfulness, physical exercise significantly enhances both sleep quality and self-control. In contrast, for individuals with higher levels of mindfulness, although physical exercise still promoted self-control, its effect on sleep quality was no longer significant.

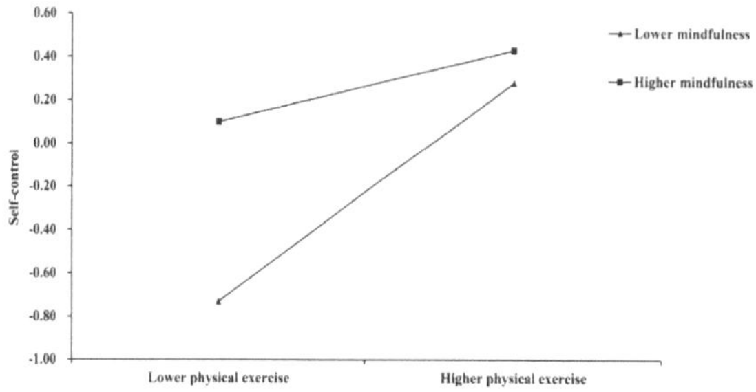

Figure 3. Mindfulness moderates the relationship between physical exercise and self-control.

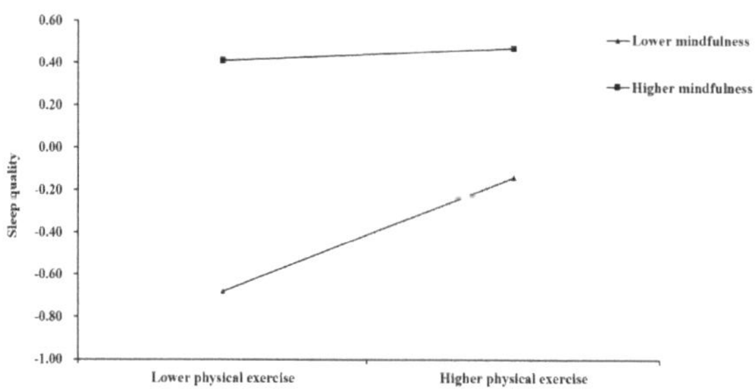

Figure 4. Mindfulness moderates the relationship between physical exercise and sleep quality.

5. Discussion

5.1. Physical Exercise and Sleep Quality

The present study demonstrates that physical exercise significantly and positively correlates with the sleep quality of college students. These findings are consistent with prior research investigating the impact of physical activity on sleep quality among college students (Bodziony & Stetson, 2024). Thus, Hypothesis 1 has been confirmed. However, our study further suggests that multiple factors may underlie the positive association between physical exercise and sleep quality among college students, with both physiological and psychological aspects providing explanatory frameworks for these results. From a physiological perspective, numerous studies have established a clear connection between body temperature regulation and sleep quality (Chang et al., 2009; Quanten et al., 2006). For example, physical exercise triggers an elevation in central, skin, and cerebral temperatures. Consequently, under the thermoregulatory mechanism, peripheral blood vessels dilate, facilitating heat emission to the periphery and resulting in a decrease in overall body temperature. Research indicates that a reduction in body temperature by 0.5–1 °C enhances the likelihood of falling asleep and promotes better sleep quality Moreover, post-exercise changes in body surface temperature, particularly the gradient between distal and proximal skin temperatures, may serve as a pivotal factor in initiating sleep onset for individuals (Kräuchi, 2007). Additionally, exercise induces alterations in serotonin, epinephrine, melatonin, and cortisol levels, all of which have been linked to variations in sleep quality (Chennaoui et al., 2015). From a psychological point of view, improving college students' emotional state through exercise has been shown to be an important additional factor in improving their sleep quality (Ghrouz et al., 2019). Specifically, many adverse psychological emotions such as anxiety, depression (Slykerman et al., 2020), and stress (Herawati & Gayatri, 2019) could affect the sleep quality of college students. Further studies have shown that improving the above-mentioned psychological emotions can enhance the sleep quality of college students (Johnston et al., 2021).

In summary, our study shows that, on the one hand, proper physical activity can help college students fall asleep faster and have a better sleep quality. Several physiological factors such as hormones, fatigue, and body temperature changes may provide an explanation for this phenomenon. On the other hand, engaging in appropriate physical activity can also alleviate the psychological distress of college students, which can im-prove their sleep quality from a psychological perspective.

5.2. The Mediating Role of Self-Control

Our study elucidates the mediating role of self-control in influencing the relationship between physical exercise and sleep quality among college students. In line with previous research, self-control has been identified as a mediator in the association between physical exercise and the adoption of healthy lifestyle habits (Kuang et al., 2023). Our investigation extends this understanding by demonstrating that self-control significantly moderates the relationship between physical exercise and sleep quality in college students. Specifically, Chinese college students who regularly participate in physical exercise exhibit higher levels of self-control, leading to enhanced sleep quality. As illustrated in the first half of this study, according to the self-control resource model, when college students conduct self-control activities during the day and consume part of their self-control resources, their self-control resources are often deficient at night. At this time, college students do not easily resist temptation (such as using mobile phones, etc.), which can disrupt sleep patterns and reduce sleep quality. However, it has been confirmed that physical exercise could improve the self-control ability of college students; that is, college students who often participate in physical exercise often have a higher level of self-control ability and more self-control resources, which makes it easier for them to resist various external temptations and improve their sleep quality. In other words, adequate sleep can improve individuals' self-control ability, and when they have more self-control resources, they are more likely to resist temptation, make sleep a higher priority, and have better-quality sleep. Our study further suggests that, through physical exercise, improved self-control ability could improve the sleep quality of college students, which may serve as a theoretical guideline for future family education and school education in improving the sleep quality of college students.

5.3. The Moderating Role of Mindfulness

One significant finding from our study was the potential moderating effect of mindfulness on the relationship between physical exercise and self-control. Specifically, both the direct effect that physical exercise itself exerted on sleep quality and the indirect effect of self-control were moderated and buffered by mindfulness, with these effects being stronger for college students with lower levels of mindfulness. This outcome suggests that mindfulness, as a positive personality trait, may enhance the self-control capacities of college students during physical exercise. As their self-control strengthens, they are better equipped to resist negative temptations, thereby potentially improving their sleep quality. This finding is consistent with the enhancing interaction hypothesis in the protective model (Wills et al., 1992), which posits that both mindfulness and self-control serve as protective factors, with each factor enhancing the effects of the other. Specifically, self-control is recognized as a protective factor that provides individuals with the executive function necessary to avoid staying up late, resist poor optimization, and pursue a healthy lifestyle. Mindfulness is also regarded as another protective factor that enhances individuals' awareness of the health risks associated with staying up late and experiencing poor sleep quality, thereby facilitating these processes. That is, individuals with higher levels of mindfulness exhibit lower sensitivity compared to those with diminished levels of mindfulness in the context of self-control's impact on sleep quality. The findings from our study reveal an intriguing result: the simple slope at low levels of mindfulness was significantly greater than that at high levels of mindfulness. This suggests that for college students exhibiting low levels of mindfulness, physical exercise serves as a highly effective means to enhance self-control, with mindfulness functioning primarily as a complementary factor in this process. This finding presented above offers a novel perspective in terms of enhancing the sleep quality of college students: it is essential to focus more on college students with low levels of mindfulness than those with high levels.

Furthermore, this finding also further supports the Metacognitive Model of Insomnia, which model contends that an individual's ability to accurately observe internal and external experiences (e.g., mindfulness) and respond appropriately to external stimuli related to sleep significantly influence sleep quality (Ong et al., 2012). This suggests that college students with higher mindfulness are more attuned to both their internal and external experiences, thereby gaining a clearer appreciation of the health benefits associated with improved sleep quality. Consequently, individuals with higher mindfulness levels tend to exhibit greater adaptability in addressing sleep disorders, often resorting to positive coping mechanisms, potentially enhancing their sleep quality. The aforementioned phenomenon further elucidates why individuals with high levels of mindfulness do not show strong sensitivity to the effects of physical exercise on sleep quality. It is particularly intriguing to observe from the simple slope graph that as levels of mindfulness increase, the impact of physical exercise on sleep quality diminishes. Notably, we encountered a counterintuitive finding indicating that physical activity did not significantly influence sleep quality in individuals with higher levels of mindfulness. This observation further underscores that the relationship between physical exercise and sleep quality among col-lege students constitutes a holistic and systematic process; thus, understanding this in-ternal dynamic cannot be fully achieved by examining each component in isolation. For instance, our results indicate that when analyzing the effects of physical exercise and mindfulness on college students' sleep quality separately, both factors exhibit positive influences. However, when exploring their interaction concerning sleep quality, we encounter inconsistent outcomes. This suggests that in both research and practical ap-plications, it is essential to avoid viewing the effects of physical exercise and sleep quality in isolation. Instead, considering their interplay is crucial for comprehensively and accurately addressing issues related to sleep quality. Thus, it is imperative for relevant authorities, such as educators and practitioners, to recognize an intriguing insight: individuals with higher levels of mindfulness were significantly less likely to have sleep risks, and encouraging them to participate in physical exercise did not improve their sleep quality. On the contrary, for individuals who do not possess a strong inclination towards physical activity, enhancing their level of mindfulness appears to be an effective strategy for improving sleep quality.

5.4. Limitations and Future Directions

Although our study contributes new evidence regarding the mediating role of self-control and the moderating effect of mindfulness on the relationship between physical exercise and sleep quality in college students, it is essential to recognize several limitations. Firstly, our study utilized a cross-sectional design, which precludes establishing definitive causal relationships between variables. Secondly, the use of convenience sampling and the restriction to participants from only Hubei Province may introduce sampling biases and limit the generalizability of our findings. Additionally, our investigation focused solely on two internal factors, namely self-control and mindfulness, without considering a broader array of external influences.

To address the limitations of our study and further explore the impact of physical exercise on college students' sleep quality, future research could be enhanced in the following ways: Firstly, given the methodological limitations, subsequent studies should employ longitudinal follow-up research to ascertain the causal relationships between variables more accurately. Secondly, considering the limitations of our sampling methods and participant selection, future research endeavors could broaden the dataset and explore the model using random or stratified sampling techniques to examine diverse and larger cohorts. Lastly, acknowledging the constraints of our current understanding of influencing mechanisms, future research could incorporate additional variables, particularly external factors such as family environment (Counts et al., 2018) and school support (Wang & Bíró, 2021). This broader scope of investigation would enable a more comprehensive exploration of how these external factors interact to influence college students' sleep quality.

6. Conclusions

The results of this study reveal a significant positive correlation between physical exercise and the sleep quality of college students, which is mediated by self-control and moderated by mindfulness. Specifically, physical exercise can not only directly improve the sleep quality of college students, but also enhance their sleep quality indirectly through self-control. In addition, mindfulness plays a crucial moderating role in both the direct and indirect pathways mentioned above. Notably, the moderating effect of mindfulness is more pronounced among individuals with lower levels of mindfulness compared to those with relatively higher mindfulness levels. Physical exercise has a beneficial impact on self-control and sleep quality among college students with low mindfulness, while mindfulness itself exerts a distinct influence among those with high mindfulness. Overall, while our study acknowledges certain limitations, it significantly contributes to the understanding of the interplay between physical exercise, sleep quality, self-control, and mindfulness among college students. Furthermore, this research offers valuable insights for parents and educators in developing programs aimed at promoting sleep quality and fostering healthy living policies for adolescents.

Author Contributions: X.L.: Data Collection, Writing—original draft, Writing—Review & Editing; C.X.: Resources and Funding, Data Collection; W.C.: Research Design, Data Analysis, Writing—Review & Editing; J.T.: Data Collection. All authors have read and agreed to the published version of the manuscript.

Funding: This research, as well as the APC, were funded by General Project of China Social Science Foundation (Grant No. 22BTY009).

Institutional Review Board Statement: Ethical review and approval were waived for this study due to the study protocol complying with the ethical guidelines of Central China Normal University, but the ethics committee of Central China Normal University considered that the study protocol was conducted by questionnaire only and no written ethical review report was required.

Informed Consent Statement: Informed consent was obtained from all subjects involved in the study.

Data Availability Statement: The data presented in this study are available on request from the corresponding author.

Acknowledgments: The authors would like to appreciate all participants, parents and the teachers for their support and cooperation during the investigation.

Conflicts of Interest: The authors declare no conflicts of interest.

References

Bajaj, B., Gupta, R., & Pande, N. (2016). Self-esteem mediates the relationship between mindfulness and well-being. *Personality and Individual Differences, 94*, 96–100. [CrossRef]

Bernecker, K., & Job, V. (2020). Too exhausted to go to bed: Implicit theories about willpower and stress predict bedtime procrastination. *British Journal of Psychology, 111*(1), 126–147. [CrossRef]

Boat, R., Williams, R. A., Dring, K. J., Morris, J. G., Sunderland, C., Nevill, M. E., & Cooper, S. B. (2024). Associations of self-control with physical activity, physical fitness, and adiposity in adolescents. *Behavioral Medicine, 50*(1), 82–90. [CrossRef]

Bodziony, V., & Stetson, B. (2024). Associations between sleep, physical activity, and emotional well-being in emerging young adults: Implications for college wellness program development. *Journal of American College Health, 72*(4), 1057–1067. [CrossRef]

Boksem, M. A., Meijman, T. F., & Lorist, M. M. (2006). Mental fatigue, motivation and action monitoring. *Biological Psychology, 72*(2), 123–132. [CrossRef]

Brown, K. W., & Ryan, R. M. (2003). The benefits of being present: Mindfulness and its role in psychological well-being. *Journal of Personality and Social Psychology, 84*(4), 822. [CrossRef]

Buysse, D. J., Reynolds, C. F., Monk, T. H., Berman, S. R., & Kupfer, D. J. (1989). The Pittsburgh sleep quality index: A new instrument for psychiatric practice and research. *Psychiatry Research, 28*(2), 193–213. [CrossRef] [PubMed]

Chang, A., Reid, K. J., Gourineni, R., & Zee, P. C. (2009). Sleep timing and circadian phase in delayed sleep phase syndrome. *Journal of Biological Rhythms, 24*(4), 313–321. [CrossRef]

Chen, X., Zhang, G., Yin, X., Li, Y., Cao, G., Gutiérrez-García, C., & Guo, L. (2019). The relationship between self-efficacy and aggressive behavior in boxers: The mediating role of self-control. *Frontiers in Psychology, 10*, 212. [CrossRef] [PubMed]

Chennaoui, M., Arnal, P. J., Sauvet, F., & Léger, D. (2015). Sleep and exercise: A reciprocal issue? *Sleep Medicine Reviews, 20*, 59–72. [CrossRef] [PubMed]

Counts, C. J., Grubin, F. C., & John-Henderson, N. A. (2018). Childhood socioeconomic status and risk in early family environments: Predictors of global sleep quality in college students. *Sleep Health, 4*(3), 301–306. [CrossRef] [PubMed]

Davis, T. J., Morris, M., & Drake, M. M. (2016). The moderation effect of mindfulness on the relationship between adult attachment and wellbeing. *Personality and Individual Differences, 96*, 115–121. [CrossRef]

Eysenck, M. W., Derakshan, N., Santos, R., & Calvo, M. G. (2007). Anxiety and cognitive performance: Attentional control theory. *Emotion, 7*(2), 336. [CrossRef] [PubMed]

Ghrouz, A. K., Noohu, M. M., Dilshad Manzar, M., Warren Spence, D., BaHammam, A. S., & Pandi-Perumal, S. R. (2019). Physical activity and sleep quality in relation to mental health among college students. *Sleep and Breathing, 23*, 627–634. [CrossRef]

Greco, L. A., Baer, R. A., & Smith, G. T. (2011). Assessing mindfulness in children and adolescents: Development and validation of the Child and Adolescent Mindfulness Measure (CAMM). *Psychological Assessment, 23*(3), 606. [CrossRef]

Hagger, M. S., Gucciardi, D. F., Turrell, A. S., & Hamilton, K. (2019a). Self-control and health-related behaviour: The role of implicit self-control, trait self-control, and lay beliefs in self-control. *British Journal of Health Psychology, 24*(4), 764–786. [CrossRef]

Hagger, M. S., Hankonen, N., Kangro, E. M., Lintunen, T., Pagaduan, J., Polet, J., Ries, F., & Hamilton, K. (2019b). Trait self-control, social cognition constructs, and intentions: Correlational evidence for mediation and moderation effects in diverse health behaviours. *Applied Psychology: Health and Well-Being*, *11*(3), 407–437. [CrossRef]

Hale, L., Troxel, W., & Buysse, D. J. (2020). Sleep Health: An opportunity for public health to address health equity. *Annual Review of Public Health*, *41*(1), 81–99. [CrossRef] [PubMed]

Hayes, A. F. (2013). *Introduction to mediation, moderation, and conditional process analysis: A regression-based approach*. Guilford.

Hayes, A. F. (2015). An index and test of linear moderated mediation. *Multivariate Behavioral Research*, *50*(1), 1–22. [CrossRef] [PubMed]

Hayes, A. F. (2017). Partial, conditional, and moderated moderated mediation: Quantification, inference, and interpretation. *Communication Monographs*, *85*(1), 4–40. [CrossRef]

Hayes, A. F., & Rockwood, N. J. (2016). Regression-based statistical mediation and moderation analysis in clinical research: Observations, recommendations, and implementation. *Behaviour Research and Therapy*, *98*, 39–57. [CrossRef] [PubMed]

Herawati, K., & Gayatri, D. (2019). The correlation between sleep quality and levels of stress among students in Universitas Indonesia. *Enfermeria Clinica*, *29*, 357–361. [CrossRef]

Jiang, C. M., Zhang, Y. M., Zhang, Y. F., & Meng, Y. Z. (2009). Identification on evaluation of participating degree in physical exercise for both urban and rural residents in China. *China Sport Science*, *29*(5), 24–31.

Johnston, S. A., Roskowski, C., He, Z., Kong, L., & Chen, W. (2021). Effects of team sports on anxiety, depression, perceived stress, and sleep quality in college students. *Journal of American College Health*, *69*(7), 791–797. [CrossRef] [PubMed]

Koyanagi, A., & Stickley, A. (2015). The association between sleep problems and psychotic symptoms in the general population: A global perspective. *Sleep*, *38*(12), 1875–1885. [CrossRef]

Kräuchi, K. (2007). The thermophysiological cascade leading to sleep initiation in relation to phase of entrainment. *Sleep Medicine Reviews*, *11*(6), 439–451. [CrossRef]

Kroese, F. M., Evers, C., Adriaanse, M. A., & de Ridder, D. T. (2016). Bedtime procrastination: A self-regulation perspective on sleep insufficiency in the general population. *Journal of Health Psychology*, *21*(5), 853–862. [CrossRef] [PubMed]

Kuang, J., Arnett, J. J., Chen, E., Demetrovics, Z., Herold, F., Cheung, R. Y., Hall, D. L., Markwart, M., Gerber, M., Ludyga, S., Kramer, A. F., & Zou, L. (2023). The relationship between dimensions of emerging adulthood and behavioral problems among Chinese emerging adults: The mediating role of physical activity and self-control. *International Journal of Mental Health Protection*, *25*(8), 937. [CrossRef]

Lentz, T. A., & Brown, C. (2019). Mindfulness and health behaviors in college students: The moderating role of sleep. *Journal of American College Health*, *67*(6), 505–514. [CrossRef]

Li, J., Zhou, K., Li, X., Liu, M., Dang, S., Wang, D., & Xin, X. (2016). Mediator effect of sleep hygiene practices on relationships between sleep quality and other sleep-related factors in Chinese mainland university students. *Behavioral Sleep Medicine*, *14*(1), 85–99. [CrossRef] [PubMed]

Liang, D. (1994). Stress levels of students in higher education and their relationship with physical activity. *Chinese Mental Health Journal*, *1*, 5–6.

Liu, J., Zhu, L., & Liu, C. (2020). Sleep quality and self-control: The mediating roles of positive and negative affects. *Frontiers in Psychology*, *11*, 607548. [CrossRef] [PubMed]

Liu, Q. Q., Zhang, D. J., Yang, X. J., Zhang, C. Y., Fan, C. Y., & Zhou, Z. K. (2018). Perceived stress and mobile phone addiction in Chinese adolescents: A moderated mediation model. *Computers in Human Behavior*, *87*, 247–253. [CrossRef]

Liu, X. (1996). Reliability and validity of the Pittsburgh sleep quality index. *Chinese Journal of Psychiatry*, *29*, 103.

Lueke, N. A., & Assar, A. (2024). Poor sleep quality and reduced immune function among college students: Perceived stress and depression as mediators. *Journal of American College Health*, *72*(4), 1112–1119. [CrossRef]

Lyddy, C. J., Good, D. J., Bolino, M. C., Thompson, P. S., & Stephens, J. P. (2021). The costs of mindfulness at work: The moderating role of mindfulness in surface acting, self-control depletion, and performance outcomes. *Journal of Applied Psychology*, *106*(12), 1921. [CrossRef]

MacLean, E. L., Hare, B., Nunn, C. L., Addessi, E., Amici, F., Anderson, R. C., Aureli, F., Baker, J. M., Bania, A. E., Barnard, A. M., Boogert, N. J., Brannon, E. M., Bray, E. E., Bray, J., Brent, L. J. N., Burkart, J. M., Call, J., Cantlon, J. F., Cheke, L. G., . . . Zhao, Y. (2014). The evolution of self-control. *Proceedings of the National Academy of Sciences*, *111*(20), E2140–E2148. [CrossRef]

Mahfouz, M. S., Ali, S. A., Bahari, A. Y., Ajeebi, R. E., Sabei, H. J., Somaily, S. Y., Madkhali, M. A., Hrooby, R. H., & Shook, R. A. N. (2020). Association between sleep quality and physical activity in Saudi Arabian University students. *Nature and Science of Sleep*, *12*, 775–782. [CrossRef]

Memon, M. A., Cheah, J., Ramayah, T., Ting, H., Chuah, F., & Cham, T. H. (2019). Moderation analysis: Issues and guidelines. *Journal of Applied Structural Equation Modeling*, *3*(1), i–xi. [CrossRef]

Ong, J. C., Ulmer, C. S., & Manber, R. (2012). Improving sleep with mindfulness and acceptance: A metacognitive model of insomnia. *Behaviour Research and Therapy*, *50*(11), 651–660. [CrossRef] [PubMed]

Patterson, M. S., Gagnon, L. R., Vukelich, A., Brown, S. E., Nelon, J. L., & Prochnow, T. (2021). Social networks, group exercise, and anxiety among college students. *Journal of American College Health, 69*(4), 361–369. [CrossRef] [PubMed]

Podsakoff, P. M., MacKenzie, S. B., Lee, J. Y., & Podsakoff, N. P. (2003). Common method biases in behavioral research: A critical review of the literature and recommended remedies. *Journal of Applied Psychology, 88*(5), 879. [CrossRef] [PubMed]

Preacher, K. J., Rucker, D. D., & Hayes, A. F. (2007). Addressing moderated mediation hypotheses: Theory, methods, and prescriptions. *Multivariate Behavioral Research, 42*(1), 185–227. [CrossRef] [PubMed]

Quanten, S., De Valck, E., Cluydts, R., Aerts, J., & Berckmans, D. (2006). Individualized and time-variant model for the functional link between thermoregulation and sleep onset. *Journal of Sleep Research, 15*(2), 183–198. [CrossRef]

Ruffault, A., Bernier, M., Juge, N., & Fournier, J. F. (2016). Mindfulness may moderate the relationship between intrinsic motivation and physical activity: A cross-sectional study. *Mindfulness, 7*, 445–452. [CrossRef]

Schlomer, G. L., Bauman, S., & Card, N. A. (2010). Best practices for missing data management in counseling psychology. *Journal of Counseling Psychology, 57*(1), 1–10. [CrossRef] [PubMed]

Shapiro, S. L., Carlson, L. E., Astin, J. A., & Freedman, B. (2006). Mechanisms of mindfulness. *Journal of Clinical Psychology, 62*(3), 373–386. [CrossRef] [PubMed]

Slykerman, R. F., Thompson, J. M., Coomarasamy, C., Wall, C. R., Waldie, K. E., Murphy, R., & Mitchell, E. A. (2020). Early adolescent physical activity, sleep and symptoms of depression at 16 years of age. *Acta Paediatrica, 109*(7), 1394–1399. [CrossRef]

Stocker, E., Englert, C., & Seiler, R. (2019). Self-control strength and mindfulness in physical exercise performance: Does a short mindfulness induction compensate for the detrimental ego depletion effect? *Journal of Applied Sport Psychology, 31*(3), 324–339. [CrossRef]

Tan, S. H., & Guo, Y. Y. (2008). Revision of self-control scale for Chinese college students. *Chinese Journal of Clinical Psychology, 16*(5), 468–470.

Tehseen, S., Ramayah, T., & Sajilan, S. (2017). Testing and controlling for common method variance: A review of available methods. *Journal of Management Sciences, 4*(2), 142–168. [CrossRef]

Wang, F., & Bíró, É. (2021). Determinants of sleep quality in college students: A literature review. *Explore, 17*(2), 170–177. [CrossRef] [PubMed]

Wills, T. A., Vaccaro, D., & McNamara, G. (1992). The role of life events, family support, and competence in adolescent substance use: A test of vulnerability and protective factors. *American Journal of Community Psychology, 20*(3), 349–374. [CrossRef] [PubMed]

World Health Organization. (2021). *Health behaviour in school-aged children (HBSC) study*. Highlights. Available online: https://www.who.int/europe/initiatives/health-behaviour-in-school-aged-children-(hbsc)-study/highlights (accessed on 9 January 2025).

World Medical Association. (2013). World medical association declaration of Helsinki: Ethical principles for medical research involving human subjects. *JAMA, 310*(20), 2191–2194. [CrossRef] [PubMed]

Wu, R., Wang, W., Li, W., Zhao, M., Dewaele, A., Zhang, W., Buysse, A., Guo, L., & Lu, C. (2021). Sexual orientation and sleep problem among Chinese college students: Mediating roles of interpersonal problems and depressive symptoms. *Journal of Affective Disorders, 295*, 569–577. [CrossRef] [PubMed]

Xiong, M., Chen, J., & Ye, Y. (2023). How relative deprivation affects the sleep quality of Chinese college students: Testing an integrated model of social anxiety and trait mindfulness. *Frontiers in Psychology, 14*, 1111845. [CrossRef]

Zhang, L., Zheng, H., Yi, M., Zhang, Y., Cai, G., Li, C., & Zhao, L. (2022). Prediction of sleep quality among university students after analyzing lifestyles, sports habits, and mental health. *Frontiers in Psychiatry, 13*, 927619. [CrossRef] [PubMed]

Zhang, X., Gu, X., Zhang, T., & Keller, J. M. (2022). The mediating roles of sleep quality and sedentary behavior between physical fitness and depression among female college freshmen. *Journal of American College Health, 70*(5), 1528–1535. [CrossRef]

Zheng, B., Li, M., Wang, K. L., & Lv, J. (2016). Analysis of the reliability and validity of the Chinese version of Pittsburgh sleep quality index among medical college students. *PubMed, 48*(3), 424–428.

behavioral sciences

MDPI

Article

Participants' Roles in Bullying Among 7–11 Year Olds: Results from a UK-Wide Randomized Control Trial of the KiVa School-Based Program

Judy Hutchings [1,*], Ruth Pearson [1], Malavika Babu [2], Suzy Clarkson [1], Margiad Elen Williams [1], Julia R. Badger [3], Rebecca Cannings-John [2], Richard P. Hastings [4], Rachel Hayes [5] and Lucy Bowes [6,7]

1 Centre for Evidence Based Early Intervention, Bangor University, Bangor LL57 2DG, UK; ruth.pearson04@outlook.com (R.P.); s.clarkson@bangor.ac.uk (S.C.); margiad.williams@bangor.ac.uk (M.E.W.)
2 Centre for Trials Research, Cardiff University, Neuadd Meirionnydd, Heath Park, Cardiff CF14 4YS, UK; babum@cardiff.ac.uk (M.B.); canningsrl@cardiff.ac.uk (R.C.-J.)
3 Department of Education, University of Oxford, Oxford OX1 2JD, UK; julia.badger@education.ox.ac.uk
4 School of Social Policy and Society, University of Birmingham, Birmingham B15 2TT, UK; r.hastings@birmingham.ac.uk
5 Department for Public Health and Sports Sciences, Faculty of Health and Life Sciences, South Cloisters, St Luke's Campus, University of Exeter, Exeter EX1 2LU, UK; r.a.hayes@exeter.ac.uk
6 Department of Experimental Psychology, Oxford University, Oxford OX2 6GG, UK; lucy.bowes@psy.ox.ac.uk
7 National Institute for Health and Care Research (NIHR), Oxford Health Biomedical Research Centre, Oxford University, Oxford OX3 7JX, UK
* Correspondence: j.hutchings@bangor.ac.uk

Abstract: This paper describes the social architecture model of school-based bullying behavior. The model proposes that the behavior of all students affects rates of bullying. Alongside self-reported victims and bullies, the model identified four bystander roles: assistant, reinforcer, outsider, and defender. The level of support for bullies varies based on school policies that address bullying and promote school connectedness. The universal components of the KiVa school-based anti-bullying program designed to teach pupils to stand against bullying are described. The Stand Together trial, a UK-based randomized controlled trial, recruited 11,000+ students from 118 schools across the UK, half of whom received the KiVa program whilst the remainder delivered usual practice to address bullying. The main trial results reported a significant reduction in victimization in favor of KiVa. This paper examines data collected on the pupil-reported Participant Role Questionnaire (PRQ), one of the secondary measures used to explore whether significant reductions in victimization were accompanied by changes in bystander behavior. The results showed reductions in the student response rates of self-identified roles as bullies, assistants, and reinforcers in favor of KiVa, but outsider roles increased, and defender roles reduced. This provides tentative support for the social architecture model as taught in the Stand Together KiVa trial but also suggests that further work needs to be conducted to support the development of defender behaviors and address this important public health challenge.

Keywords: bullying; victimization; children; intervention; KiVa; school; participant roles

1. Introduction

School-based bullying is a major international health concern requiring action at a policy level, in the wider community, and in schools (Iati, 2019; Srabstein & Leventhal, 2010; Currie et al., 2012) In the UK, schools are required to have anti-bullying policies, although there is considerable variability in terms of their content and the ways in which schools implement them (Smith et al., 2012, 2008).

The most widely used definition of bullying (Olweus, 1994) has three components: intention, repetition, and the involvement of a higher status of individual or individuals.

> *"a student is being bullied or victimized when he or she is exposed, repeatedly and over time, to negative actions on the part of one or more other students" (and where there is) "an imbalance of strength (an asymmetric power relationship)"* (Olweus, 1994, p. 1173).

Experience of bullying in school, for both victims and perpetrators, can have significant negative effects in childhood and through adolescence and is linked to a range of difficulties into adulthood (Camodeca & Nava, 2020; Ttofi et al., 2011; Rigby, 2003; Smith, 2016; Wolke & Lereya, 2015; Arseneault et al., 2010) with evidence of different effects on victims than perpetrators (Brown & Taylor, 2008; Wolke et al., 2013). The impact of victimization is associated with depression and anxiety (Arseneault et al., 2006; Eastman et al., 2018; Ttofi et al., 2011; Zhang et al., 2020), poor academic achievement, sleep disturbances, somatic and psychosomatic complaints, night terrors, the loss of self-esteem, absenteeism, poor life satisfaction, loss of appetite, poor physical health (Fisher et al., 2017; Hawker & Boulton, 2000; Smith & Brain, 2000; Smith, 2016; Wang, 2023), and thoughts of suicide and suicide attempts in later life (Moore et al., 2017; Ttofi et al., 2011). Perpetrating bullying can also contribute to detrimental short- and longer-term difficulties (Smith, 2016; Grennan & Woodhams, 2007; Zuckerman, 2016). This can include an increased risk of low academic attainment, employment difficulties, lower socioeconomic status, a higher risk of being involved in domestic violence (Brown & Taylor, 2008), and involvement in criminal behavior in young adulthood (Fergusson et al., 2014). Those students who assist bullies by joining in but not initiating bullying can also experience an increased risk of aggressive externalizing problems, low academic achievement, involvement in criminal activity, and substance misuse (Clark et al., 2022; Evans et al., 2019; Riffle et al., 2021). Even witnessing bullying may contribute to subsequent depressive and anxiety symptoms (Camodeca & Nava, 2020; Midgett & Doumas, 2019).

The school environment contributes to bullying perpetration, with bullying norms playing a large role in rates of school bullying. School connectedness matters and can be defined as the cohesiveness between diverse groups in the school community, including students, families, school staff, and the wider community (Rowe et al., 2007). Feelings of school connectedness have a positive impact on children (McNeely et al., 2002), and are associated with lower levels of school bullying (Espelage et al., 2014; Glew et al., 2005; Merrin et al., 2018), whereas insufficient adult supervision, inadequate anti-bullying policies, and/or a permissive attitude toward bullying within a school setting are associated with an increased risk of bullying behaviors (Liu et al., 2020; Espelage & Swearer, 2003). Types of bullying have been categorized in different ways. Olweus (1993) describes bullying as a sub-form of aggressive behavior, which he classified as direct and indirect (Olweus, 1993), with direct identification being verbal and physical. Other researchers, e.g., Orpinas and Horne (2006), identified three categories—direct, indirect, and relational or psychological—which include damaging or vandalizing possessions, writing threatening or frightening notes, and social isolation. Other classification systems have been suggested, including the addition of sexual bullying (Pepler et al., 2006). Salmivalli and colleagues identified nine categories of bullying: physical, verbal, social, cyber, social manipulation, material, threat, racist, and sexual (Menesini & Salmivalli, 2017; Salmivalli et al., 2011a; Smokowski & Kopasz, 2005). However, as many as 25% of teachers often do not recognize some types of bullying (Boulton, 1997) with teachers being more likely to identify physical bullying incidents than relational ones (Chen et al., 2018) and several indirect forms of bullying are often dismissed (Maunder et al., 2010) Consequently, teachers also need help to both recognize and intervene effectively when bullying occurs (Ey & Campbell, 2022; Campbell et al., 2019).

1.1. Roles in Bullying

Bullying is increasingly recognized as a group process with all students contributing to the maintenance, escalation, and potential of the reduction in bullying in schools (Salmivalli et al., 1996; Salmivalli, 2001; Twemlow et al., 2004; Goodstein, 2013; Twemlow & Sacco, 2013; Swearer & Hymel, 2015). Alongside bullies and victims, including bully victims, children who both bully and are bullied, Salmivalli et al.'s (1996) social architecture model describes a range of bystander roles, suggesting that bullying behaviors provide social reward for the perpetrator by fulfilling a need such as social attention, and improved social status among, or power over, their peers (Salmivalli et al., 1996, 2011b; Saarento & Salmivalli, 2015). The presence and behavior of others during a bullying incident can reinforce the bullying behavior by actively joining in, laughing, or watching, or conversely reducing its occurrence by removing the social reward. Salmivalli et al. (1996) identified four bystander roles that influence the bullying situation: being an assistant to the bully, the reinforcer of the bully, the outsider, and the defender of the victim (Salmivalli et al., 1996; Salmivalli et al., 2011b). Assistants take an active role, but they follow the perpetrator's lead and/or take instruction from them. They do not initiate the attack but are seen by victims as bullies (Salmivalli et al., 1996). Reinforcers provide social support for the bully by laughing or shouting encouragement. Their actions can have an adverse effect on the victim, leaving them feeling socially isolated and lowering their self-esteem (Salmivalli et al., 1996). Outsiders remain neutral, which may be due to the fear of becoming a target themselves but can be seen by victims and others as approving of the bullying by being silently complicit (Salmivalli et al., 1996). Defending can take different forms, including confronting the bully (bully-oriented defending) and comforting the victim (victim-oriented defending) (Reijntjes et al., 2016). Their support by telling the bully to stop, letting an adult know what is happening, comforting the victim, or other supportive behaviors reduce the victim's feeling of social isolation (Salmivalli et al., 1996). Knowledge of the way in which bystander behavior impacts school-based bullying guided the development of the KiVa school-based bullying program (Espelage et al., 2013; Guo, 2021). There is evidence that students in KiVa schools perceive a significant increase in the number of classmates acting as defenders of victims and also see an increase in their own defending behavior (e.g., Saarento & Salmivalli, 2015). Less is known about changes in other participants' roles that may influence bullying.

1.2. Kiva in Finland

Finnish comprehensive schools provide for children aged 7 to 15 and are non-selective, and Finish children perform very highly in terms of academic outcomes (Niemi, 2023). As in UK schools, Finnish schools are required to have an anti-bullying policy, but over a 10-year period this had no impact on reported rates of bullying (Salmivalli et al., 2011a). Professor Salmivalli had, for many years, been undertaking research on bullying and as a result, in 2006, the Finnish government funded her and her team at the University of Turku to develop a program for schools. The program, KiVa, has all the tools needed to address bullying, and has achieved extremely good outcomes in terms of reduced reported bullying and victimization in Finland. Following the success of the original randomized controlled trial (Kärnä et al., 2011), KiVa was offered to all Finnish comprehensive schools, achieving a 90% take up and showing year-on-year reductions in reported bullying over a seven-year period (Herkama et al., 2017).

1.3. The Components of the KiVa Program

KiVa has a set of universal school-wide activities to impact the behavior and attitudes of all students and a specific targeted intervention strategy to address bullying (the indicated action plan).

The universal component is as follows:

i. Staff materials, including a PowerPoint presentation, are provided to ensure that all members of school staff are familiar with the definition of bullying, the program, and the process of referral to the KiVa team.
ii. Materials to be shared with all parents, including a presentation for a launch meeting with parents, are provided. Parents are informed that the school is a KiVa school and stands against bullying and are also provided with a booklet that describes ways to talk with their child about bullying.
iii. Staff supervise break times and lunch times and wear a hi-visibility vest with a KiVa symbol on it to remind students that they are in a KiVa school.
iv. Posters are distributed throughout the school to remind everyone that they are in a KiVa school and that they have a responsibility to make the school a happy place.
v. KiVa has three sets of lesson units for ages 7 to 9 (Unit 1), 10 to 12 (Unit 2), and 13 to 15-year-olds (Unit 3). For units 1 and 2, there are ten 90 min lessons. Lessons are scripted and include videos, small and large group discussions, role-play, written assignments, and other play activities and KiVa games. Lessons start with components to promote prosocial behavior, learning to identify emotions, how to be a member of the team, and how to make the classroom a happy place. As they progress throughout the year, students and their teachers address issues related to bullying, how to define it, how to recognize it, and safe ways to stand against it. Throughout the year, students identify the KiVa rules. The aim is to encourage students away from behaviors that support bullying and towards behaviors that promote defense of victims.
vi. The annual anonymous student survey enables children to report, annually, on their own behavior in terms of whether or not they have experienced or perpetrated bullying. The overall result is reported back to their school, along with information regarding the responses of KiVa schools in general.

The indicated action component is as follows:

This is used when a confirmed bullying incident is identified. To achieve this, every member of the school staff is taught the definition of bullying and what to do if they believe that bullying may have taken place. The incident is recorded and sent to the trained KiVa Team within the school. The team reviews the information and decides whether it meets the criteria to be considered bullying. If it does not, it is dealt with through normal school procedures for resolving disagreements, fallouts, accidents, and misunderstandings. If it is identified as a bullying incident, there is a structured process for the KiVa Team to follow. This does not require blaming the bully but the commitment to finding a solution; the no-blame approach has been shown to achieve equally good results, particularly with the younger age range. As a result of this process, 78% of incidents ceased altogether, and a further 19.5% were reduced; in other words, it has an impact on 97.5% of all cases addressed (Garandeau et al., 2014).

1.4. KiVa in the UK

UK schools are required to have an anti-bullying policy, but, as in Finland before the introduction of KiVa, it is left to individual schools to decide what goes into it and how to implement it (Smith et al., 2012), and no specific evidence-based advice is provided.

Whilst the results from Finland are very convincing, the system of education in the UK is very different from that of Finland and, therefore, evidence of transportability was required. An analysis of the required curriculum for compulsory personal social education in both England and Wales showed that the KiVa curriculum covered 50% of the required topics, and in 2013, with the Welsh Government's support, KiVa was introduced in Wales. Promising reductions in bullying-related behavior were reported from the first 17 schools to implement the program (Hutchings & Clarkson, 2015). At that point, a license to disseminate KiVa across the UK was obtained from Finland, and it was implemented in the first 41 UK schools to trial the program (Clarkson et al., 2019) and again reported significant reductions in both bullying and victimization at a reasonable ongoing implementation cost. Following the Hutchings and Clarkson (2015) and Clarkson et al. (2019) papers, both reporting significant benefits from early implementer schools, a small lottery grant was obtained for a pilot RCT with 22 schools. This did not demonstrate significant benefits but reported considerable variability in its implementation across the schools (Axford et al., 2020).

1.5. The Stand Together Trial

Based on the initial pre-post evidence that KiVa reduced victimization and bullying in UK primary schools (Hutchings & Clarkson, 2015; Clarkson et al., 2019), in 2019, the National Institute for Health and Care Research (NIHR) funded a randomized controlled trial (RCT), the UK Stand Together Trial, to establish outcomes based on one year of KiVa delivery compared to usual practice. With collaboration across five universities (Bangor, Oxford, Exeter, and Warwick for recruitment and Cardiff for data analysis), 118 state-maintained primary schools and over 11,000 students were recruited from across four areas (North Wales, Oxfordshire, Devon, and Birmingham). Each of the four sites recruited 28 or 29 schools. Parents were given an opt-out option for their child's participation. Children provided their written assent via e-tablets for self-reported outcomes at each data collection point. From a potential of 11,922 students, 11,111 (93.2%) students completed a baseline questionnaire. Child questionnaires were administered via e-tablets, with researchers reading the questions aloud to the whole class. Further information about recruitment and methods is reported in the main outcome paper (Bowes et al., 2024). Rates of free school meals (FSMs) ranged from 7 to 28%, and the number of 7–11-year-old pupils ranged from 64 to 224. Schools were randomized on a 1:1 basis, taking into account school size, rurality, and the level of free school meal eligibility. Data were collected on levels of victimization using the self-reported Olweus Bully Victimization Questionnaire (OBVQ, Olweus, 2006). Secondary outcomes included self-reported bullying (OBVQ), empathy towards victims (Pöyhönen et al., 2010), and roles in bullying situations as measured using the "Participant Role Questionnaire" (PRQ) (Salmivalli & Voeten, 2004). Teachers rated children based on the Teacher Strengths and Difficulties Questionnaire (TSDQ), which records behavioral and emotional problems as well as pro-social behavior. They also collected data on lesson administration. At baseline, 21.6% of students reported being bullied in the usual-practice group and 20.3% in the KiVa-intervention group, which were broadly comparable with reports from other studies.

Parental consent was not required for children to participate in KiVa school-based activities as it formed part of the compulsory Personal Social Educational curriculum in both England and Wales. The trial was funded to undertake the evaluation of KiVa, which was delivered by randomized intervention schools whilst control schools continued with the usual anti-bullying practice. Ethical approval for the collection of trial data was obtained from the Bangor University Psychology Research Ethics and Governance Committee (reference: 2019-16592). This included giving parents an option to remove their children from the collection of trial data.

All analyses were pre-registered and performed blind by statisticians at the Centre for Trials Research, a UKCRC Registered Trials Unit at Cardiff University. Details on recruitment, data collection, statistical analysis procedures, and hypotheses were reported in a protocol paper (Clarkson et al., 2022).

1.6. Training and Support for KiVa Trial Schools

Funding was obtained for schools to deliver KiVa, and in order to address some of the implementation challenges experienced during the Axford et al. (2020) trial, KiVa trainers were appointed for each site. During the trial year, trainers met each term with the schools and were also available to schools for consultation if requested. Two school staff from each allocated KiVa school attended a two-day training coordinated through the Children's Early Intervention Trust Charity (CEIT) that holds the UK KiVa dissemination license. At the KiVa training session, the roles of the school coordinator and KiVa team lead were explained, and the participants planned for the launch of Kiva in their school. The KiVa coordinator was responsible for ensuring that all school staff were aware of the definition of bullying, how to recognize it, and what to do when it is identified. They also oversaw the implementation generally, ensuring that class teachers delivered the KiVa lessons and oversaw the annual online KiVa pupil survey. The KiVa team lead was responsible for training identified staff as members of the KiVa team that was set up to address confirmed bullying incidents.

Despite considerable disruption in schools returning from the COVID-19 shutdown and with high levels of post-COVID-19 absenteeism, the UK Stand Together KiVa RCT results (Bowes et al., 2024) showed that after one year of implementation, the KiVa program had significantly reduced the odds of bullying victimization among students by 13% compared with students from schools continuing with usual practice. In addition, KiVa students demonstrated significantly higher levels of empathy, and fewer teachers reported peer relationship problems. The defender scale of the Participant Role Questionnaire (PRQ), reported as a secondary outcome, indicated that students in the KiVa arm had 24% lower odds of defending bullying compared to the usual-practice arm (significant at the p = 0.03 level). Exploratory findings indicated that the effectiveness of KiVa was consistent across different levels of the school's socioeconomic status, school size, and gender, and the economic evaluation reported that KiVa was a low-cost intervention compared to many other UK school-based interventions. Together, these results suggest that KiVa is a feasible and efficient strategy for reducing bullying in schools.

The positive outcome from the trial in favor of KiVa provided the opportunity to explore possible changes in children's responses to the Participant Role Questionnaire (PRQ) (Salmivalli et al., 1996).

1.7. Aims

The PRQ was included in the main RCT as one of the exploratory objectives. The PRQ data provide an opportunity to establish whether the anticipated participant roles changed, with reductions in assisting, reinforcing, and being an outsider and increases in defending, occurring, as implied by the social architecture model (Salmivalli et al., 1996).

2. Methods

School recruitment is described in the Clarkson et al. (2022) protocol paper and the Bowes et al. (2024) main results paper. It involves circulating information about the trial in each of the trial areas and recruiting mainstream primary schools with at least two classes of pupils aged between 7 and 11 on a first-come-first-served basis. One hundred and eighteen schools and 11,922 students were recruited, either 29 or 30 schools, at each of the four sites. Baseline questionnaires were completed by 11,111 (93.2%) students aged between 7 and 11 years, and 9981 (90.1%) completed follow-up questionnaires one year later, including 5321 (90.0%) students in the KiVa schools and 4660 (90.2%) in usual-practice schools. Questionnaires were administered in person using e-tablets, with researchers reading the questions and answering options aloud to the whole class. The KiVa program was implemented in the academic year September 2021 to July 2022, and survey outcomes were measured between April and June 2022. Baseline student and teacher characteristics were well balanced across the trial arms.

2.1. Materials

The PRQ (Salmivalli et al., 1996) provides a measurement of the multifaceted roles of bullying, which range from direct participation to defending. An accurate assessment of these roles is critical for developing targeted interventions. In its initial form, the PRQ was a peer-report measure. Initially comprising 50 items, it has since undergone adaptations, with subsequent versions including the 15-item version (Demaray et al., 2016), which was developed to address concerns about the length and complexity of the original questionnaire. The 15-item version preserves the core structure and includes the original five roles: the bully, assistants to the bully, reinforcers of the bully, outsiders, and defenders of the victim. The PRQ has been shown to have good internal consistency with Cronbach's alpha coefficients of 0.93 for the bully scale, 0.95 for the assistant scale, 0.90 for the reinforcer scale, 0.89 for the defender scale, and 0.88 for the outsider scale (Salmivalli et al., 2011b).

Although developed as a peer-report measure, the PRQ was subsequently revised as a self-report measure, in part due to ethical concerns about asking students to nominate/report on their peers (Espelage & Holt, 2001; Verlinden et al., 2015) and there were concerns from both teachers and researchers about parent opt-out from peer ratings, allowing pupils to rate others as bullies, which might significantly reduce recruitment. The self-report version involves participants reporting on their own behavior and experiences (Felix et al., 2011) and has become a preferred approach due to its time and cost-effectiveness (Espelage & Swearer, 2003; Furlong et al., 2010; Vivolo-Kantor et al., 2014). In Salmivalli et al.'s (1996) study, both peer nominations and self-report versions of the PRQ were collected, and the self-estimated scores on the bully, assistant, reinforcer, outsider, and defender scales were positively correlated with the corresponding peer-estimated scores.

The 15-item self-report version was used in the current trial. In the self-report version, the wording and language of the items ask only how the person completing the survey behaves. Each of the 15 items is rated on a 3-point Likert scale (0 = never, 1 = sometimes, 2 = often). An extra response was added to all questions in the Stand Together trial to give students the option to not answer the questions as required for ethical approval (3 = I'd rather not say).

- Bully scale: "I bully other children", "I make other people bully other children with me", and "I always find new ways to annoy the bullied pupil". Higher scores indicate more frequent bullying behavior (negative).
- Assistant scale: "I join in with bullying when someone else starts it", "When someone is bullying other children, I help the bully", and "When someone is bullying other children, I help them, maybe by catching the bullied child". Higher scores indicate more frequent assistant behavior (negative).
- Reinforcer scale: "When someone is being bullied, I go and see what's happening", "When someone is being bullied, I laugh", and "When someone is being bullied, I tell the bully to keep on doing it". Higher scores indicate more frequent reinforcer behavior (negative).

- Outsider scale: "I am around when other people get bullied", "When someone is being bullied, I stay away from where it is happening", and "When someone is being bullied, I don't take sides with either the bully or the pupil being bullied". Higher scores indicate more frequent outsider behavior (positive).
- Defender scale: "When someone is being bullied, I try and make the bullied pupil feel better and say they should tell a teacher", "When someone is being bullied, I tell the bullies to stop", and "I try and make the bullies stop bullying other people". Higher scores indicate more frequent defender behavior (positive).

The PRQ was administered as part of a group of measures completed by children and included the 22-item version of the Olweus Bullying and Victimization Questionnaire (OBVQ; Olweus, 2006), which provided data for the main hypothesis regarding reduction in victimization (see Clarkson et al., 2022; Bowes et al., 2024).

2.2. Statistical Analysis

Pupils' self-reported results on the bully, assistant, reinforcer, outsider, and defender scales were assessed by averaging scores from the corresponding three items of the PRQ to a single measure. Each subscale was categorized into two categories for analysis (never = 0 if the subscale score was zero; sometimes/often = 1 if the subscale score was greater than zero) and reported as frequencies alongside percentages. A logistic regression model was used to assess the impact of KiVa training on the PRQ scales. Results were presented as the odds ratio (ORs) alongside the 95% confidence interval (CI). All analyses were intended to treat without imputation (a complete case analysis restricted to students with responses at both baseline and follow-up), with outcomes compared between KiVa and usual-practice groups using three-level regression models (allowing for clustering between students within school and between schools within sites). Analyses controlled for school-level stratification variables (school size, proportion of students eligible for FSM), key student characteristics (age, sex), and baseline outcome measures. The statistical analyses took into account clustering by school and site using random effects. All analyses controlled for the school-level stratification variables (site, school size, proportion of children eligible for FSM), the age and gender of the pupils, and the baseline measure of the outcome. Data analysis was conducted in IBM SPSS Statistics version 26 (IBM Corporation, Armonk, NY, USA), R software (R Core Team (2021)), and Stata® version 17 (StataCorp LP, College Station, TX, USA).

3. Results

One hundred and eighteen schools were recruited across the four trial sites between October 2020 and February 2021, with 11,111 students (5944 KiVa arm; 5167 usual practice) completing a baseline questionnaire (from a potential of 11,922 students). Twelve months of follow-up data were collected from 5321 (90.0%) students in the KiVa schools compared to 4660 (90.2%) in usual-practice schools. A total of 263 (KiVa) and 202 (usual practice) additional questionnaires were completed by students who had not completed a baseline questionnaire. Hence, the final numbers at 12 months were 5584 (KiVa) and 4862 (usual practice). The total number of students available for the complete case analysis (baseline and 12-month follow-up) was 9981. Student characteristics recorded at baseline were similar between arms; 49% of students were female, and the majority self-reported their age as being between 8 and 10 years of age (Table 1).

Table 1. Student characteristics.

	KiVa N = 5944	Usual Practice N = 5167
Trial site n (%)		
North Wales	1556 (57.5)	1148 (42.5)
Devon	1225 (52.6)	1106 (47.5)
Oxfordshire	1168 (50.2)	1161 (49.9)
Birmingham	1995 (53.2)	1752 (46.8)
Student-reported characteristics		
Females n (%)	2905 (49.0)	2560 (49.6)
Missing	10 (0.2)	1 (0.02)
Age (in years) n (%)		
6/7 years old	517 (8.9)	566 (11.0)
8 years old	1918 (32.9)	1650 (32.6)
9 years old	1913(32.8)	1702 (33.6)
10/11 years old	1417 (23.9)	1157 (22.4)
Missing	7 (0.12)	2 (0.04)

3.1. The PRQ Bully Scale

Most respondents reported never having bullied other children at both baseline and 12-month follow-up; however, for those that did report bullying other children, there was a greater reduction in the KiVa arm at 13.9% to 9.7% and a reduction of 4.2 percentage points (Table 2) compared with a reduction of 0.6 percentage points (from 12.7% to 12.1%) in the usual-practice arm. When rates of bullying at 12 months follow-up were compared between arms, the adjusted odds ratio (AOR) was 0.72 (95% confidence interval (CI) = 0.53 to 0.99, *p*-value 0.041), indicating a statistically significant 13% reduction in the odds of victimization among students attending schools randomized to receive KiVa when compared to those attending schools receiving usual practice.

Table 2. Participant Role Questionnaire domains at baseline and 12-months follow-up by study arm.

	Baseline		12-Month Follow-Up				
	KiVa (N = 5944)	Usual Practice (N = 5167)	KiVa (N = 5584)	Usual Practice (N = 4862)	Trial Arm	Adjusted [a] OR (95% CI)	*p* Value
Bully Scale [b], n (%)							
Never	4541 (86.1)	4017 (87.3)	4640 (90.3)	3871 (87.9)	Usual Practice	Reference	
Sometimes/Often	735 (13.9)	586 (12.7)	499 (9.7)	535 (12.1)	KiVa	0.72 (0.53, 0.99)	0.041
Assistant Scale [c], n (%)							
Never	4340 (81.4)	3729 (81.5)	4255 (83.5)	3486 (79.4)	Usual Practice	Reference	
Sometimes/Often	995 (18.6)	846 (18.5)	841 (16.5)	902 (20.6)	KiVa	0.79 (0.62, 0.99)	0.046
Reinforcer Scale [d], n (%)							
Never	1026 (19.1)	947 (20.3)	1031 (20.4)	831 (19.0)	Usual Practice	Reference	
Sometimes/Often	4342 (80.9)	3722 (79.7)	4020 (79.6)	3535 (81.0)	KiVa	0.90 (0.73, 1.12)	0.358

Table 2. *Cont.*

	Baseline		12-Month Follow-Up				
	KiVa (N = 5944)	Usual Practice (N = 5167)	KiVa (N = 5584)	Usual Practice (N = 4862)	Trial Arm	Adjusted [a] OR (95% CI)	p Value
Outsider Scale [e], n (%)							
Never	274 (5.8)	262 (6.4)	215 (4.8)	154 (3.9)	Usual Practice	Reference	
Sometimes/Often	4432 (94.2)	3864 (93.6)	4255 (95.2)	3808 (96.1)	KiVa	0.73 (0.59, 0.90)	0.003
Defender Scale [f], n (%)							
Never	108 (2.1)	116 (2.5)	148 (3.0)	127 (2.9)	Usual Practice	Reference	
Sometimes/Often	5173 (97.9)	4515 (97.5)	4784 (97.0)	4190 (97.1)	KiVa	0.76 (0.59, 0.97)	0.030

CI = confidence interval, OR = odds ratio. For all PRQ domains, Score 0 = never, Score > 0 = sometimes/always. [a] Adjusted for corresponding baseline measure, FSM and KS2 size, and age and sex of pupils. [b] Higher scores indicate more frequent bullying behavior (negative); [c] Higher scores indicate more frequent assistant behavior (negative). [d] Higher scores indicate more frequent reinforcer behavior (negative). [e] Higher scores indicate frequent outsider behavior (positive). [f] Higher scores indicate more frequent defender behavior (positive).

3.2. The PRQ Assistant Scale

The rates of sometimes/often assisting a bully were comparable at baseline (18.6% KiVa vs. 18.5% usual practice). The KiVa arm experienced a reduction in assistance of 2.1 percentage points over the 12 months (from 18.6% to 16.5%), with usual-practice schools experiencing an increase of 2.1 percentage points (from 18.5% to 20.6%). When rates of assistance at 12 months follow-up were compared between arms, the AOR was 0.79 (95% CI = 0.62 to 0.99, *p*-value 0.046), indicating a statistically significant lower rate of assistance among the students attending schools that were randomized to receive KiVa, when compared to students attending schools receiving usual practice.

3.3. The PRQ Reinforcer Scale

Higher rates of reinforcing bullying were observed across both arms at baseline (80.9% KiVa vs. 79.7% usual practice), with a small decrease in the KiVa arm of 1.5 percentage points and a small increase of 1.3 percentage points in children sometimes or often reinforcing bullying in the usual-practice arm. The difference of 1.4% between arms did not achieve statistical significance (AOR = 0.90 (95% CI = 0.73, 1.12), $p = 0.358$).

3.4. The PRQ Outsider Scale

The majority of children from both trial arms reported being an outsider sometimes or often at baseline (94.2% KiVa vs. 93.6% usual practice). At follow-up, the percentage of children reporting being an outsider to bullying increased by 1 percentage point in the KiVa arm and by 2.5 percentage points in the usual-practice arm. The difference between arms at follow-up of 0.9 percentage points achieved statistical significance (AOR = 0.73 (95% CI = 0.59, 0.90), $p = 0.003$).

3.5. The PRQ Defender Scale

The defender scale was reported as a secondary outcome in the main outcomes paper (Bowes et al., 2024). A high proportion of children reported defending bullying at baseline (97.9% KiVa vs. 97.5% usual practice), which reduced over time. There was evidence to suggest a difference between the arms at follow-up (AOR 0.76 (95% CI 0.59 to 0.97), $p = 0.03$).

4. Discussion

The KiVa curriculum was built on the social architecture model (Salmivalli et al., 1996) with the aim of the universal components being to change the responses of all children to bullying. The Stand Together trial was successful at achieving its main outcome of reducing victimization (Bowes et al., 2024). The present paper explored students' responses to the Participant Role Questionnaire (PRQ) to see whether, and if so how, the significant reduction in victimization reported for the KiVa arm of the UK Stand Together trial (Bowes et al., 2024) was reflected in the responses of students to other bullying roles.

All schools in the UK are required to have an anti-bullying policy and to address cases of bullying, and this forms part of the compulsory PSE curriculum for UK schools. The main trial result is important, particularly given that it was achieved during the post-COVID-19 return to school period in a year that had significant teacher and pupil absenteeism. However, addressing bullying is an ongoing process. In Finland, the program showed year-on-year reductions in victimization over a seven-year period when, following the results from the initial randomized controlled trial, the Finnish government rolled the program out across Finland (Kärnä et al., 2011; Herkama et al., 2017).

Having established that the program was effective in reducing bullying in UK primary schools, the data from the PRQ enabled us to explore whether the UK KiVa intervention significantly reduced participant roles associated with increased bullying (bullying, assisting, reinforcing, and outsiders) and increased those intended to help reduce bullying (defending). Whilst most children are not involved in bullying as victims or bullies, the social architecture model implies that all children have a role to play in bullying. Our results provide tentative support for this model, demonstrating some changes in the responses of all children to the PRQ, not just those directly involved in bullying.

The OBVQ reduction in bullying behavior, based on a single question reported in the main trial paper, favored KiVa but did not achieve significance ($p = 0.08$; Bowes et al., 2024). However, the PRQ bullying response, based on three questions, demonstrated a significant reduction in bullying relative to usual-practice schools ($p = 0.041$), providing evidence that the reductions in the odds of victimization (13%, Bowes et al., 2024) were accompanied by a reduction in the self-reported rates of bullying alongside the significant reported reduction in victimization.

The result for the assistance scale—students who do not initiate bullying but join in when it is occurring—showed an increase in never assisting for the KiVa condition and a decline in the usual-practice condition ($p = 0.046$) and suggested that KiVa worked in the way intended.

The results from the reinforcer scale, which refers to students who stand by and contribute with laughter or other overt forms of support for the bully, also favored KiVa with the response of never reinforcing, reducing slightly in the usual-practice condition and increasing in the KiVa condition; however, this did not achieve significance ($p = 0.358$).

The result from the outsider scale showed that the number of students reporting sometimes or always being an outsider increased for both KiVa (94.2–95.2%) and usual practice (93.6 and 96.1%), but this increase was significantly greater in usual-practice schools than KiVa schools ($p = 0.003$).

The result for the defender scale showed that the high rates of baseline self-reported defender behavior (97.9% KiVa and 97.5% usual practice) reduced during follow-up (97% KiVa and 97.1% usual practice), and this was significantly greater in the KiVa condition.

Pupil self-reported bullying, assistance, and reinforcer ratings were all reduced, significantly in favor of KiVa in the case of bullying and assistance to bullies and non-significantly in the case of reinforcers. However, the increases in outsider behavior require explanation, particularly given that the reported rates of bullying and bully-supporting behaviors were reduced. The questions on the outsider scale report the actual behavior of outsiders at the time of bullying, "I am around when other people get bullied", "When someone is being bullied, I stay away from where it is happening", and "When someone is being bullied, I don't take sides with either the bully or the pupil being bullied". Their interpretation is not entirely clear as the motivation for behaving as if bullying is not happening can be varied, including a positive decision to avoid reinforcing bullying behavior or a fear of being bullied oneself. Whilst outsider behavior increased for the KiVa group, there was a significantly greater increase for the control children. Nevertheless, the fact that the result in the KiVa intervention arm was significantly less than the usual-practice arm is encouraging. However, given that the reported rates of defending behavior also reduced, the increase in outsider rates and reduction in defender behavior suggest that research and practice need to focus on how to support children to become active defenders and not outsiders. The added challenge that may have impacted this result was that data were collected before the end of the school year. In order to obtain data from the same class of children, the follow-up data were collected between March and June when, for some classes, only two-thirds of the class lessons were delivered. Initial lesson topics address working as a team, making the classroom a happy place, giving compliments, and learning to detect and understand feelings of self and others. Dealing with bullying comes later in the curriculum. This meant that some aspects of the program to address bullying would not have been delivered. Nevertheless, whilst there is material in the KiVa lessons designed to teach children how to do this, either by challenging bullies when it is safe to do so or by informing an adult or showing support to victims, these results may suggest that more work needs to be carried out in this regard.

Limitations

In addition to the data collection timetable requiring that data were collected before the end of the school year, the post-COVID-19 year was affected by increased levels of both teacher and pupil absenteeism, and it is not known how many pupils were present when lessons were delivered. Absenteeism could have contributed to the lower levels of reduced victimization achieved due to reduced access/exposure to material for some children. Future trials should identify ways of collecting data on each child's exposure to the KiVa lessons, such as through attendance registers for these lessons. The trial team now has access to the National Pupil Database, and analysis of pupil absenteeism will become available.

It is important to acknowledge that there is likely to have been significant variation in the delivery of bullying policies in usual-practice (UP) schools, as previously identified in other studies (Smith & Brain, 2000). The variation in school practice and lack of evidence-based guidance was one of the reasons for initially opting for the trial of KiVa in the UK. However, schools that registered for the trial are likely to be those that are more proactive in addressing bullying. Future papers (Bowes et al., 2025) should analyze and report on the data collected for the process evaluation on delivery in both KiVa and UP schools.

A limitation of the findings is that since the PRQ collects data on each question individually, students can report themselves as active on more than one of the scales, and further work is being undertaken to explore patterns of responses across the scales, which will provide an opportunity to establish the other response patterns of students who reported less support for bullies and more outsider and less defending behavior.

5. Conclusions

The trial took place during a very difficult post-COVID-19 period. The delivery of the program during the year 2021/22 was one in which teachers were struggling to address the challenges of students returning from lockdown and was also accompanied by significant absenteeism on the part of both pupils and teachers. Therefore, although the evidence suggests that the program was generally delivered as intended (Bowes et al., 2024), it is not known how much of the program individual students accessed. Nevertheless, despite these limitations, the evidence presented suggests that some changes in response to bullying fit with the social architecture model and show that the program influenced some behaviors in all children involved.

The findings add to the evidence for the importance of measuring bystander effects and implementing evidence-based whole-school approaches to address bullying. The results provide a valuable foundation for further research on the mechanisms by which KiVa changes rates of victimization, bullying, and the behavior of the whole school population. It has implications for longer-term integration and the embedding of KiVa into school practices.

Author Contributions: Conceptualization, J.H., L.B., S.C. and R.P.H.; Methodology, J.H., L.B., S.C., R.P.H., R.H., R.C.-J. and M.B.; Formal Analysis, R.C.-J. and M.B.; Investigation, J.H., L.B., S.C., R.P.H., R.H., M.E.W. and J.R.B.; Data Curation, R.C.-J. and M.B.; Writing—Original Draft Preparation, J.H. and R.P.; Writing—Review and Editing, J.H., L.B., S.C., R.P.H., R.H., R.C.-J., M.B., R.P., M.E.W. and J.R.B.; Funding Acquisition, J.H., L.B., S.C., R.P.H. and R.C.-J. All authors have read and agreed to the published version of the manuscript.

Funding: This research was funded by the National Institute for Health Research Public Health Research Grant (PHR 17/92/11).

Institutional Review Board Statement: This study was conducted in accordance with the Declaration of Helsinki and approved by the Psychology Research Ethics and Governance Committee of Bangor University (2019-16592, 13 November 2019).

Informed Consent Statement: Informed consent was obtained from all subjects involved in this study.

Data Availability Statement: The data presented in this study are available on request from the corresponding author (the data are not yet publicly available due to privacy and ethical restrictions).

Conflicts of Interest: The authors declare no conflicts of interest.

References

Arseneault, L., Bowes, L., & Shakoor, S. (2010). Bullying victimization in youths and mental health problems: 'Much ado about nothing'? *Psychological Medicine, 40*(5), 717–729. [CrossRef] [PubMed]

Arseneault, L., Walsh, E., Trzesniewski, K., Newcombe, R., Caspi, A., & Moffitt, T. E. (2006). Bullying victimization uniquely contributes to adjustment problems in young children: A nationally representative cohort study. *Pediatrics, 118*(1), 130–138. [CrossRef] [PubMed]

Axford, N., Bjornstad, G., Clarkson, S., Ukoumunne, O. S., Wrigley, Z., Matthews, J., Berry, V., & Hutchings, J. (2020). The effectiveness of the KiVa bullying prevention program in Wales, UK: Results from a pragmatic cluster randomized controlled trial. *Prevention Science, 21*, 615–626. [CrossRef] [PubMed]

Boulton, M. J. (1997). Teachers' views on bullying: Definitions, attitudes and ability to cope. *British Journal of Educational Psychology, 67*(2), 223–233. [CrossRef] [PubMed]

Bowes, L., Babu, M., Badger, J. R., Broome, M. R., Cannings-John, R., Clarkson, S., Coulman, E., Edwards, R. T., Ford, T., Hastings, R. P., Hayes, R., Lugg-Widger, F., Owen-Jones, E., Patterson, P., Segrott, J., Sydenham, M., Townson, J., Watkins, R. C., Whiteley, H., . . . Hutchings, J. (2024). The effects and costs of an anti-bullying program (KiVa) in UK primary schools: A multicenter cluster randomized controlled trial. *Psychological Medicine, 54*(15), 4362–4373. [CrossRef]

Bowes, L., Seagrott, J., Williams, M., Hutchings, J., & The Stand Together Team. (2025). *A process evaluation of the delivery of antibullying support in the UK Stand Together trial* [Manuscript in preparation].

Brown, S., & Taylor, K. (2008). Bullying, education and earnings: Evidence from the national child development study. *Economics of Education Review, 27*(4), 387–401. [CrossRef]

Camodeca, M., & Nava, E. (2020). The long-term effects of bullying, victimization, and bystander behavior on emotion regulation and its physiological correlates. *Journal of Interpersonal Violence, 37*(3–4), 088626052093443. [CrossRef] [PubMed]

Campbell, M., Whiteford, C., & Hooijer, J. (2019). Teachers' and parents' understanding of traditional and cyberbullying. *Journal of School Violence*, *18*(3), 388–402. [CrossRef]

Chen, L.-M., Wang, L. C., & Sung, Y. H. (2018). Teachers' recognition of school bullying according to background variables and type of bullying. *Journal of Educational, Cultural and Psychological Studies*, *18*, 147–164. [CrossRef]

Clark, K. N., Eldridge, M. A., Dorio, N. B., Demaray, M. K., & Smith, T. J. (2022). Bullying, victimization, and bystander behavior: Risk factors across elementary—Middle school transition. *School Psychology*, *37*(1), 37. [CrossRef]

Clarkson, S., Bowes, L., Coulman, E., Broome, M. R., Cannings-John, R., Charles, J. M., Edwards, R. T., Ford, T., Hastings, R. P., Hayes, R., Patterson, P., Segrott, J., Townson, J., Watkins, R., Badger, J., Hutchings, J., & Stand Together Team. (2022). The UK stand together trial: Protocol for a multicentre cluster randomised controlled trial to evaluate the effectiveness and cost-effectiveness of KiVa to reduce bullying in primary schools. *BMC Public Health*, *22*(1), 608. [CrossRef] [PubMed]

Clarkson, S., Charles, J. M., Saville, C. W. N., Bjornstad, G. J., & Hutchings, J. (2019). Introducing KiVa school-based anti-bullying programme to the UK: A preliminary examination of effectiveness and programme cost. *School Psychology International*, *40*(4), 347–365. [CrossRef]

Currie, C., Zanotti, C., Morgan, A., Currie, D., de Looze, M., Roberts, C., Samdal, O., Smith, O. R. F., & Barnekow, V. (2012). *Social determinants of health and well-being among young people. Health Behaviour in School-aged Children (HBSC) study: International report from the 2009/2010 survey*. WHO Regional Office for Europe.

Demaray, M. K., Summers, K. H., Jenkins, L. N., & Becker, L. D. (2016). Bullying Participant Behaviors Questionnaire (BPBQ): Establishing a reliable and valid measure. *Journal of School Violence*, *15*(2), 158. [CrossRef]

Eastman, M., Foshee, V., Ennett, S., Sotres-Alvarez, D., Reyes, H. L. M., Faris, R., & North, K. (2018). Profiles of internalizing and externalizing symptoms associated with bullying victimization. *Journal of Adolescence*, *65*, 101–110. [CrossRef]

Espelage, D. L., & Holt, M. K. (2001). Bullying and victimization during early adolescence: Peer influences and psychosocial correlates. *Journal of Emotional Abuse*, *2*(2–3), 123–142. [CrossRef]

Espelage, D. L., Polanin, J. R., & Low, S. K. (2014). Teacher and staff perceptions of school environment as predictors of student aggression, victimization, and willingness to intervene in bullying situations. *School Psychology Quarterly*, *29*(3), 287. [CrossRef]

Espelage, D. L., Rao, M. A., & De La Rue, L. (2013). Current research on school-based bullying: A social-ecological perspective. *Journal of Social Distress and the Homeless*, *22*(1), 21–27. [CrossRef]

Espelage, D. L., & Swearer, S. M. (2003). Research on school bullying and victimization: What have we learned and where do we go from here? *School Psychology Review*, *32*(3), 365–383. [CrossRef]

Evans, C. B. R., Smokowski, P. R., Rose, R. A., Mercado, M. C., & Marshall, K. J. (2019). Cumulative bullying experiences, adolescent behavioral and mental health, and academic achievement: An integrative model of perpetration, victimization, and bystander behavior. *Journal of Child and Family Studies*, *28*(9), 2415–2428. [CrossRef]

Ey, L. A., & Campbell, M. (2022). Australian early childhood teachers' understanding of bullying. *Journal of Interpersonal Violence*, *37*(15–16), NP13766–NP13790. [CrossRef] [PubMed]

Felix, E. D., Sharkey, J. D., Green, J. G., Furlong, M. J., & Tanigawa, D. (2011). Getting precise and pragmatic about the assessment of bullying: The development of the California bullying victimization scale. *Aggressive Behavior*, *37*(3), 234–247. [CrossRef]

Fergusson, D. M., Boden, J. M., & Horwood, L. J. (2014). Bullying in childhood, externalizing behaviors, and adult offending: Evidence from a 30-year study. *Journal of School Violence*, *13*(1), 146–164. [CrossRef]

Fisher, K., Cassidy, B., & Mitchell, A. M. (2017). Bullying: Effects on school-aged children, screening tools, and referral sources. *Journal of Community Health Nursing*, *34*(4), 171–179. [CrossRef]

Furlong, M., McGilloway, S., Bywater, T., Hutchings, J., Donnelly, M., Smith, S. M., & O'Neill, C. (2010). Behavioural/cognitive-behavioural group-based parenting interventions for children age 3–12 with early onset conduct problems. *The Cochrane Library*, *1*, 1–14.

Garandeau, C. F., Poskiparta, E., & Salmivalli, C. (2014). Tackling acute cases of school bullying in the KiVa anti-bullying program: A comparison of two approaches. *Journal of Abnormal Child Psychology*, *42*, 981–991. [CrossRef]

Glew, G., Fan, M.-Y., & Katon, W. (2005). Bullying, psychosocial adjustment, and academic performance in elementary school. *Archives of Pediatrics & Adolescent Medicine*, *159*(11), 1026–1031.

Goodstein, P. K. (2013). *How to stop bullying in classrooms and schools: Using social architecture to prevent, lessen, and end bullying*. Routledge.

Grennan, S., & Woodhams, J. (2007). The impact of bullying and coping strategies on the psychological distress of young offenders. *Psychology, Crime & Law*, *13*(5), 487–504. [CrossRef]

Guo, S. (2021). A comparison of traditional victims, cyber victims, traditional-cyber victims, and uninvolved adolescents: A social-ecological framework. *Child & Youth Care Forum*, *50*(5), 925–945. [CrossRef]

Hawker, D. S. J., & Boulton, M. J. (2000). Twenty years' research on peer victimization and psychosocial maladjustment: A meta-analytic review of cross-sectional studies. *Journal of Child Psychology and Psychiatry*, *41*(4), 441–455. [CrossRef]

Herkama, S., Saarento, S., & Salmivalli, C. (2017). KiVa antibullying program: Lessons learned and future directions. In P. Sturmey (Ed.), *Handbook on Aggression and Violence* (Vol. 3). Wiley.

Hutchings, J., & Clarkson, S. (2015). Introducing and piloting the KiVa bullying prevention programme in the UK. *Educational and Child Psychology*, *32*(1), 49–61. [CrossRef]

Iati, M. (2019, December 5). *An 8-year-old killed himself after being bullied, lawsuit says. The school district wants immunity*, Washington Post. Available online: https://www.washingtonpost.com/education/2019/12/05/an-year-old-killed-himself-after-being-bullied-police-say-school-district-wants-immunity/ (accessed on 24 January 2025).

Kärnä, A., Voeten, M., Little, T. D., Poskiparta, E., Kaljonen, A., & Salmivalli, C. (2011). A large-scale evaluation of the KiVa antibullying program: Grades 4–6. *Child Development*, *82*(1), 311–330. [CrossRef] [PubMed]

Liu, X., Peng, C., Yu, Y., Yang, M., Qing, Z., Qiu, X., & Yang, X. (2020). Association between sub-types of sibling bullying and mental health distress among Chinese children and adolescents. *Frontiers in Psychiatry*, *11*, 368. [CrossRef] [PubMed]

Maunder, R. E., Harrop, A., & Tattersall, A. J. (2010). Pupil and staff perceptions of bullying in secondary schools: Comparing behavioural definitions and their perceived seriousness. *Educational Research*, *52*(3), 263–282. [CrossRef]

McNeely, C. A., Nonnemaker, J. M., & Blum, R. W. (2002). Promoting school connectedness: Evidence from the national longitudinal study of adolescent health. *Journal of School Health*, 138–146. [CrossRef]

Menesini, E., & Salmivalli, C. (2017). Bullying in schools: The state of knowledge and effective interventions. *Psychology, Health & Medicine*, *22*(Suppl. S1), 240–253. [CrossRef]

Merrin, G. J., Espelage, D. L., & Hong, J. S. (2018). Applying the social-ecological framework to understand the associations of bullying perpetration among high school students: A multilevel analysis. *Psychology of Violence*, *8*(1), 43–56. [CrossRef]

Midgett, A., & Doumas, D. M. (2019). Witnessing bullying at school: The association between being a bystander and anxiety and depressive symptoms. *School Mental Health*, *11*(3), 454–463. [CrossRef] [PubMed]

Moore, S. E., Norman, R. E., Suetani, S., Thomas, H. J., Sly, P. D., & Scott, J. G. (2017). Consequences of bullying victimization in childhood and adolescence: A systematic review and meta-analysis. *World Journal of Psychiatry*, *7*(1), 60. [CrossRef] [PubMed]

Niemi, M. (2023, June 16). *What is behind the PISA test results? Case Finland.* TAMKjournal.

Olweus, D. (1993). *Bullying at school.* Blackwell Publishing.

Olweus, D. (1994). Bullying at school: Basic facts and effects of a school based intervention program. *Journal of Child Psychology and Psychiatry*, *35*(7), 1171–1190. [CrossRef]

Olweus, D. (2006). *Revised olweus bully/victim questionnaire (OBVQ). APA PsycTests.* [CrossRef]

Orpinas, P., & Horne, A. M. (2006). *Bullying prevention: Creating a positive school climate and developing social competence.* American Psychological Association.

Pepler, D. J., Craig, W. M., Connolly, J. A., Yuile, A., McMaster, L., & Jiang, D. (2006). A developmental perspective onbullying. *Aggressive Behavior*, *32*, 376–384. [CrossRef]

Pöyhönen, V., Juvonen, J., & Salmivalli, C. (2010). What does it take to stand up for the victim of bullying? The interplay between personal and social factors. *Merrill-Palmer Quarterly*, *56*(2), 143–163. [CrossRef]

R Core Team. (2021). *R: A language and environment for statistical computing.* R Foundation for Statistical Computing. Available online: https://www.R-project.org/ (accessed on 24 January 2025).

Reijntjes, A., Vermande, M., Olthof, T., Goossens, F. A., Aleva, L., & Van der Meulen, M. (2016). Defending victimized peers: Opposing the bully, supporting the victim, or both? *Aggressive Behavior*, *42*(6), 585–597. [CrossRef] [PubMed]

Riffle, L. N., Kelly, K. M., Demaray, M. L., Malecki, C. E., Santuzzi, A. M., Rodriguez-Harris, D. J., & Emmons, J. D. (2021). Associations among bullying role behaviors and academic performance over the course of an academic year for boys and girls. *Journal of School Psychology*, *86*, 49–63. [CrossRef] [PubMed]

Rigby, K. (2003). Consequences of bullying in schools. *The Canadian journal of psychiatry*, *48*(9), 583–590. [CrossRef]

Rowe, F., Stewart, D., & Patterson, C. (2007). Promoting school connectedness through whole school approaches. *Health Education*, *107*(6), 524–542. [CrossRef]

Saarento, S., & Salmivalli, C. (2015). The role of classroom peer ecology and bystanders' responses in bullying. *Child Development Perspectives*, *9*(4), 201–205. [CrossRef]

Salmivalli, C. (2001). Feeling good about oneself, being bad to others? Remarks on self-esteem, hostility, and aggressive behavior. *Aggression and Violent Behavior*, *6*(4), 375–393. [CrossRef]

Salmivalli, C., Kärnä, A., & Poskiparta, E. (2011a). Counteracting bullying in Finland: The KiVa program and its effects on different forms of being bullied. *International Journal of Behavioral Development*, *35*(5), 405–411. [CrossRef]

Salmivalli, C., Lagerspetz, K., Björkqvist, K., Österman, K., & Kaukiainen, A. (1996). Bullying as a group process: Participant roles and their relations to social status within the group. *Aggressive Behavior*, *22*(1), 1–15. [CrossRef]

Salmivalli, C., & Voeten, M. (2004). Connections between attitudes, group norms, and behaviour in bullying situations. *International Journal of Behavioral Development*, *28*(3), 246–258. [CrossRef]

Salmivalli, C., Voeten, M., & Poskiparta, E. (2011b). Bystanders matter: Associations between reinforcing, defending, and the frequency of bullying behavior in classrooms. *Journal of Clinical Child & Adolescent Psychology*, *40*(5), 668–676. [CrossRef]

Smith, P. K. (2016). Bullying: Definition, types, causes, consequences and intervention: Bullying. *Social and Personality Psychology Compass*, *10*(9), 519–532. [CrossRef]

Smith, P. K., & Brain, P. (2000). Bullying in schools: Lessons from two decades of research. *Aggressive Behavior*, *26*(1), 1–9. [CrossRef]

Smith, P. K., Kupferberg, A., Mora-Merchan, J. A., Samara, M., Bosley, S., & Osborn, R. (2012). A content analysis of school anti-bullying policies: A follow-up after six years. *Educational Psychology in Practice*, *28*(1), 47–70. [CrossRef]

Smith, P. K., Smith, C., Osborn, R., & Samara, M. (2008). A content analysis of school anti-bullying policies: Progress and limitations. *Educational Psychology in Practice*, *24*(1), 1–12. [CrossRef]

Smokowski, P. R., & Kopasz, K. H. (2005). Bullying in school: An overview of types, effects, family characteristics, and intervention strategies. *Children & Schools*, *27*(2), 101–110. [CrossRef]

Srabstein, J. C., & Leventhal, B. L. (2010). Prevention of bullying-related morbidity and mortality: A call for public health policies. *Bulletin of the World Health Organization*, *88*(6), 403. [CrossRef] [PubMed]

Swearer, S. M., & Hymel, S. (2015). Understanding the psychology of bullying: Moving toward a social-ecological diathesis–stress model. *American Psychologist*, *70*(4), 344–353. [CrossRef]

Ttofi, M. M., Farrington, D. P., Lösel, F., & Loeber, R. (2011). Do the victims of school bullies tend to become depressed later in life? A systematic review and meta-analysis of longitudinal studies. *Journal of Aggression, Conflict and Peace Research*, *3*(2), 63–73. [CrossRef]

Twemlow, S. W., Fonagy, P., & Sacco, F. C. (2004). The role of the bystander in the social architecture of bullying and violence in schools and communities. *Annals of the New York Academy of Sciences*, *1036*(1), 215–232. [CrossRef] [PubMed]

Twemlow, S. W., & Sacco, F. C. (2013). How & why does bystanding have such a startling impact on the architecture of school bullying and violence? *International Journal of Applied Psychoanalytic Studies*, *10*(3), 289–306.

Verlinden, M., Jansen, P. W., Veenstra, R., Jaddoe, V. W. V., Hofman, A., Verhulst, F. C., Shaw, P., & Tiemeier, H. (2015). Preschool attention-deficit/hyperactivity and oppositional defiant problems as antecedents of school bullying. *Journal of the American Academy of Child & Adolescent Psychiatry*, *54*(7), 571–579. [CrossRef]

Vivolo-Kantor, A. M., Martell, B. N., Holland, K. M., & Westby, R. (2014). A systematic review and content analysis of bullying and cyber-bullying measurement strategies. *Aggression and Violent Behavior*, *19*(4), 423–434. [CrossRef] [PubMed]

Wang, Q. (2023). Exploring the nature and impact of school bullying: The effects of individual and environmental factors. *SHS Web of Conferences*, *171*, 01012. [CrossRef]

Wolke, D., Copeland, W. E., Angold, A., & Costello, E. J. (2013). Impact of bullying in childhood on adult health, wealth, crime, and social outcomes. *Psychological Science*, *24*(10), 1958–1970. [CrossRef]

Wolke, D., & Lereya, S. T. (2015). Long-term effects of bullying. *Archives of Disease in Childhood*, *100*(9), 879–885. [CrossRef] [PubMed]

Zhang, S., Gong, M., Li, W., Wang, W., Wu, R., Guo, L., & Lu, C. (2020). Patterns of bullying victimization and associations with mental health problems in Chinese adolescents: A latent class analysis. *International Journal of Environmental Research and Public Health*, *17*(3), 779. [CrossRef]

Zuckerman, D. (2016). Bullying harms victims and perpetrators of all ages. *Health Progress*, *97*(4), 63–66.

MDPI AG
Grosspeteranlage 5
4052 Basel
Switzerland
Tel.: +41 61 683 77 34

Behavioral Sciences Editorial Office
E-mail: behavsci@mdpi.com
www.mdpi.com/journal/behavsci